Atkins Diabetes Revolution

Atkins Diabetes Revolution

The Groundbreaking Approach to
Preventing and Controlling
Type 2 Diabetes

Based on the teachings of
ROBERT C. ATKINS, M.D.
with
Mary C. Vernon, M.D., C.M.D.,
and Jacqueline A. Eberstein, R.N.

wm

WILLIAM MORROW
An Imprint of HarperCollinsPublishers

The information presented in this work is in no way intended as medical advice or as a substitute for medical treatment. This information should be used in conjunction with the guidance and care of your physician, especially if you are taking medications, including diuretics or medication for blood pressure or diabetes. Whether or not you are at your goal weight, consult your physician before beginning this program as you would with any nutritional plan. Your physician should perform baseline laboratory tests to allow for proper follow-up and to individualize your maintenance level of carbohydrate intake. As with any plan, the weight-loss phases of the Atkins Blood Sugar Control Program should not be used by patients on dialysis or by pregnant or nursing women.

HarperCollins books may be purchased for educational, business, or sales promotional use. For information please write: Special Markets Department, HarperCollins Publishers Inc., 10 East 53rd Street, New York, NY 10022.

FIRST EDITION

Designed by Katy Riegel

Printed on acid-free paper

Library of Congress Cataloging-in-Publication Data

Vernon, Mary C.
    Atkins diabetes revolution : the groundbreaking approach to preventing and controlling
    Type 2 diabetes / by Mary C. Vernon and Jacqueline A. Eberstein.—1st ed.
      p. cm.
      ISBN 0-06-054008-7
     1. Diabetes—Diet therapy.   2. Low-carbohydrate diet.   3. Non-insulin-dependent
    diabetes.   4. Glycemic index.   5. Insulin resistance.   I. Atkins, Robert C.
    II. Eberstein, Jacqueline A.   III. Title.

RC662.V47 2004
616.4'620654—dc22   2004047470

04   05   06   07   08   DIX/RRD   10 9 8 7 6 5 4 3 2 1

There is only one person to whom we could have dedicated this book: Bob Atkins. His vision inspired us and influenced our professional careers. His courage, passion, steadfastness, and willingness to think outside the box have galvanized us—and many others—to carry on his legacy.

Contents

Acknowledgments

In true Atkins tradition, producing this complex book was a team effort, led by Michael Bernstein, senior vice president of Atkins Health and Medical Information Services at Atkins Nutritionals, Inc. (ANI). Olivia Bell Buehl, vice president and editorial director, coordinated the day-to-day operations. Paul D. Wolff, chairman and chief executive officer of our company, and Scott Kabak, president and chief operating officer, were both instrumental in getting this project off the ground.

To ensure the accuracy of the nutritional information, nutritionist Colette Heimowitz, M.S., vice president and director of education and research, reviewed the manuscript and worked closely with us throughout the project. Dietitian Marlene Koch, R.D., developed all the meal plans and accompanying recipes that allow even individuals who have to severely restrict their carbs to enjoy tasty, varied, and easy-to-prepare meals. Nutritionist and coordinator of education and research Eva Katz, M.P.H., R.D., spent untold hours tracking down often elusive scientific references and ensuring the accuracy of all the references. Leyla Muedin and Shannah Johnson, R.D., assisted her. Leyla also reviewed Dr. Atkins' patient files to find those whose clinical experiences included in these pages represent the thousands who consulted Dr. Atkins for blood sugar disorders and related issues.

Contributing writer Sheila Buff put our thoughts into words, patiently reworking the manuscript as we refined the content. Contributing editor Lynn Prowitt-Smith gave the manuscript a final polish to help simplify an often complex subject.

Nutritionist and executive editor Christine Senft, M.S., and Web site content manager Rachel Fireman helped find many of the individuals whose experiences are related in this book, assisted by Kathy Maguire. Freelance writers Janet Cappiello Blake, Catherine Censor, and Mary Selover interviewed them and wrote the case studies. Special thanks also to the individuals who shared their personal stories with us. Senior food editor Allison Fishman reviewed all the meal plans and made valuable suggestions. Associate food editor Kelly Staikopoulos oversaw the testing of all recipes.

Atkins Nutritionals medical director Stuart L. Trager, M.D., reviewed the entire manuscript. As a triathlete, he also gave valuable assistance on the fitness program. Likewise, pediatrician, researcher, and member of the Atkins Physicians Council Stephen Sondike, M.D., vetted the chapters on childhood obesity and diabetes. Food scientist and vice president for product development at Atkins Nutritionals Matt Spolar and his associate Paul Bruns, Ph.D., contributed valuable expertise on the intricacies of sugar alcohols and were always ready to answer the most arcane questions.

Finally, this project would not have occurred had it not been for the superb efforts of our editor, Sarah Durand, and her team at William Morrow. Special thanks to Jane Friedman, Cathy Hemming, Michael Morrison, Libby Jordan, Lisa Gallagher, Debbie Stier, Kristen Green, Kim Lewis, Chris Tanigawa, Lorie Young, Juliette Shapland, Betty Lew, Richard Aquan, Barbara Levine, and Jeremy Cesarec.

—M.C.V. and J.A.E.

I would like to thank Tricia Thomann, R.N., Melissa Transue, R.N., and Heather Yates, P.A., as well as the rest of my dedicated staff, whose support allows me to pretend to be in three places at once. I am also indebted to my family, patients, and partners for their support. Eric Westman, M.D., was always just a telephone call away when I had a question that needed an immediate answer.

—M.C.V.

I would like to thank my husband, Conrad, for his patience and understanding of all the late nights and weekends this project consumed.

—J.A.E.

Foreword

For 29 years I worked side by side with Bob Atkins in a variety of roles, including nutrition counselor and director of medical education at the Atkins Center for Complementary Medicine, until his death in April 2003. From the very beginning of our relationship, it was obvious to me that Bob's mission was to put an end to the twin epidemics of obesity and Type 2 diabetes. His desire to address this dual crisis became even more immediate in the last decade of his life as he was diagnosing more people—and more younger people—with diabetes.

But first let me tell you a little bit about myself. In the five years after I graduated from nursing school, my experience was primarily in a conventional medical setting, including intensive care and the recovery room. I began to work with Bob quite by accident. In my initial interview I told him bluntly that I was highly skeptical of his dietary approach. As I reluctantly accepted his offer to work as a staff nurse in his medical practice, I doubted that I would stay long.

Within a few short weeks, I was surprised to observe firsthand the benefits his patients experienced. Not only did they lose weight without experiencing hunger, they also invariably reported improvements in an array of symptoms. As Bob was not yet using complementary therapies, these improvements were clearly related solely to diet.

Like many young women, I was always concerned about my

weight. I began to put on extra pounds at age 12 and struggled for years to keep my weight under control by skipping meals and low-calorie dieting. I never let myself gain more than ten pounds before I took action, because my family history of diabetes and morbid obesity scared me. As a nurse, I knew where I was headed.

Even though I was able to lose those extra ten pounds easily, when I was dieting I was always hungry and fighting carbohydrate cravings. I also experienced symptoms such as irregular heartbeats, palpitations, tremors in my hands, insomnia, weakness, and a host of other symptoms that no 25-year-old should have.

Never once did any of the doctors I consulted ask me about what I ate or my family history. Nor did it ever occur to *me* that my symptoms were related to my weight-loss efforts. After ruling out an overactive thyroid and an adrenal tumor, doctors treated my symptoms with cardiac drugs. I was convinced my problem wasn't with my heart, and I soon stopped taking them.

A few months after beginning to work with Bob, I experienced a recurrence of the symptoms. When I told Bob about my medical history and the tests I had been given, he asked me why I had never had a glucose tolerance test (GTT). I didn't have an answer. In those days, hypoglycemia—the only reason someone would take a GTT—was considered a "fad" diagnosis and not taken seriously, so the test was never even suggested.

Bob routinely ordered a GTT as a part of his new-patient workup, so I joined the next group of new patients and finally had my diagnosis: severely unstable blood sugar that by today's definition would fit the diagnosis of diabetes—at the ripe old age of 25.

I have Bob to thank for the good health I enjoy today. I am grateful for his courage, commitment, and perseverance in his beliefs. I share this personal information because I know what it is like to confront the health issues we talk about in this book—and I want you to know that you can succeed just as I have.

When Bob's widow, Veronica, approached me about completing this book, I was deeply honored. And although Bob's shoes are very large ones to fill, I am confident that I can transmit the message, as he would have expressed it himself. In fact, after working closely with him for many years, I find that I use the same words and phrases he so often used because I intimately know his approach to both obesity and diabetes. The basics were set forth in *Dr. Atkins' New Diet Revolution*, as well as in the many, many newsletter articles he penned, presentations he made at medical conferences, radio shows he hosted, and, most important, the records he left behind.

I am fortunate that my partner in this endeavor is Mary Vernon, M.D., C.M.D., a family practitioner and vice president of the American Society of Bariatric Physicians. Bob had a significant influence on the way Mary practices medicine. He was a larger-than-life character, but in many ways Mary reminds me of him. She shares his enthusiasm for caring for and interacting with patients. Like him, she has a natural curiosity and is willing to learn from her patients and other practitioners. Mary is equally open to exploring complementary approaches and began to use Bob's controlled-carbohydrate approach because she could see that it worked for her patients. Last but not least, not only is Mary as intelligent as Bob was, but like him she loves going to work each day and helping people get better.

This book is the natural extension of Bob's clinical practice. Over decades, although it was not conventional medical practice, he ordered thousands of insulin and blood sugar tests for patients who came to him with a variety of medical problems. Along with his patients' symptoms, their test results allowed him to see the relationship between blood sugar and lipid values and the deterioration of the blood sugar mechanism that ultimately results in diabetes. He foresaw the epidemics of obesity and Type 2 diabetes before it was fashionable to talk about them. He was especially concerned with what he saw happening to the health of young people.

Bob believed he had the answer—not just for treatment—but also, more important, for prevention. Even if diabetes was already established, Bob believed he could effectively treat it—if the patient was willing to do what it takes to achieve and maintain a reasonable weight. In most cases, the pancreas could recover, protecting what function it still possessed. Controlling carbohydrate intake was always essential to this goal.

His more important mission was to partner with his patients to educate them about their risks, so that they could prevent the onset of diabetes and its potentially serious results. It is this philosophy that is explored in detail in this book. Despite having already authored more than a dozen books, Bob often spoke of writing one about preventing diabetes, which would be the culmination of his life's work. Although he did not live long enough to complete *Atkins Diabetes Revolution*, those of us who worked with him and understood his commitment and courage have done that. This is that book, and I believe it is an appropriate legacy for this man of vision.

Bob had clearly conceptualized this book and had mapped out the contents. His excitement about the project was infectious, and he and I spent many hours talking about how he envisioned it. While Dr. Mary Vernon and I wrote this book, the dietary advice and nutritional principles come directly from Bob's teachings and my decades of experience working with him. We may be the authors, but we want you to realize that it is really *his* voice speaking loud and clear. Most case histories are taken directly from Bob's patient records. (For clarity, the case studies that come from Dr. Vernon's practice are indicated in italics, followed by her name.) We have used pseudonyms in case histories in which only a first name is used. We owe a debt of gratitude to all the individuals who have shared their personal stories in this book.

Bob Atkins' teachings can help you be a partner in your health care and health maintenance. You too can learn about your risks for diabetes and what to do about them. You can practice prevention for yourself and your family. Making lifestyle changes is not as easy as taking a drug, yet the results are immeasurably better and will positively impact all aspects of your life.

I know that Bob would feel his mission was accomplished if you, with the help of your health care provider, are able to use the information in this book to make permanent lifestyle changes—changes that become the framework of your personal health solution. In doing so, you will become part of the larger solution to the epidemics of obesity and diabetes that are fast becoming a public health nightmare.

—Jacqueline A. Eberstein, R.N.
Director of Nutrition Information
Atkins Health & Medical Information Services

Introduction

Let me share with you some frightening facts that could have a devastating effect on your life:

- One of every three children born in the year 2000 will develop diabetes.[1]
- Diabetes is the leading cause of heart disease.[2]
- About 75 percent of people who have diabetes will die of heart disease.[3]
- In the United States, diabetes has increased nearly 50 percent in the past ten years alone, according to estimates of the Centers for Disease Control and Prevention (CDC), and the incidence of the disease is expected to grow another 165 percent by 2050 under current trends.[4]
- Diabetes prescription costs create such a financial burden that one in five older adults with diabetes reports cutting back on prescription medication.[5]
- Total medical cost of diabetes in the United States in 2002 was $92 billion; add in indirect costs of $40 billion—disability payments, days of work lost, and premature death—and the total comes to $132 billion.[6]
- Overall, the risk of death for people with diabetes is about twice that for people without it.[7]

Behind all these numbers are millions of people and their families. My practice is simply a microcosm of the impending health care crisis. Every day I see in my patients' lives the devastating impact of these statistics—which, as you will learn from this book, is intimately linked to being overweight or obese. Excess weight and its associated metabolic imbalances—resulting in diabetes, coronary artery disease, and hypertension—are costing them their health and, in some cases, even their lives.

I have been interested in controlled-carbohydrate nutrition for years. As a family physician, I saw my patients fail in their attempts to use the standard recommendations I was schooled to give them. I could see that they needed to control their weight and metabolism. I felt helpless, with nothing to offer them that would make a significant impact. The ubiquitous low-fat, low-calorie approach to weight loss was difficult for my overweight patients to use. They complained of hunger and irritability. I needed an effective tool to help them control their appetite so they could achieve long-term success in losing weight and keeping it off.

Back to the books I went to reeducate myself about effective ways to manage weight and metabolism. I was eventually driven to pursue my interest in bariatric medicine, the treatment of obesity and its associated conditions. (I am now board certified in bariatrics.) Like every physician, I studied metabolism in medical school, including the role carbohydrates play in fat storage. But this time around, I saw how the information applied directly to my patients. I now wanted to make it clear to them, too. Much of this book is devoted to conveying in the simplest terms possible the complex biochemical functions of insulin production and blood sugar regulation.

I decided to examine the available tools for carbohydrate control, rather than reinvent the wheel. I reviewed all the popular plans that control carbohydrate intake. The Atkins Nutritional Approach appealed to me because it was simple (no calculator or food scale required) and because it could be individualized. Using controlled-carbohydrate nutrition, which has its own natural appetite-suppressing effect, I was able to help my patients.

I was amazed at their significant improvements in lipid and cardiovascular risk factors, as well as insulin and blood sugar control. I also began to hear my patients say the very things that Dr. Atkins had written about in his books. They told me that their energy levels had increased, their moods were more stable, and they had fewer aches and pains, less acid reflux and indigestion, and an improved sense of well-being. My patients' results convinced me I was on the right track.

I met Bob for the first time in 2000 at a continuing-medical-education conference on low carbohydrates in New York City. There, I spoke with other clinicians whose patients were experiencing the same success. I also met researchers, including Dr. Eric Westman and Dr. William S. Yancy Jr., both of Duke University. They were among those who had been conducting clinical trials and whose findings demonstrated the safety and efficacy of the Atkins Nutritional Approach both for weight management and improvement in cardiovascular risk factors. As I related my own experiences, Dr. Westman agreed to analyze my patient data, which confirmed my observations. My successful clinical experiences with Type 2 diabetic patients were published in the fall 2003 edition of *Metabolic Syndrome and Related Disorders.*

Other researchers at equally prestigious institutions were also taking an unbiased look at the Atkins Nutritional Approach (ANA). By 2002, the first two studies supportive of the ANA were published in peer-reviewed journals or presented at conferences. (As I write this introduction, there are now 27 studies supportive of the ANA,* two of which I am proud to say I authored.) Although many people had experienced success doing Atkins and had long embraced this approach, the publication of an article by science writer Gary Taubes in the *New York Times Magazine* in July 2002 was a major turning point. Entitled "What If It's All Been a Big Fat Lie?" the article made clear that the low-fat approach had minimal scientific underpinnings and that, in fact, emerging research was supportive of controlling carbs. For this kind of information, written by a respected science writer, to appear in the *New York Times* was a watershed moment.

In September 2002, I met Bob again when he lectured at the American Society of Bariatric Physicians conference. Dr. Westman and I presented our data on the Atkins Nutritional Approach, showing the benefits of the ANA compared with a low-fat, calorie-restricted diet.

---

* For a list of the studies supporting controlled-carbohydrate nutrition published to date, see page 448.

Overall, there was huge interest in the emerging science validating the Atkins approach as well as personal support for Bob. He clearly felt vindicated by this reception. "You see?" he said. "I've known for years how amazing this is!" Over several meals with Bob and Veronica Atkins, he and I shared our clinical experiences. He came to realize that I had a full understanding of his approach and shared his commitment to patient care.

Our conversations continued over the ensuing months. Bob followed my presentations and reviewed my clinical results with excitement. He then paid me the ultimate compliment: When I visited The Atkins Center for Complementary Medicine in November 2002, he asked me to join his practice. Coincidentally, during that visit I had the thrill of being with Bob the day that Dr. Westman's research comparing the Atkins Nutritional Approach with the American Heart Association (AHA) recommendations was presented at the association's annual meeting. Finally, AHA members were presented with an excellent, randomized, controlled trial that confirmed results similar to those Bob had long put forward. He relished the scientific confirmation of his clinical experience.

Bob and I continued to discuss the possibility of my joining his practice up until the accident that resulted in his death. Things did not turn out as planned. Now, instead of working as his colleague at the Atkins Center, I am a member of the Atkins Physicians Council (APC), whose members have expertise in fields such as diabetes, pediatrics, women's health, bariatrics, and orthopedics. As part of Atkins Health and Medical Information Services, this group is committed to educating the medical community, health consumers, and policy makers on the merits of controlled-carbohydrate nutrition, which can play a major role in addressing the epidemics of obesity and diabetes. As part of that effort, the APC has already presented the Atkins Lifestyle Food Guide Pyramid (see page 473) as an alternative dietary guideline. As a member of the APC, I am honored to be a co-author of this book—helping to impart the knowledge Bob acquired in his lifetime of work. I take on this task with deep respect. I could have spent a lifetime learning from Bob. Instead, I honor his legacy by helping to complete his last and most important work. It is anticipated that the other members of the APC will also write future publications under the Atkins banner.

I would not presume to tackle this important task alone. With Jacqueline Eberstein as my partner, this book has come to fruition. Since Jackie lived those years of discovery with Bob, she can translate decades of clinical practice into the words he would have used. Everything about how to implement controlled-carbohydrate nutrition is imprinted in her mind. And as we have worked together on this book, we have often been amazed by the similarities in our day-to-day clinical experiences using this approach.

Another person who is integral to carrying on Bob's legacy is, of course, his wife, Veronica. During their time together, she was not just his helpmate, but was also intimately involved in many aspects of his work, including collaborating on a cookbook. Together, they were committed to furthering independent research on controlled-carb nutrition and to that end established the ongoing Dr. Robert C. Atkins Foundation, of which Veronica is chairperson. Grant money has already been used to fund research at institutions such as Duke University, Albert Einstein College of Medicine, Ball State University, the University of Connecticut, Pennsylvania Hospital, the University of Kansas, and Beth Israel–Deaconess Medical Center.

As a bariatrician, I recognize the need to personalize each patient's program. Individuals with chronic diseases such as diabetes, hypertension, and cardiovascular disease should work with their physician to find a treatment plan that specifically benefits them. The contents of this book provide information about a program that many have found effective. Although this book is written in language most nonprofessionals can understand, it is by no means intended as a replacement for the physician-patient relationship.

I take great joy in offering my patients lifestyle choices that empower them to improve their health. Jackie and I believe that this book will provide *you* and *your* health care practitioner with information that will empower you in the same way. After all, as a pioneer in complementary medicine, Bob's most enduring legacy is the gift of knowledge. He truly practiced the "art of medicine," a skill that is the foundation of inspired patient care.

—Mary C. Vernon, M.D., C.M.D.
Member, Atkins Physicians Council

Part One

Blood Sugar and Your Health

Chapter 1

THE DIABETES CROSSROADS

It's a frustrating fact of life: We don't have much say over whether we fall victim to life-threatening diseases such as cancer, Alzheimer's, or, to a large extent, some types of heart disease. However, there is one, all-too-common killer disease over which we have a great deal of say. Most people do have a choice when it comes to Type 2 diabetes. Astonishing as it sounds, this epidemic disease is almost entirely preventable. Of course, no one consciously chooses to get diabetes. Various factors—some in our control and some not—combine to create the unfortunate scenario. But if we all took proper care of our bodies and kept vigilant rein on the factors that are within our control, there would be no diabetes epidemic. Do you think we're overstating things? No way. In fact, what we hope we have created with this book is a realistic and practical guide to wiping out Type 2 diabetes, one individual at a time.

According to the National Institutes of Health, in 2002, a record number of Americans—18.2 million, or 6.3 percent of the population—were thought to have diabetes. Of these, 13 million were already diagnosed, while 5.2 million probably have diabetes but haven't been diagnosed yet.[1] That means many millions of Americans are blindly chugging down this dangerous road. Sadly, in our experience, many well-meaning health care professionals give their patients the standard information, some of which perpetuates the very disease it's supposed to cure or prevent. That's why Dr. Atkins felt it was crucial to write this book.

In 2002 and 2003, the American Diabetes Association redefined and standardized the criteria for blood sugar abnormalities. Unfortunately, none of these changes were implemented in order to find patients earlier in the process. Our interest is in *identifying* patients with these metabolic problems long before they advance to the "official" blood sugar level defined as diabetes.[2-4]

If you know what to look for, you can identify the metabolic signposts that signal trouble even earlier in the process—and intervene immediately. If you are reading this book, you are clearly concerned about your health or perhaps it's someone you love about whom you're concerned. Either way, congratulations to you for picking up this book. Let's not waste another minute.

We will show you how to make relatively simple lifestyle changes that can significantly reduce your risk of ever getting diabetes, even if you already have some of the preliminary symptoms. And if you have already been diagnosed with diabetes, this book can help you mitigate its effects or maybe even stop further progression.

We can be your guides on the road to better health, but it is you who must take control of your destiny by making and implementing the right choices. Imagine that you are standing at a crossroads in the map of your life. Ahead of you lie two paths. One almost inevitably leads to diabetes and its accompanying health problems; the other leads to optimal health. Which will you choose?

THE RIGHT ROAD

Let us tell you about the path that Dr. Atkins recommended to his patients for decades. It differs dramatically from the treatment with drugs most health care practitioners have been taught. Instead, his path identifies risks for diabetes as early as possible, focuses on prevention, and involves *permanent* lifestyle changes to address the underlying metabolic problems that lead to diabetes. These lifestyle changes can be as simple as changing what you put on your plate—a better option, we think you'll agree, than swallowing an array of expensive and potentially dangerous drugs. Those of you who have read Dr. Atkins' other books will recognize a point he hammered home for decades: Instead of treating the *symptoms*, his approach can correct the *problem* itself.

Finally, for individuals whose blood sugar abnormalities are further advanced or who already have diabetes, this path decreases or eliminates the need for drugs to treat these conditions. (Did you know that some of these drugs actually make it harder to lose weight? Talk about a vicious cycle.) Whether you're just beginning to be concerned about diabetes or you've already been handed the official diagnosis, controlling carbohydrates is the vehicle that will take you off the rutted road of self-destruction and onto the smooth one of recovery and excellent health.

The decision to improve your health is an obvious one, but to follow this "right road"—and stay on it—you need clear directions and a good map. That's what the Atkins Blood Sugar Control Program (ABSCP) gives you. The ABSCP is a highly individualized approach to weight control and permanent management of the risk factors for diabetes and cardiovascular disease. And it works.

I've witnessed these life-changing improvements in patients such as this 45-year-old woman. Ruth L. weighed 375 pounds, with a body mass index (BMI) of 60.5 and uncontrolled Type 2 diabetes. Although Ruth took three medications daily in an effort to control her blood sugar, her glycated hemoglobin (A1C) was 11 (more than two times the norm, demonstrating very poor blood sugar control). The day she began the program, I had her stop all her blood sugar medications. After two months, her A1C was down to 7.7. After 18 months, she had lost 132 pounds, her lab values were normal, with an A1C of 5.4, and she remained off blood sugar medications. —MARY VERNON

The ABSCP builds on the basic controlled-carbohydrate concepts of the famed Atkins Nutritional Approach and individualizes it specifically for people like Ruth who have—or are at risk for—blood sugar abnormalities and diabetes.

Once you're heading in the right direction, the program helps you to stay with it and map your progress as you pass milestones along the

A WORLDWIDE PROBLEM

The diabetes epidemic is growing by leaps and bounds around the world. According to the World Health Organization, in 2000, the total number of people worldwide with Type 2 diabetes was 176 million plus. By the year 2030, that number is estimated to rise to some 370 million people. In 2025, the worldwide prevalence of diabetes in adults will have increased by 35 percent, and the number of people with diabetes will have increased by 122 percent.[5] The countries with the largest number of diabetics in 2030 will be India (an estimated 80.9 million), China (an estimated 42 million), and the United States (an estimated 30 million).[6]

way. The ABSCP includes controlled-carbohydrate nutrition; supplementation with vitamins, minerals, and other nutrients; and exercise—all of which are customized to your needs.

To begin, you need to understand more about this insidious disease. Let's start with the basics.

WHAT IS DIABETES?

Diabetes is defined as a condition in which blood sugar (glucose) levels are above the normal range. In a minority of cases, this happens because your body is no longer producing the hormone insulin, which carries glucose into your cells where it can be converted into energy. This is known as Type 1 diabetes, sometimes called juvenile diabetes or insulin-dependent diabetes mellitus (IDDM). In Type 1 diabetes, the specialized beta cells of the pancreas stop producing the hormone insulin, which is necessary for moving glucose into the cells, where it is burned for energy. Type 1 diabetes usually starts in childhood; currently people with this form of diabetes require lifelong insulin administration and careful dietary management to survive. Recently, it has been reported that stem-cell transplants have been successful in curing this disease. Type 1 diabetes accounts for about 5 to 10 percent

GESTATIONAL DIABETES

Each year some 4 percent of pregnant women, or about 135,000 women in the United States, develop gestational diabetes.[7] If you're over age 25, are obese, have blood sugar or blood pressure problems, a family history of diabetes, or belong to certain ethnic groups, you may be at risk for gestational diabetes.

Gestational diabetes can be a serious problem, because it can result in an infant with a dangerously high birth weight, which causes difficulties during labor, including a higher risk for cesarean delivery. These women are also more likely to develop hypertension during pregnancy and have it persist after delivery.[8] There is also risk to the infant. Babies exposed to high concentrations of glucose before birth may have problems maintaining their blood sugar in the first few days after delivery. They are also more likely to have breathing problems and require oxygen supplementation if born early.

Gestational diabetes can generally be controlled by diet and sensible exercise during pregnancy. Blood sugar levels usually return to normal after delivery. If you had gestational diabetes, however, you have about a 20 to 50 percent chance of developing Type 2 diabetes within the next five to ten years.[9] Also, your baby may be more likely to become overweight and develop diabetes later in life because he or she has inherited your metabolic tendencies.

of all cases of diabetes.[10] The cause of Type 1 diabetes is in most cases an autoimmune disease in which the body mistakenly attacks and destroys the cells in the pancreas that produce insulin. Type 1 diabetes usually strikes very suddenly—the person may appear fine one day and be very sick just a few weeks or even days later.

Because Type 2 diabetes is by far the most common type of diabetes, and because it can be prevented and treated through diet and lifestyle changes, it will be the focus of this book. Although some of the advice in this book can be helpful for people with Type 1 diabetes

POLYCYSTIC OVARY SYNDROME

Women who have polycystic ovary syndrome (PCOS) have a high risk of developing Type 2 diabetes. Like diabetes, PCOS is associated with increased insulin resistance and high insulin secretion.[11]

PCOS is a hormonal imbalance that can cause irregular menstruation, infertility, weight gain, and excessive hair growth. PCOS is surprisingly common—estimates are as high as 11 percent of all women aged 20 to 40.[12] Fortunately, PCOS responds extremely well to a controlled-carbohydrate approach. Many of our PCOS patients return to normal blood sugar levels within a few months of doing Atkins, and their other symptoms often improve as well. Some patients even report being able to conceive when following this approach.

Of women who have PCOS, 35 percent have been shown to progress to diabetes five to ten times faster than women without this condition.[13]

as well, in general, whenever we talk about diabetes we are referring to Type 2 diabetes.

Ninety to 95 percent of the people with diabetes have Type 2, a disease that is quite different from Type 1.[14] In the large majority of cases of the Type 2 variety, the individual still makes insulin—in fact, he or she may make large amounts of it—but the cells respond more slowly to its presence. This slowed response is called *insulin resistance.* If you have Type 2 diabetes, over time, as your cells become more resistant to the insulin signal, blood sugar rises above normal levels. What's happening? It's as if the insulin knocks at the doors of the cells and asks that the glucose be let in, but the cells don't answer the door. So the amount of glucose circulating in the blood increases—you become hyperglycemic—and that causes a lot of damage. To force the glucose to enter the cells, your pancreas pours out more insulin. Eventually, the pancreas becomes unable to produce such high levels of insulin; as a result, insulin must be administered in order to control the blood sugar level.

Kids and Diabetes

Until recently, Type 2 diabetes was primarily a problem for older adults. It was very rare for children and people in their twenties or even thirties to have Type 2 diabetes. Today, even children are being diagnosed with this disease. Some experts now suggest that as much as 45 percent of all children with newly diagnosed diabetes have Type 2.[15] The causes are similar to those for adults: obesity, a sedentary lifestyle,

THE LOW-DOWN ON LIPIDS

The term *blood lipids* (lipid is another word for fat) is used as an overall way to describe the various types of cholesterol and fat that are normally found in the bloodstream. People with blood sugar abnormalities or diabetes typically have characteristic abnormalities in their blood lipid profiles. We'll be discussing lipids in detail in other parts of this book, especially Chapter 9 on heart disease, but for now let's go over the main types:

Cholesterol. Technically, cholesterol isn't a fat. It's a waxy substance that's a sort of kissing cousin to fat—the main difference is that you don't burn cholesterol for energy in your cells as you do fat. Cholesterol is essential for your health. Among the many other functions it serves in your body, it's used to make the membranes of your cells, to form the insulating layer of your nerve cells, and to manufacture many hormones, including the sex hormones testosterone, estrogen, and progesterone.

Low-Density Lipoprotein, or LDL Cholesterol. To move the waxy cholesterol around in your watery blood to where it needs to go, your liver coats it with protein. LDL cholesterol is often simplistically called the "bad" cholesterol, because high levels of it in the blood are statistically associated with an increased risk of heart disease.

High-Density Lipoprotein, or HDL Cholesterol. This is often called the "good" cholesterol, because it carries cholesterol back to your liver, where it can be processed into bile and excreted.

Triglycerides. These are tiny droplets of fat found in your bloodstream. Triglycerides are stored as body fat.

and a high-carbohydrate diet. Kids with Type 2 diabetes are more likely also to have a family history of the disease. Children with this disease face a future of serious health problems that will likely shorten their life spans and significantly affect their quality of life. Fortunately, as we'll explain in Chapter 25, the Atkins Blood Sugar Control Program is very effective for young people.

The Human Cost

Over the long run, the metabolic imbalance that raises your blood sugar causes a host of other very serious health problems, including high blood pressure, abnormal blood lipids, and a sharply increased risk of heart disease. Other complications include kidney disease, blindness, gangrene of the extremities (leading to amputation), and an increased risk of cancer.[16] In fact, the dangerous duo of high insulin and high blood sugar has the potential to damage every cell in your body, which is why diabetes and its complications are the sixth leading cause of death in the United States.[17]

The Financial Cost

Diabetes is also expensive. In 2002, the direct costs of treating the disease in the United States alone were $92 billion. The indirect costs of disability, lost work, and premature death were an additional $40 billion, bringing the total cost for diabetes in just that one year to $132 billion.[18] In addition to the monetary cost is the devastating price paid in quality of life by people with diabetes and their families.

RISK FACTORS FOR TYPE 2 DIABETES

The gradual accumulation of several risk factors leads down a long road that results in diabetes. Those risk factors are:

Obesity. Of all the different risk factors for diabetes, being overweight or obese tops the list. The risk is much greater if the excess weight settles around your abdomen, but in general, the heavier you are, the greater your risk.

Diet. A diet high in poor-quality, high-glycemic carbohydrates, especially sugary and starchy foods, contributes strongly to both obesity and diabetes.

Sedentary Lifestyle. Lack of exercise and poor physical condition are major risk factors for diabetes. A sedentary lifestyle increases insulin resistance and contributes to obesity and loss of muscle mass.

Heredity. Having a close relative, especially a parent or sibling, with Type 2 diabetes increases your risk. But don't think you're safe if you have no family history. We have seen numerous patients, even very young ones, well on their way to diabetes because of unhealthy diet and lifestyle alone.

Ethnicity. Some ethnic groups, including African Americans, Asian Americans, Hispanic Americans, Native Americans, and Pacific Islanders, have a high incidence of Type 2 diabetes.

History of Gestational Diabetes. Women who have had gestational diabetes or who have given birth to a baby weighing more than nine pounds are more likely to develop Type 2 diabetes later in life.

Metabolic Syndrome. Also known as syndrome X, this group of signs includes abdominal obesity, hypertension, and abnormal lipids, signaling a major risk for heart disease, prediabetes, and diabetes.

Elevated Blood Sugar. If your blood sugar is already on the high side, but not yet high enough to constitute a diagnosis of diabetes, you're at a much greater risk of developing the disease as time goes on. In the meantime, damage to your body from the process that raises your blood sugar has already begun its insidious progression.

Abnormal Blood Lipids. The combination of high triglycerides and low HDL cholesterol is a major warning sign of abnormal blood sugar metabolism.

High Blood Pressure. High blood sugar and high blood pressure often go hand in hand. Each is a warning sign of the same underlying metabolic problem.

Age. Simply growing older increases the risk of Type 2 diabetes, especially in combination with any of the other risk factors.

In later chapters of this book, we will explore these risk factors and what you can do about them in greater detail. For now, the most important things to remember are that Type 2 diabetes almost always develops over a period of years and that it is almost always related to being overweight. Most people have more than one risk factor, and the early warning signs are present long before full-blown diabetes is diagnosed. That's both the tragedy and the hope of this metabolic problem. It's a tragedy, because all too often the early signs are ignored until diabetes develops—and by that time, the process leading to Type 2 diabetes may well have resulted in serious damage. But it's also the hope, because the sooner you recognize those early signs and put the Atkins Blood Sugar Control Program into action, the sooner you can increase your chances of arresting this devastating disease.

WHAT IS YOUR RISK FOR GETTING DIABETES?

Take this quiz to get an idea.

I am overweight.	Yes ❑	No ❑
I have excess weight around my waist.	Yes ❑	No ❑
My diet is high in carbohydrates such as bread, potatoes, and pasta.	Yes ❑	No ❑
I eat starchy snack foods/sweets every day.	Yes ❑	No ❑
I exercise fewer than three hours a week.	Yes ❑	No ❑
I am African American, Hispanic American, Asian American, Native American, or Pacific Islander.	Yes ❑	No ❑
My mother, father, sister, or brother has/had diabetes.	Yes ❑	No ❑
I had gestational diabetes.	Yes ❑	No ❑
My blood sugar is high.	Yes ❑	No ❑
My blood pressure is high.	Yes ❑	No ❑
I have high triglycerides.	Yes ❑	No ❑
I am over age 45.	Yes ❑	No ❑

Count up your yes answers. The more yes answers you have, the greater the likelihood you will get diabetes—or that you have it already. If you have more than five yes answers, discuss your risk of diabetes with your doctor as soon as possible.

Chapter 2

WRONG TURN: THE LONG ROAD TO DIABETES

The long, slow process of developing Type 2 diabetes can take years. The symptoms can develop so gradually that you don't really notice them, at least not at first. In fact, many cases of diabetes are diagnosed only because the person went to the doctor for another ailment. Long before you might notice any symptoms of diabetes, your body may already be having trouble regulating your insulin and blood sugar levels.

UNDERSTANDING BLOOD SUGAR

We've already used the terms *blood glucose* and *blood sugar* a lot, and we're going to use them a lot more in this book. Let's take a closer look at glucose and how your body puts it to use. Glucose is a simple form of sugar that is one of your body's primary fuels for energy; glucose is derived primarily from carbohydrates. (Fat is your body's backup energy source.) Blood glucose, then, is the amount of sugar that's in your bloodstream at any given time. That amount can vary quite a bit over the course of the day—it's generally higher shortly after you eat something and lower between meals. Under normal circumstances, your body can also manufacture glucose from dietary protein so that your blood sugar level can be maintained.

Although the words *blood glucose* and *blood sugar* are often used interchangeably, glucose and sugar aren't exactly the same thing. But because *blood glucose* and *blood sugar* are so commonly used to describe the same thing—the amount of glucose in your bloodstream—we'll use the two terms interchangeably as well.

If your blood sugar mechanism is functioning normally and you eat a high-carbohydrate food such as a bowl of spaghetti, your body starts to break the starchy pasta down into glucose the moment it enters your mouth. (You can prove this to yourself by chewing a strand of plain cooked spaghetti and holding it in your mouth. As enzymes in your saliva start to break down the carbohydrate, you'll notice a faintly sweet taste.) The carbohydrate continues to be broken down further in your digestive system, but some glucose enters your bloodstream almost immediately.

HOW IT SHOULD BE

As your blood sugar begins to rise, the pancreas releases enough insulin to handle it. The body likes to keep its glucose level within a fairly narrow range, so it quickly releases insulin to carry the glucose into your cells, where it can be converted into energy. If there's more glucose than the cells can handle, the body can store the extra amount as glycogen in the liver and muscle cells for future energy needs. Once the glycogen storage areas are full, any glucose remaining is then stored as body fat.

Normally, after you eat a meal that contains protein, fat, and carbohydrates, you would expect that the glucose and insulin in your blood would first go up steadily within the proper range and then slowly go down again over the next several hours, without wide swings, which cause stress hormone release.

That's how it *should* function. However, if you're at risk for diabetes, your blood sugar and insulin balance can gradually start to get out of sync. It's a slow process that happens in stages that almost imperceptibly merge into each other.

MILESTONES ON THE ROAD TO DIABETES

Though the progression to diabetes is slow and insidious, Dr. Atkins observed, through decades of evaluating patients with blood sugar abnormalities, that it can nonetheless be divided into six distinct stages. His observations are similar to those of other researchers in this area.[1] The first four stages are milestones on the road to diabetes:

1. Insulin resistance of cells
2. Insulin resistance with hyperinsulinism (the production of large amounts of insulin)
3. Insulin resistance with hyperinsulinism and reactive hypoglycemia (low blood sugar)
4. Insulin resistance and hyperinsulinism with impaired glucose tolerance (now called prediabetes)
5. Type 2 diabetes with insulin resistance and high insulin production
6. Type 2 diabetes with low or virtually no insulin production

We'll be discussing the six stages in more detail as we progress through this book, starting with the first three stages of insulin resistance as it gradually worsens and leads to excessive insulin production and hypoglycemia.

THE PROGRESSION OF INSULIN RESISTANCE

The first steps on the diabetes road usually begin with excessive consumption of carbohydrates (or a high-calorie diet) that leads to excess glucose being stored as fat. The result? Weight gain. As you put on the pounds, you gradually become insulin resistant—meaning your cells begin to be less responsive to the effects of insulin. Why? That's a very good question, and despite its importance, it's a question for which the medical profession still doesn't have a good answer. (Today many researchers believe that one of the underlying causes is inflammation, but we're just starting to understand what causes the inflammation.)[2-4]

As you gain fat, your insulin resistance increases. Though not everyone who is overweight is insulin resistant, the heavier you are, the more likely you are to become insulin resistant. On the other hand, in some people, insulin resistance begins at normal body weight and can worsen due to a high-carb diet even if their body weight stays normal. For these people, insulin resistance may be due to genetic factors or other factors not yet well understood. Fortunately, a controlled-carbohydrate lifestyle benefits just about everyone with insulin resistance, whether or not they are overweight. That's because controlling carbs alone helps your cells regain their ability to respond properly to insulin, even if weight loss isn't needed.[5, 6]

To compensate for insulin resistance, your pancreas pours out extra insulin in an attempt to force your cells to take in glucose and to maintain your blood sugar within the normal range. You now have what doctors call *hyperinsulinemia* or *hyperinsulinism*—meaning excess insulin in the blood. What happens then is that the smooth rise and fall of glucose and insulin in your bloodstream becomes unbalanced after a meal. To clear away the glucose, your pancreas produces a big spike of extra insulin.

As time goes on, your blood sugar and insulin production get increasingly out of sync. Your blood sugar rises, but now the insulin surge takes longer to occur, and when it does happen, you produce more insulin than is needed. When the insulin finally does kick in, your glucose then drops below its normal level, causing reactive *hypoglycemia,* or low blood sugar.

When hypoglycemia occurs, you may suffer from numerous symptoms, including ups and downs in energy level, shakiness, irritability, and even trouble thinking clearly. You'll probably also feel cravings for your favorite carbs as your body instinctively tries to bring your blood sugar level back up—which puts you right back on the blood sugar roller coaster. A dramatic case of this among Dr. Atkins' patients was Warren S., a 35-year-old who came to him because blood sugar swings were causing panic attacks, dizziness, headaches, and an array of other unpleasant symptoms. Within two weeks of starting on the controlled-carb approach, he told Dr. Atkins, "I'm a different person." And he was—his symptoms had improved almost immediately.

ONWARD TO PREDIABETES

The earliest three stages of the progression to diabetes can go on for months or even years before you move on to the next stage. After a while, however, even all that extra insulin can't force enough glucose to enter your cells. The amount of sugar in your blood begins to peak at higher than the normal range. You now have reached the fourth stage: You have not only hyperinsulinemia but also *hyperglycemia*— elevated levels of blood sugar. What some people will then develop is what Dr. Atkins called a high-low curve. One to two hours after a high-carb meal, the blood sugar goes higher than it should, provoking symptoms such as sleepiness or a strong desire to nap. This is followed by the belated insulin spike, which causes hypoglycemia with the symptoms described above. This stage, in which the temporary elevation of blood sugar two hours after a glucose challenge during a glucose tolerance test goes above 140 mg/dL (milligrams per deciliter) but is still less than 200 mg/dL, is called impaired glucose tolerance. (We'll explain more about how we measure blood sugar levels and what they mean in Chapter 6, Diagnosis: Diabetes.)

As the condition progresses, your fasting blood sugar (the amount of sugar in your blood after not eating for 8 to 12 hours) will slowly begin to rise. Once your fasting blood sugar hits a level of 100 mg/dL to 125 mg/dL, you have impaired fasting glucose, or prediabetes. Dr. Atkins observed that individuals with this condition could also have above-normal levels of blood sugar after eating a high-carbohydrate meal. Florence S. is a good example. At 61 years old and five feet three inches tall, she weighed 141 pounds. Florence had signs of metabolic syndrome and was taking a number of medications for high blood pressure and abnormal lipids. During her glucose tolerance test (GTT), her fasting blood sugar was 114, revealing prediabetes; at the half-hour point of the GTT, her blood sugar was 198; at one hour, 215; at two hours, 173; at three hours, 83; at four hours, 76; and at five hours, 89. As you'll learn in a later chapter, this blood sugar pattern is the "high-low curve."

If you have progressed to impaired glucose tolerance or if you have reached the point of impaired fasting glucose, you have what is called *prediabetes.* Now things are getting really serious—so serious that we'll have to spend all of Chapter 5 discussing prediabetes and what it means for your health.

Unless action is taken to stop the underlying cycle of insulin resistance and hyperinsulinism, then the body's compensatory mechanism of overproduction of insulin will continue. As your insulin resistance becomes more severe, your blood sugar levels become increasingly difficult to control and your pancreas becomes increasingly stressed. Without proper intervention, you'll move from prediabetes to the next stage of full-blown Type 2 diabetes.

ARRIVING AT DIABETES

Stage 5 represents the early phase of true diabetes. In this stage, your fasting blood sugar is usually 126 mg/dL or higher, and your blood sugar after meals will consistently be even higher above the normal range. At this point, most people continue to have high levels of insulin production combined with severe insulin resistance.

Unless dramatic intervention occurs, the huge amounts of insulin your pancreas is forced to produce will eventually lead to a loss of pancreatic beta cell function. Indeed, you may lose so much beta cell function that your pancreas is making little or no insulin. By now, to survive, you will require the daily administration of insulin. When this happens, you have reached stage 6—insulin-dependent diabetes.

Oftimes, it is only when you have reached these last two stages that a diagnosis of Type 2 diabetes is finally made. Now the diagnosis is hard to miss. Your fasting blood sugar is in the diabetic range of 126 mg/dL or higher, and the classic symptoms of increased thirst, increased hunger, and increased urination occur. In some cases, unexplained weight loss and blurred vision also occur. By now, insulin resistance, hyperinsulinism, and hyperglycemia have been present for a long time, perhaps years, silently causing damage.

ARE YOU AN UNDIAGNOSED DIABETIC?

According to the American Diabetes Association, of the 18 million Americans with Type 2 diabetes, somewhere between 5 million and

8 million don't know they have it. Here's one reason that early diagnosis is so important: Retinopathy, blood vessel damage to the eyes, begins to develop at least seven years before clinical diagnosis of Type 2 diabetes is made based either on symptoms or standard blood tests.[7, 8] Some undiagnosed diabetics will find out the hard way: when they end up in the emergency room with a heart attack, a stroke, kidney disease, or other vascular conditions. Others will learn the truth when they visit the doctor for something else and a routine blood test reveals their disease. Could you be one of them?

BLOOD SUGAR BY THE NUMBERS

According to the American Diabetes Association, the definitions of normal and impaired blood sugar are:

Normal Fasting Blood Sugar (FBS). Although there may be some variation among testing labs, normal FBS ranges from 65 to 99 mg/dL (milligrams per deciliter) after a fast of 8 to 12 hours. The measurement is accurate only if you haven't eaten for at least 8 hours before your blood is drawn.

Impaired Fasting Glucose (IFG). A blood glucose level between 100 and 125 mg/dL (5.5 to 6.9 mmol/L [millimoles per liter]) after a fast of at least eight hours. If you have IFG, you have prediabetes.

Impaired Glucose Tolerance (IGT). You have impaired glucose tolerance if two hours after eating a carbohydrate test meal your blood sugar has risen to above 140 mg/dL but stays below 200 mg/dL. If you have impaired glucose tolerance, you have prediabetes, whether or not you also have impaired fasting blood sugar.

Diabetes. Fasting blood sugar of 126 mg/dL or higher on two readings after fasting for at least eight hours indicates diabetes. An alternative measurement is a postprandial (after a meal) blood sugar of 200 mg/dL or higher two hours after a high-carbohydrate meal on two different days, or similar results at the two-hour point during an oral glucose tolerance test.[9]

Being diagnosed with high fasting blood sugar is like being told you're a little bit pregnant—things will become more apparent very soon. That's what happened with a patient named Donna G. Less than a year passed from the time her doctor told her she had high fasting blood sugar to the time she came to see Dr. Atkins to treat her full-blown Type 2 diabetes. If only she had started on the Atkins program when she was first diagnosed with high blood sugar, she might well never have gone on to that point. As it is, following the program has helped her quite a bit. Her fasting blood sugar over the past several years has always been steady at around 100 mg/dL.

Current medical guidelines say that if you have *any* of the risk factors for diabetes, your doctor should regularly check your fasting blood sugar level. But if you've been paying attention, you now know that by the time your fasting blood sugar is high, the damage has already started. (We'll discuss tests to detect blood sugar abnormalities in Chapter 6, Diagnosis: Diabetes.)

The onward march toward diabetes and steadily worsening health might seem inevitable. Not so! At any point along the way it is possible to stop the progression. The sooner the better, of course, but even if you have reached stage 6 of diabetes, the Atkins Blood Sugar Control Program can help you manage the disease and help you to stave off some of its worst consequences. Please read on—that's what the rest of this book is all about.

DO YOU HAVE A BLOOD SUGAR PROBLEM?

The effects of the blood sugar roller coaster on your health and well-being are fairly predictable. Compare your symptoms to the following list of the most common symptoms of abnormal blood sugar. Score each symptom according to how you experience it:

0 = never
1 = mild and/or rarely
2 = moderate and/or up to twice a week
3 = severe and/or more than twice a week

	0	1	2	3
Hunger between meals				
Craving sweets				
Craving starchy foods				
Waking with a headache				
Thirsty all the time				
Frequent urination				
Irritable before meals				
Shaky feeling, especially when hungry				
Constant tiredness				
Daytime sleepiness				
Sleepiness after meals				
Difficulty concentrating				

Add up each column and then multiply the sum by the number at the top of that column. Now add all the numbers together. Remember, all the answers in the 0 column = 0. If your score is 12 or more, you're probably experiencing some blood sugar abnormalities. Please see your doctor to explore the issue further, especially if you also have any risk factors for diabetes.

A NEW PATH WITHOUT PILLS

After a 30-year hiatus, Ann McKay has returned to the very same program with which she initially experienced success. It is now helping her restore her health.

NAME: **Ann McKay**
AGE: **57**
HEIGHT: **5 feet 0 inches**
WEIGHT BEFORE:
247 pounds
WEIGHT NOW:
205 pounds

I've had a serious weight problem all my life. In fact, I did Atkins for the first time 32 years ago when Dr. Atkins' original book, Dr. Atkins' Diet Revolution, *was published. I am a registered nurse and, at the time, I was working on a surgical unit. Although I was doing well on Atkins—losing weight and feeling good—the surgeons I worked with were vehemently against it. They told me I was going to get sick and that it would ruin my kidneys. They were on me about it every day. Atkins was a brand-new concept at the time, and I thought, "Well, what if they're right?" So I did go off the program after about 12 weeks. During the 30 years since then, I have been on every conceivable diet there is, never with any real success.*

In 1996, I was placed on the drug Lupron and had a hysterectomy. From that point on, my weight problem only got worse. No mat-

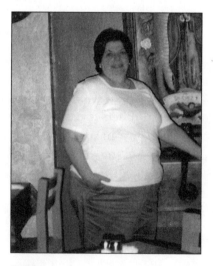

BEFORE

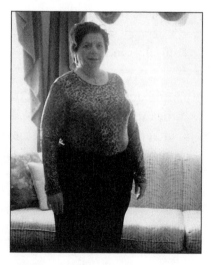

AFTER

ter how little I ate, no matter what diet I tried, I simply could not lose any weight.

About two years ago, I found myself at a depressing 247 pounds—I'm only 5 feet tall—and wearing a size 26. I also discovered that my blood sugar level was going up—it was around 170 mg/dL. When I spoke to my primary-care doctor about it, he wanted me to go on a 1,500-calorie-a-day American Diabetes Association (ADA) diet. I told him, "Well, I've been on a 1,000-calorie diet pretty much my whole life, one way or another, and it hasn't worked."

I had even been hospitalized in the 1970s for my weight problem, where I was placed on a 700- to 800-calorie-a-day diet. I remember waiting for my eight o'clock snack of Tab soda and celery sticks. It was really sad. I was there for three and a half weeks and I gained 5 pounds.

All these years later, not wanting to be put on yet another low-calorie diet, I asked my doctor, "What about Atkins?" And he said, "Oh, I just lost 40 pounds on Atkins! But I don't want you on it." He was apparently concerned about my medical history—I've had some serious health problems. I don't think he wanted to do the close monitoring that he thought would be necessary if I went on Atkins. So, he handed me the 1,500-calorie ADA diet and said, "Try this for two weeks and then come back and we'll see what we're going to start you on." I knew what that meant: He was going to put me on diabetes medication.

When I got home, I was very upset. I knew I had the phone number for The Atkins Center somewhere in my house and began madly sifting through my papers to find it. When I called the number, a nurse answered the phone and I spilled my guts to her. "I just left my doctor's office and I'm very angry and upset," I said. "I know where's he's heading. He wants to put me on medication. Also, I've been seeing him for hypothyroidism, and I feel he's not looking at it properly. All my hormone levels are normal but I know there's something wrong with my thyroid. I was just wondering if Dr. Atkins still sees patients?" I was told he did. I breathed a sigh of relief. She faxed me a questionnaire that day, I filled it out and, three weeks later, I had my appointment. I did one day of lab work and then saw Dr. Atkins the very next day.

I liked Dr. Atkins right away. He reminded me of the old-time GP I had as a child. He was solid and confident. "You've got a complex medical situation here," he said, "and it could have been straightened out years *ago." He asked me several questions, went through the eating plan with me, and told me I'd need to come to The Atkins Center once a month for follow-up. So for the next six months, I went every month—a big commitment when you have to drive three and a half hours to get there. Fortunately, my husband was willing to get up at six a.m. and drive with me each time.*

When I first saw Dr. Atkins, my blood sugar level was 179, my cholesterol was 215, my triglycerides were 158, my HDL was 41 and my LDL was 142, and other lab results were also out of whack. As I'd suspected, my thyroid was not okay. Dr. Atkins took me off my medication and put me on natural alternatives. As of my last visit, my thyroid was normal, my cholesterol was down to 160, my blood sugar was within the normal range, and all of my other lab results had dropped from high-risk levels to within a normal range. My weight is 205 pounds—42 pounds less than I was—and I'm still losing about a quarter of a pound each week. I have lost 72 inches and am wearing a size 16 or 18. It's a very slow process, but I have to look at the big picture. It's not so much the change in my weight that matters, it's the improvements in my blood sugar and my cholesterol. Recent labs measured a fasting blood sugar level of 96, cholesterol of 164, triglycerides of 72, HDL of 55, and LDL of 95. Dr. Atkins said that when I first came to him, I was three months away from a heart event.

Thanks to Atkins, I now exercise and can walk up and down the stairs of my house without becoming out of breath. Best of all, at age 57, I have a general, overall sense of well-being that I never had before. I also like what I see in the mirror. Recently, I was packing for a trip to Florida and I tried on a top that was a size 2X or something. I turned to my husband and said, "Look how big this is on me!" He smiled at me and said, "You just lit right up when you said that." I'm going to save that top forever as a reminder to never go back to that size again.

Note: Your individual results may vary from those reported here.

Chapter 3

WEIGHING IN: THE NUMBER ONE RISK FACTOR

As we have stressed, the road to diabetes is a long one and at any point along the way, you can tip the balance back in your favor and stop the progression. That's because you have a good deal of control over most of the risk factors for diabetes. The warning signs are there, if you have the knowledge and awareness to recognize them. In fact, if all this book does is help you notice these signs before you—or your doctor— would have otherwise, it will have been well worth the purchase price.

The number one risk factor for both men and women for developing diabetes is obesity, although you do not have to be overweight to become diabetic.[1] There is a clear relationship among weight gain, age, and the risk of developing Type 2 diabetes in women. The younger a woman is when she begins to gain weight, the higher her lifetime risk of getting diabetes. The good news is that studies show that overweight women who slimmed down were able to lower their risk.[2]

Research findings on men show the same trends. The long-running Health Professionals Study looked at the relationship between obesity and weight gain and Type 2 diabetes in more than 51,000 men, ages 40 to 75. Researchers found that men with a BMI of 35 or greater were 42.1 times more likely to develop diabetes compared with men at their ideal weight with a BMI of 23 or less.[3]

Preventing normal individuals in certain populations from becoming overweight has also been shown to prevent diabetes. Maintaining a healthy weight would result in a 62 percent reduction in the incidence of Type 2 diabetes in Mexican Americans and a 74 percent reduction in non-Hispanic whites.[4] Genetics and other factors—which we'll discuss later—can lead to Type 2 diabetes in people whose weight is within the normal range.

WHAT DOES OVERWEIGHT MEAN?

How heavy do you need to be to be at risk? That depends. The terms *normal weight, overweight,* and *obese* are really ways of describing weight ranges, not exact weights. That's why the medical profession has stopped using the old weight-for-height charts to determine a person's level of excess weight. The charts took a one-size-fits-all approach that defined the normal range too broadly and did not take body composition into consideration.

Since 1998, doctors have used the body-weight guidelines issued by the National Institutes of Health. These guidelines are based on body mass index (BMI). The BMI uses a mathematical formula to compare your height to your weight. (There's a separate BMI formula for kids and teens, discussed in Chapter 24.) To find your BMI, use the table on pages 28–29.

According to the chart, a woman who is 64 inches tall (5 feet 4

WHAT YOUR BMI MEANS

Doctors use the BMI to classify an individual's weight as follows:

Normal weight range: BMI of between 20 and 24.9
Overweight: BMI of between 25 and 29.9
Obese: BMI of 30 or more
Extremely or morbidly obese: BMI of 40 or more[5]

inches) and weighs between 110 and 144.9 pounds is within the normal weight range for her height. As a general rule, however, you want your BMI to be in the 20 to 22 range—so in this case, she would ideally weigh between 116 and 128 pounds. The difference in pounds across BMI levels takes into account different builds and body types. If this same woman weighed between 145 and 173 pounds, she would be overweight; if she weighed 174 pounds or more, she would be obese. To qualify as morbidly obese, she would need to weigh more than 232 pounds. (The terms *extreme* and *morbid obesity* are used for people who are so overweight that their weight interferes with basic physical functions such as breathing.) The BMI chart lets you see quickly and accurately where you stand in weight range for your height. If you're overweight or obese, it also gives you a good idea of what a healthier weight range would be for you.

Still, there are some limitations to the BMI chart. If you're very muscular, your BMI might fall into the overweight category, even though you're very fit and have a normal to low percentage of body fat. A more worrisome problem is that you might fall into the normal BMI weight range even though poor health has left you frail and you should actually weigh more. For those over 65, desirable BMI ranges are slightly higher.[6] However, the BMI is a pretty good indication how your weight compares with the normal range.

A more accurate way to figure out if you're overweight is to ascertain your percentage of body fat. Body-fat measurement is not a standard test at a typical doctor's office. It requires special equipment and it's usually not an exact science. It's most useful for tracking the trend of your weight, especially if you are exercising, to see if you are losing fat and gaining muscle.[7]

DIABETES AND BMI

An individual's risk of getting diabetes increases proportionally to the increase in his or her BMI. In the United States, two-thirds of the adult men and women diagnosed with diabetes have a BMI above 27. As you can see by the chart on pages 28–29, a BMI of 27 qualifies a person as overweight but not yet obese.[8, 9]

To use this chart, find your height in inches in the left-hand column, and then look across to find your weight in pounds. The number at the top of the column is your body mass index.

BODY MASS INDEX (BMI) TABLE

	NORMAL						OVERWEIGHT					OBESE				
BMI	19	20	21	22	23	24	25	26	27	28	29	30	31	32	33	34	35
HEIGHT (INCHES)							BODY WEIGHT (POUNDS)										
58	91	96	100	105	110	115	119	124	129	134	138	143	148	153	158	162	167
59	94	99	104	109	114	119	124	128	133	138	143	148	153	158	163	168	173
60	97	102	107	112	118	123	128	133	138	143	148	153	158	163	168	174	179
61	100	106	111	116	122	127	132	137	143	148	153	158	164	169	174	180	185
62	104	109	115	120	126	131	136	142	147	153	158	164	169	175	180	186	191
63	107	113	118	124	130	135	141	146	152	158	163	169	175	180	186	191	197
64	110	116	122	128	134	140	145	151	157	163	169	174	180	186	192	197	204
65	114	120	126	132	138	144	150	156	162	168	174	180	186	192	198	204	210
66	118	124	130	136	142	148	155	161	167	173	179	186	192	198	204	210	216
67	121	127	134	140	146	153	159	166	172	178	185	191	198	204	211	217	223
68	125	131	138	144	151	158	164	171	177	184	190	197	203	210	216	223	230
69	128	135	142	149	155	162	169	176	182	189	196	203	209	216	223	230	236
70	132	139	146	153	160	167	174	181	188	195	202	209	216	222	229	236	243
71	136	143	150	157	165	172	179	186	193	200	208	215	222	229	236	243	250
72	140	147	154	162	169	177	184	191	199	206	213	221	228	235	242	250	258
73	144	151	159	166	174	182	189	197	204	212	219	227	235	242	250	257	265
74	148	155	163	171	179	186	194	202	210	218	225	233	241	249	256	264	272
75	152	160	168	176	184	192	200	208	216	224	232	240	248	256	264	272	279
76	156	164	172	180	189	197	205	213	221	230	238	246	254	263	271	279	287

Source: Adapted from *Clinical Guidelines on the Identification, Evaluation, and Treatment of Overweight and Obesity in Adults: The Evidence Report.*

Dr. Atkins used to say that he rarely saw a patient with a BMI above 30 who wasn't already well on the way to diabetes, or there already. One patient, Larry H., really stands out in that regard. Several years before he came to see Dr. Atkins, Larry was told by his doctor that he was borderline diabetic and put him on a variety of drugs. Larry, who

	OBESE							EXTREME OBESITY										
36	37	38	39	40	41	42	43	44	45	46	47	48	49	50	51	52	53	54
							BODY WEIGHT (POUNDS)											
172	177	181	186	191	196	201	205	210	215	220	224	229	234	239	244	248	253	258
178	183	188	193	198	203	208	212	217	222	227	232	237	242	247	252	257	262	267
184	189	194	199	204	209	215	220	225	230	235	240	245	250	255	261	266	271	276
190	195	201	206	211	217	222	227	232	238	243	248	254	259	264	269	275	280	285
196	202	207	213	218	224	229	235	240	246	251	256	262	267	273	278	284	289	295
203	208	214	220	225	231	237	242	248	254	259	265	270	278	282	287	293	299	304
209	215	221	227	232	238	244	250	256	262	267	273	279	285	291	296	302	308	314
216	222	228	234	240	246	252	258	264	270	276	282	288	294	300	306	312	318	324
223	229	235	241	247	253	260	266	272	278	284	291	297	303	309	315	322	328	334
230	236	242	249	255	261	268	274	280	287	293	299	306	312	319	325	331	338	344
236	243	249	256	262	269	276	282	289	295	302	308	315	322	328	335	341	348	354
243	250	257	263	270	277	284	291	297	304	311	318	324	331	338	345	351	358	365
250	257	264	271	278	285	292	299	306	313	320	327	334	341	348	355	362	369	376
257	265	272	279	286	293	301	308	315	322	329	338	343	351	358	365	372	379	386
265	272	279	287	294	302	309	316	324	331	338	346	353	361	368	375	383	390	397
272	280	288	295	302	310	318	325	333	340	348	355	363	371	378	386	393	401	408
280	287	295	303	311	319	326	334	342	350	358	365	373	381	389	396	404	412	420
287	295	303	311	319	327	335	343	351	359	367	375	383	391	399	407	415	423	431
295	304	312	320	328	336	344	353	361	369	377	385	394	402	410	418	426	435	443

was overweight, dutifully took the drugs but didn't change his high-carb diet. When he arrived at the office, he had gained even more weight and his BMI was around 37. Dr. Atkins took one look at Larry and just knew he already had diabetes. His fasting blood sugar confirmed his hunch—it came in at 201 mg/dL.

RESEARCH REPORT: WOMEN, WEIGHT GAIN, AND DIABETES

In an article published in 1995, researchers studied weight and weight gain among women as risk factors for developing Type 2 diabetes. They looked at more than 114,000 women, ages 30 to 55, who had taken part in the long-running Nurses' Health Study between 1976 and 1990.[10]

Not surprisingly, the researchers found that among these women, body mass index was the dominant predictor of diabetes. The higher their BMI, the greater the risk. Even women who were at the high end of *normal* weight, with a BMI of 24, had an elevated risk.

The heavier a woman is, the greater her risk of diabetes, as shown in the following chart:

BMI	DIABETES RISK
22	<1
25–26.9	8.1 times greater
29–30.9	27.6 times greater
35+	93.2 times greater

The researchers also looked at the women's weight gain over the 14 years of the study. Compared with women whose weight stayed pretty much the same or went up by fewer than 11 pounds, women who experienced more weight gain had a greater risk of diabetes, as shown in the following chart:

14-YEAR WEIGHT GAIN	RELATIVE RISK OF DIABETES
Up to 11-lb. gain	(no change)
11- to 17-lb. gain	1.9 times greater
17- to 24-lb. gain	2.7 times greater
44-lb. gain	12.3 times greater

Even among the women who fell into the normal BMI category, modest amounts of weight gain increased the risk of diabetes. The women who started the study with BMIs between 22 and 25 and gained only 11 to 15 pounds (5 to 6.9 kg) over 14 years still had 1.6 times the risk of diabetes. In other words, even though at the end of the study period they were still within the guidelines for normal weight, the weight they did gain was enough to nearly double their risk of diabetes.[11]

THE HEALTH RISKS OF BEING OVERWEIGHT

If you are carrying around extra pounds, you are tempting fate in more ways than one. Overall, being obese significantly increases your risk of developing the metabolic syndrome and all its potential complications. It is so important that you understand this condition that we have devoted an entire chapter to it. Without an understanding of the abnormal changes in your chemistry, it will be impossible for you to comprehend why controlling carbs is a key to prevention of diabetes. Being overweight also is implicated in gallbladder disease, a number of forms of cancer, osteoarthritis, asthma, sleep apnea, breathing difficulties, complications of pregnancy, polycystic ovary syndrome (PCOS), and increased surgical risk.[12]

If you're overweight and also have low HDL cholesterol and high triglycerides, there's a pretty good chance that you're also insulin resistant and could be well on your way to prediabetes or diabetes. Add in high blood pressure or any other diabetes risk factor and the odds are even greater. Even if you're not yet insulin resistant and have normal cholesterol and blood pressure, you're still not immune to diabetes and other health problems. The following table gives you a good idea of exactly how your risk for a number of chronic diseases increases if you're overweight or obese, compared with your risk if your weight is normal (BMI of 24.9 or less).

INCREASED RISK OF WEIGHT-RELATED DISEASES

DISEASE	BMI 25 OR LESS	BMI 25–30	BMI 30–35	BMI 35+
Arthritis	1.00	1.56	1.87	2.39
Heart disease	1.00	1.39	1.86	1.67
Type 2 diabetes	1.00	2.42	3.35	6.16
Gallstones	1.00	1.97	3.30	5.48
Hypertension	1.00	1.92	2.82	3.77
Stroke	1.00	1.53	1.59	1.75

Source: The Lewin Group, "Costs of Obesity," September 2000, available at: http://www.lewin.com/Lewin_Publications/Uncategorised/Publication-8.htm

THE INFAMOUS LOVE HANDLES

Strange as it sounds, carrying most of your excess weight in the abdominal area—sometimes described as having an "apple" shape—gives you a higher risk of diabetes. This very important risk factor is discussed in the next chapter. Study after study has shown that having a high waist-to-hip ratio or a large waist is a powerful predictor of diabetes risk. Even if your weight is within the norm for your height, how your body fat is distributed plays an important role. The more abdominal fat you have, the greater your risk of diabetes.[13–15]

Also, when researchers compare people with the same BMI—in other words, those who are roughly the same weight and height—they invariably find that the ones who have the most abdominal fat have the worst lipid profiles.

STRESS-RELATED OVERINDULGING

Everyone knows stress is bad, but the myriad ways it sabotages your health might surprise you. Many people overeat when they're stressed, so high stress levels can lead to obesity, which in turn can lead to diabetes. But there is another, insidious factor at work when you're under a lot of stress: Your body produces large amounts of stress hormones, such as cortisol. Among other things, stress hormones increase your appetite and raise your insulin levels. High insulin levels often lead to cravings for carbohydrates and sweets. And the cycle goes on. What's worse, the weight you put on as a result tends to accumulate in your abdominal area—which, as we've said, further increases your risk of moving on to diabetes.[16] Some people eat when they get stressed. Some people drink more alcohol. Some do both. Alcohol abuse is yet another risk factor that can nudge you toward diabetes.[17]

One reason is that heavy alcohol consumption increases your cortisol levels. Another is that long-term alcohol abuse can damage your pancreas and disrupt the normal production of insulin. Alcohol abuse also damages your liver—and because your liver plays an important role in controlling your blood sugar, this can contribute to developing diabetes. Adding to the unhealthy cycle is that abusing alcohol can also pile on the excess pounds.

Being overweight may be the biggest risk factor pushing you toward Type 2 diabetes, but it's not the only one. Having any one risk factor is a warning sign that you're probably already on the diabetes path. However, the more risk factors you combine, and the longer you have them, the greater the likelihood that you will eventually develop diabetes. In the next chapter, we'll look at a cluster of other disease risk factors that are likely to accompany you as you continue down the path to diabetes.

DO YOU UNDERSTAND THE BMI?

1. You're in the normal weight range when your BMI is: ___
2. You're in the overweight range when your BMI is: ___
3. You're in the obese range when your BMI is: ___
4. You're in the morbidly obese range when your BMI is: ___

Answers
1. 20–24.9, 2. 25–29.9, 3. 30–39.9, 4. 40 or more.

(continued)

Where do you stand on the BMI chart?
My weight: _____
My height: _____
My BMI is:
Normal _____
Overweight _____
Obese _____

Chapter 4

A DEADLY QUINTET: MEET THE METABOLIC SYNDROME

The metabolic syndrome is a group of five garden-variety risk factors that, when combined, indicate you are likely to develop diabetes, hypertension, and coronary artery (heart) disease.[1] If you have this syndrome and do nothing about it, you are almost guaranteed to end up with a life-threatening illness. Because current medical practice does not recommend, as Dr. Atkins believed it should, the earliest possible comprehensive testing for insulin/blood sugar imbalances, each of you needs to take action now and be vigilant on your own behalf. We all must be active partners in our health care if we are to effectively confront the epidemic of what Dr. Atkins called "diabesity." The symptoms of the metabolic syndrome must be identified early and taken seriously. If we can teach you to recognize the warning signs of this perilous syndrome, you can take action to stop it in its tracks. After you finish reading this book we're confident that you will understand why controlling carbohydrates with the Atkins Blood Sugar Control Program (ABSCP) is really the best—and only—solution.

HOW IT ALL BEGINS

Like diabetes, weight gain is a gradual process. The pounds of fat can creep up over the years, virtually unnoticed. Even before you've let your belt out a couple of notches, however, those extra pounds have started to damage your health.

We tend to think of excess weight as simply the body's way of storing extra fat—and we think of those rolls of flesh as soft storage banks. In fact, your body fat doesn't quietly sit there; it's metabolically active, continually secreting chemicals such as hormones and cytokines. These chemical messengers are innocent members of your body's normal cell-to-cell communication system. In large amounts, however, they can cause inflammation in your cells. Just as an infection on your finger causes swelling, warmth, and redness in the area, this overload of chemical secretions from excess body fat does the same to your *endothelium*—the cells that line your blood vessels. The difference is that you can't see or feel the inflammation. The process is complex and happens slowly at first, but it begins almost as soon as you start to put on extra pounds.

The cells of the endothelium regulate how nutrients and other substances in your bloodstream get into your cells. When the endothelium becomes inflamed, normal body processes start to get out of whack. As you continue to gain weight—especially from an inactive lifestyle and a high-carb diet—the inflammation worsens and the effect on your endothelium becomes more severe. You develop endothelial dysfunction. And what goes hand in hand with endothelial dysfunction? Insulin resistance. In fact, it's the chicken-or-the-egg scenario: endothelial dysfunction and insulin resistance are so intertwined that it's extremely difficult to tell which triggers which.[2, 3]

COINING A TERM

For decades doctors noticed a pattern in a large percentage of patients. People who were overweight tended also to have high blood pressure, diabetes, and heart disease. As a cardiologist, Dr. Atkins long ago saw a link between excess fat, insulin resistance, heart disease, and diabetes. It wasn't until the early 1980s, however, that some perceptive researchers, particularly Dr. Gerald Reaven of Stanford University, started connecting more of the dots. What they noticed was that patients who had abdominal obesity, high blood pressure, high triglycerides, low HDL cholesterol, and sometimes high fasting blood sugar were more likely to develop Type 2 diabetes, hypertension, and coronary artery disease.[4]

Doctors call a group of related signs and symptoms a syndrome, so Dr. Reaven coined the term for this cluster of signs *syndrome X*. It's still sometimes called that, but today most researchers and doctors call it the metabolic syndrome. Although many nutritionally oriented doctors have been diagnosing this syndrome, with or without a name, for years, the American medical establishment accepted its existence only in 2001, when the third Adult Treatment Panel (ATP III) of the National Cholesterol Education Program (NCEP) officially defined it. In keeping with the drug treatment approach to disease, which is the hallmark of Western medicine, the ATP III stated that control of the metabolic syndrome was secondary to the goal of controlling LDL cholesterol. This approach misses the point of correcting the underlying imbalance leading to the metabolic syndrome. We'll discuss this further in the chapter on heart disease.[5]

Another definition for the metabolic syndrome had been released by the World Health Organization (WHO) in 1999. The two definitions are somewhat different, but because the ATP III definition is the one used in the United States, that's what we'll use here.[6] (See page 38 for the WHO definition.)

DEFINING THE METABOLIC SYNDROME

You officially have the metabolic syndrome if you have *three or more* of these signs:

- Abdominal obesity: a waist circumference greater than 40 inches (102 cm) in men and 35 inches (88 cm) in women (more on this important risk factor on page 114)
- High triglycerides: 150 mg/dL or more
- Low HDL cholesterol: under 40 mg/dL for men and under 50 mg/dL for women
- High blood pressure: 135/85 mmHg or greater
- High fasting blood sugar: 110 mg/dL or greater[7]

How many people fit those criteria? Far too many. Today, about 25 percent of all American adults have the metabolic syndrome. The older you get, the more likely you are to have it: Forty-four percent of the U.S. population over the age of 50 meets the criteria.[8]

In reality, even more than 44 percent of the population probably has it. The ATP III definition doesn't include insulin resistance as a symptom—only high fasting blood sugar counts. Unfortunately, by the time you develop noticeably high blood sugar, you've probably had insulin resistance for many years—and the damage to your body

THE WHO DEFINITION

In 1998, the World Health Organization proposed a definition of the metabolic syndrome that is now widely used outside the United States.[9] There are some significant differences among the components in the WHO definition and the ATP III definition used in the United States. The WHO definition puts more emphasis on blood sugar, uses a higher cutoff point for high blood pressure, and includes the presence of small amounts of protein in the urine, known as *microalbuminuria.*

According to the WHO definition, you have the metabolic syndrome if you have impaired glucose tolerance, impaired fasting glucose, diabetes, or insulin resistance, along with two or more of these other signs:[10]

- High blood pressure: 140/90 mmHg or higher
- High triglycerides: 150 mm/dL or greater (1.7 mmol/L or greater)
- Low HDL cholesterol: 35 mg/dL or less (0.9 mmol/L or less) for men; 39 mg/dL (1.0 mmol/L) for women
- Central obesity: waist-to-hip ratio greater than 0.90 for men; 0.85 or greater for women and/or a BMI greater than 30
- Microalbuminuria: urinary albumin excretion rate of 20 μg/min or more or an albumin-to-creatinine ratio of 30 mg/g or more

has been ongoing for those many years. Dr. Atkins saw countless patients who were slightly overweight, had mild high blood pressure, and only slightly elevated triglycerides. Although they didn't yet meet the formal definition of the metabolic syndrome, they already exhibited the early stages. He recommended intervention at this stage to avoid progression to diabetes and its complications.

THE METABOLIC SYNDROME AND PREDIABETES

The metabolic syndrome and prediabetes are essentially interchangeable. Both are precursors to full-blown diabetes. Only about 13 percent of people who go on to develop diabetes *don't* meet the formal definition of the metabolic syndrome.[11] As a cardiologist, Dr. Atkins long ago recognized the link between gaining fat, insulin resistance, and the ultimate development of diabetes and heart disease. If you don't have high blood sugar, the other criteria for the metabolic syndrome still put you at higher risk for heart disease and stroke. When you consider that the elevated triglycerides and low HDL that are part of the metabolic syndrome are a result of abnormal insulin/glucose metabolism, the link is clear.[12] These warning signs are all intertwined and interdependent, and when you combine a few of them, the resulting scenario is like a ticking bomb.

LIFESTYLE CAUSE AND EFFECT

The two main lifestyle factors that cause the metabolic syndrome are exactly the same as those that can lead to diabetes: a high-carb diet combined with physical inactivity. But just as lifestyle plays the most important role in causing the metabolic syndrome, lifestyle can play the most important role in preventing or reversing it. Therefore, with lifestyle in mind, let's take a closer look at the five symptoms of the metabolic syndrome:

Abdominal Obesity

You might call it love handles, a spare tire, a potbelly, or even a beer gut. Doctors call it truncal obesity, abdominal obesity, central obesity, or visceral adiposity. Whatever the name, your protruding abdominal outline is caused by fat stored around your intestines and abdominal organs as well as right under your skin. Fat stored in this way is much more dangerous to your health than fat stored under the skin of your buttocks and thighs.[13–15] Doctors use the waist-to-hip ratio (WHR) or waist circumference to define the point at which your abdominal fat stores are posing a health risk. This is because excessive abdominal fat makes the circumference of your waist bigger than that of your hips. To find your WHR, measure your waist at the navel and measure your hips, then divide the waist number by the hip number. For example, if your waist is 36 inches and your hips are 40 inches, your WHR is 0.9. The higher your WHR, the more "apple-shaped" you are. A less scientific way to evaluate yourself is to look at your body profile in a mirror. If your silhouette is bigger around the middle than around the hips, you have an "apple" shape. If your silhouette is larger at the hips, you have a "pear" shape. If you're apple-shaped, you have greater risk of health problems related to blood sugar than someone who's pear-shaped, even if you're both the same height and weight.[16]

Now, all you pear-shaped folks, don't think you're off the hook. Even if your weight settles below the belt, you still have a greater risk of health problems than those who are normal weight, especially if your BMI is above 30.[17] No matter where it is on your body, the more fat you have, the more likely you are to develop the metabolic syndrome.

The powerful effect of abdominal fat can lead to a paradoxical condition: You could be of normal weight for your height and build, or just slightly heavier than ideal, but nonetheless be what's called *metabolically obese*.[18]

I have a patient who is a very good example of metabolic obesity. Selma M. was 48 years old, five feet three inches tall, and weighed 158 pounds, giving her a BMI of 28, when she came to me. Selma was overweight but not obese; still, she already had the worst lipid profile imaginable. Her HDL cholesterol was only 20, while her triglycerides were a sky-high

2,208! I put her on the Atkins Nutritional Approach—and the changes over the next year were remarkable. Her weight only dropped one pound, but her HDL cholesterol rose to 31 and her triglycerides dropped to just 147. Even better, her body fat dropped from 36 percent to 27.5 percent. After almost five years, she has lost a total of ten pounds, has a total cholesterol of 149, triglycerides of 84, and an HDL of 39. I should add that she did not begin an exercise program until 2002, so these remarkable outcomes were due to her dietary treatment alone.

—Mary Vernon

We don't understand exactly why abdominal fat is so detrimental. Nor do we understand why some people are more sensitive to abdominal fat. But, like Selma, some folks will develop dramatic and dangerous blood sugar and lipid problems despite only a moderate amount of excess weight—when that weight is concentrated in the torso. It's important to realize that even being on the high end of normal is sometimes enough to trigger the metabolic syndrome, especially if that excess weight is in your midsection.

The good news is that the ABSCP can reverse the metabolic syndrome, regardless of how much weight you're carrying or where you carry it. Numerous studies have shown that modest weight loss and moderate daily exercise, which builds muscle mass, can be enough to help you lose some of that abdominal fat and pull back from the brink of the metabolic syndrome.

Dr. Atkins often saw this happen with his patients. Marty K. is a typical example. When first seen, Marty carried 208 pounds on a five-foot-eight-inch frame and had already been diagnosed with the metabolic syndrome and insulin resistance. His primary-care doctor put him on a low-fat, low-protein diet (which by definition is a high-carbohydrate diet). All that did for Marty was sap his energy to the point that he could hardly get around at all, much less exercise. When he found that he not only wasn't losing weight but was now starting to have hypoglycemic episodes, he decided the time had come to visit Dr. Atkins for a different approach. Marty was immediately placed on the controlled-carb program. Within five weeks, he had lost weight and his hypoglycemic episodes stopped, his blood sugar and lipids improved markedly, and he soon felt energetic enough to begin an exercise program. That accelerated his weight loss and improved his blood sugar and lipids even more.

RESEARCH REPORT: THE PERILS OF POTBELLIES

How much does having the metabolic syndrome increase your risk of heart disease and diabetes? A lot, according to the results of numerous studies. Let's look at just one recent one, the West of Scotland Coronary Prevention Study. This study followed a group of more than 12,000 men who had slightly elevated LDL cholesterol. When the study began, none of the men had diabetes or had had a heart attack, but about 26 percent of them had the metabolic syndrome, based on the NCEP (National Cholesterol Education Program) definition. When it ended nearly five years later, the men with the metabolic syndrome had developed heart disease at nearly twice the rate as that for the men without it. In other words, their risk of heart disease because they had the metabolic syndrome was the equivalent of being ten years older than their actual age, or of being a smoker. The rate for diabetes was even more shocking. The men with the metabolic syndrome had 3.5 times the risk of developing diabetes as the men without the syndrome. When the researchers looked at the men who had four of the five signs of the metabolic syndrome (instead of the minimum of three), the risk of diabetes soared to 24.5 times higher than that for the men without the metabolic syndrome.[19]

This was no surprise to Dr. Atkins, who had observed this connection for many years because of his standard evaluation of insulin and glucose abnormalities using tests more extensive than those currently recommended. He developed the ABSCP to address this problem at its source, since it only makes sense to intervene as early as possible, especially when the consequences are severe, as this study so clearly demonstrates. Avoiding these disastrous outcomes benefits not only the patients themselves but also our whole society, by allowing more people to be productive longer and avoiding the astronomical costs of treating heart attacks, strokes, and diabetes.

High Triglycerides

The triglycerides in your blood are nothing more than tiny droplets of fat. The more of them you have floating around in your bloodstream, the greater your risk of a heart attack. If your triglyceride level is 150 mg/dL or more, your risk is definitely elevated; as your triglyceride level goes up, so does your risk. Dr. Atkins believed that the danger from high triglycerides is so serious that the optimum level should be below 100 mg/dL. Fortunately, triglycerides respond well to lifestyle

HIGH CARBS, HIGH TRIGLYCERIDES

It's an accepted truth: A high-carbohydrate diet causes high triglycerides—and this effect is independent of how heavy you are or whether your insulin levels are abnormal.[20, 21] We know from treating thousands of patients that triglycerides drop quickly and consistently in response to a decrease in carbohydrate consumption. Control your carbs, and your triglyceride number will drop sharply.

According to the American Heart Association, substituting carbohydrates for fats may raise triglyceride levels and may decrease HDL ("good") cholesterol in some people.[22] Yet most doctors persist in telling patients who gain weight easily to cut down on fat and meat. For some, this advice is a recipe for disaster. Why? Decreasing fat and protein in the diet inevitably means increasing carbohydrates. This shifts the metabolism toward fat storage—and higher triglycerides. Not only that, it also leaves the person feeling hungry all the time and subject to blood sugar swings. When the situation is reversed, however—when carbs are cut and replaced with dietary fat and protein—the opposite happens. Blood sugar metabolism normalizes, triglycerides go down, HDL cholesterol goes up, and body fat is lost.[23–26]

All of these benefits occur without the hunger and irritability that are trademarks of low-fat, reduced-calorie diet plans. Add in exercise, and you optimize HDL levels and accelerate fat burning.

changes. Remember Selma M., who was an extreme case with a triglyceride count of over 2,000?

A more typical situation will respond equally well to controlling carbs. One that really stands out is that of Muriel R. When Dr. Atkins first saw Muriel, she weighed 150 pounds at five feet tall. With a 30-year history of Type 2 diabetes, she was taking five medications. Her initial lipids showed a total cholesterol of 318, triglycerides of 1,455, an HDL of 63, and a fasting blood sugar of 196. After three months, her cholesterol had dropped significantly to 202, her triglycerides had dropped to 101, her HDL was 56, and her fasting blood sugar was 143.

Low HDL Cholesterol

High-density lipoprotein (HDL) cholesterol is often called the "good" cholesterol, because it carries cholesterol out of your arteries and other storage sites and back to your liver, where it is recycled. The more HDL cholesterol you have, the better. People with the metabolic syndrome usually have levels that are too low: 40 mg/dL or less for men and 50 mg/dL or less for women. Lifestyle factors that lower HDL include smoking, sedentary lifestyle, and, of course, a high-carb diet.[27–29]

LDL, STATINS, AND THE METABOLIC SYNDROME

You might have noticed that having a high level of low-density lipoprotein (LDL) cholesterol, many times called the "bad" cholesterol because high levels of it are associated with heart disease, isn't one of the signs of the metabolic syndrome. Even though the advertising for statin drugs, which lower LDL cholesterol, would have you believe that high LDL is a near guarantee of a heart attack, that's not always the case. A more likely near guarantee of a cardiac event, as shown by numerous studies, is the combination of low HDL and high triglycerides.

Despite all the hype, statin drugs do very little to lower triglycerides or raise HDL. What does improve these numbers is a controlled-carbohydrate eating plan along with exercise. Controlling carbs will stabilize blood sugar levels first. During this time your weight may not diminish rapidly. After blood sugar metabolism has normalized, triglycerides drop. HDL rises at the same time, although in Dr. Atkins' experience it may take three to six months for the HDL to reach the optimal level you can achieve. In many patients, LDL also drops. Sometimes, however, there is a temporary increase in LDL and total cholesterol; these levels typically drop later as your metabolism regains its normal balance.[30-38]

As you'll learn in Chapter 9, however, LDL, HDL, and total cholesterol do not tell the whole story. By controlling your carbs, you influence the complex feedback loops in the hormones and enzymes that control your blood lipids. For example, controlling carbs puts a stop to the overproduction of insulin. When less insulin is circulating in your bloodstream, the enzymes in your liver react in a way that affects the production of lipids. Theoretically, this is the same mechanism targeted by statin drugs, but enabling this mechanism through diet alone means no worrisome side effects induced by drugs. In addition to avoiding side effects and the considerable cost of drugs, you're getting the benefit of lower triglycerides and higher HDL cholesterol—factors that may be the most important predictors of heart disease.

High Blood Pressure

Because your doctor routinely checks your blood pressure at every office visit, and because you can easily check it yourself, high blood pressure (hypertension) might be the first symptom of the metabolic syndrome you notice. The latest medical guidelines for diagnosing high blood pressure, according to the National Heart, Blood and Lung Institute, say that slightly elevated blood pressure—between 120/80 mmHg and 139/89 mmHg—is now considered prehypertension.[39] It's a warning sign that hypertension may be in your future unless you start taking better care of yourself. How? Blood pressure is generally very responsive to fat loss and increased exercise. Is this beginning to sound familiar?

Blood pressure is also responsive to the Atkins Blood Sugar Control Program. It does this by normalizing your high insulin levels, which decreases sodium retention, which in turn releases excess fluid. For many of you, this means your blood pressure will probably come down quickly. As more progress is made with fat loss and exercise, your blood pressure may well return to normal even without medication.

High Fasting Blood Sugar

High fasting blood sugar (100 mg/dL or higher) first thing in the morning after not eating for at least eight hours is a sign of the metabolic syndrome and an independent warning that diabetes could lie in your future. Of all the signs of the metabolic syndrome, it's the one that's most likely to alarm your doctor, especially now that prediabetes has been established as an official diagnosis. (See Chapter 5 on prediabetes for more on this.) If you are really paying attention, you will note that the criterion for the metabolic syndrome is a blood sugar of 110 mg/dL or higher; however, the more recent definition of prediabetes is actually lower at 100 mg/dL.

High fasting blood sugar (FBS), however, is usually a fairly late development among people who have the metabolic syndrome—most people develop all the other signs first. In those with the metabolic syndrome, only about 13 percent had either elevated fasting blood sugar or were being treated for diabetes.[40]

Yet Dr. Atkins found that the vast majority of his patients had evidence of abnormal insulin/blood sugar metabolism when tested with his protocols (see Chapter 6, Diagnosis: Diabetes). The FBS alone doesn't detect this problem in many patients until late in their disease, when the damage has already begun.

If the metabolic syndrome is so closely associated with diabetes, why is high blood sugar often the last sign to develop? Because the process of inflammation, insulin resistance, and the changes in your metabolic profile begin long before blood sugar abnormalities can be easily detected by the standard recommended blood test. That's why you only need to have three of the five signs to be diagnosed with the metabolic syndrome—and that's why high blood sugar doesn't have to be one of them. Dr. Atkins spent decades measuring his patients' blood sugar and insulin levels for five hours after a glucose load and observed firsthand how long you can have a potentially dangerous imbalance of blood sugar and insulin before your fasting blood sugar goes up.

OTHER SIGNALS OF THE METABOLIC SYNDROME

High levels of an important marker for inflammation called C-reactive protein (CRP) are nearly three times as common in people who show signs of the metabolic syndrome as in people without any such signs.[41] The more signs of metabolic syndrome you have, the higher your CRP level is likely to be. Because it's now easy and inexpensive to test CRP levels in the blood, this important marker shouldn't be overlooked, especially if you have other components of the metabolic syndrome. (We'll discuss this marker more in Chapter 9, The Cardiac Connection.)

Another important risk factor associated with the metabolic syndrome is what doctors call the *prothrombotic* state. If you have this, your blood is more likely to form a clot inside a blood vessel. If this happens in an artery that nourishes your heart, it causes a heart attack. If it happens in an artery that nourishes your brain, you'll have a stroke. If it happens in a leg vein, it's called *deep venous thrombosis,* or DVT, and the clot can break off and go to your heart, lungs, or brain. We can now use blood tests to detect markers of the prothrombotic state (see Chapter 9).

YOUR CHOICE: LIFESTYLE CHANGES OR DRUGS?

You've probably noticed that throughout this chapter we've discussed two contributors to the metabolic syndrome: a high-carb diet and a lack of exercise. The standard medical advice for the metabolic syndrome is the reduced-calorie, low-fat diet based on the flawed food pyramid. (The Atkins Lifestyle Food Pyramid, which has been presented to the USDA, the Department of Health and Human Services, and White House staffers as one alternative, appears in Appendix 5, page 470.) Although portion-controlled diets such as the American Heart Association diet may work for some people, they fail for many others. Because these diets emphasize carbohydrates and frown on dietary fat, they may actually make the metabolic syndrome worse, unless one is able to lose weight on such a program.[42]

Even increasing your activity level probably won't offset the negative effects of such a diet. In fact, low-calorie, low-fat diets can actually cause you to lose both muscle and fat, while decreased dietary carbohydrates and increased protein can actually enhance muscle mass.[43, 44] Here's the scenario that is likely to unfold after you visit your doctor and get diagnosed with the metabolic syndrome. You follow your doctor's conventional dietary and fitness advice to the letter, but your health fails to improve. You may even gain weight and see a worsening of other metabolic syndrome signs.

The next thing you know, your doctor is whipping out the prescription pad and showering you with samples of statin drugs and medications for high blood pressure. You find yourself swallowing four or five expensive pills several times a day. Your blood pressure and LDL cholesterol may come down a bit, but your weight stubbornly stays the same or even climbs. Your triglycerides and HDL cholesterol hardly budge. But there's more. All those drugs, plus the carbohydrates in your diet, make you feel tired and weak, so you don't have the energy or even the inclination to exercise.

However, because your blood pressure is down and your LDL cholesterol is slightly better, your doctor is pleased. Unfortunately, you probably aren't. You feel worse—and because you're not dealing with the underlying problem, you're getting worse. Your conventional high-carb, low-fat diet, along with medications, is simply *not* the path to good health.

THE ATKINS WAY

A surprisingly small step can be enough to slow the progression of the metabolic syndrome. A very modest amount of fat loss—as little as 7 to 10 percent of your body weight—can bring about significant improvement. Changing your metabolism from fat storage to fat burning can stop the progressive damage to your body. Add in just 30 to 60 minutes a day of moderate exercise, and you're likely to step even farther away from that downward spiral.

How can you make this happen? As we've said, the metabolic syndrome can be stopped or reversed through a controlled-carbohydrate program combined with exercise: the Atkins Blood Sugar Control Program. This program has been specifically designed to combat the metabolic syndrome and its predictable outcomes. If you have already crossed the diabetes threshold, the program can help you stop the otherwise inevitable descent into heart disease, stroke, and other problems—and bring you back to better health.

DO YOU HAVE THE METABOLIC SYNDROME?

Agree or disagree with the following statements to determine if you have the metabolic syndrome.

1. My waist is greater than 40 inches
   (men) or 35 inches (women).   Yes ❑   No ❑
2. My triglycerides are 150 mg/dL or more. Yes ❑   No ❑
3. My HDL cholesterol is 40 mg/dL or less
   (men) or 50 mg/dL or less (women).   Yes ❑   No ❑
4. My blood pressure is 130/85 or more.   Yes ❑   No ❑
5. My fasting blood sugar is 110 mg/dL
   or more.   Yes ❑   No ❑

If you answered yes three or more times, you may well have the metabolic syndrome. Please read on in this book for more information to discuss with your doctor.

A HEALTHY LIFESTYLE IS MUSIC TO HIS EARS

No other man in his family has made it past the age of 50. So when it comes to praising the Atkins Nutritional Approach, 51-year-old deejay Ralph Drake gives his listeners an earful: Atkins helped him lose 100 pounds and take back his life.

NAME: Ralph Drake
AGE: 51
HEIGHT: 6 feet 1 inch
WEIGHT BEFORE:
280 pounds
WEIGHT AFTER:
175 pounds

BLOOD PRESSURE BEFORE: 110/70
BLOOD PRESSURE AFTER: 92/56
BLOOD SUGAR BEFORE: 88
BLOOD SUGAR AFTER: 84
TOTAL CHOLESTEROL BEFORE: 230
TOTAL CHOLESTEROL AFTER: 172
LDL CHOLESTEROL BEFORE: 170
LDL CHOLESTEROL AFTER: 118
HDL CHOLESTEROL BEFORE: 39
HDL CHOLESTEROL AFTER: 43
TRIGLYCERIDES BEFORE: 232
TRIGLYCERIDES AFTER: 69

My father died of a heart attack when he was 49, and with my history of obesity and severe asthma, I know I wouldn't be here today if it weren't for Dr. Atkins.

Since committing to the Atkins lifestyle on April 1, 2000, I have never been in better health. Finally, after years of being sickly and severely overweight, I found out why low-fat diets don't work! On Atkins I lost a total of 105 pounds and my asthma, shortness of breath, and heart palpitations simply disappeared.

In my job as a deejay at WDVR-FM in Hunterdon County, New Jersey, I play a song for Dr. Atkins during my show. My listeners know my story and I get enormous pleasure from teaching people how to adopt the Atkins lifestyle. I wish everyone with weight and health problems would take the same path.

I first became aware of Dr. Atkins in 1977. I was 25, working as a hospital food service director, and I weighed between 295 and 300 pounds. When I saw a picture of myself, I looked like I was 40! Then I thought about my father and headed to my doctor, who put me on a calorie-restricted diet.

My limit was 1,800 calories a day, and I almost went out of my mind. I cheated all the time. The more I cheated, the angrier I got with myself

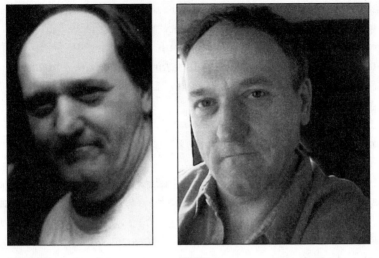

BEFORE   **AFTER**

for being weak and out of control. Then one day, I saw Dr. Atkins on television talking about how controlling carbohydrates was the key to good health and a normal weight. This was at a time when nobody believed what he was saying. But it made sense to me, so I bought a carbohydrate gram counter, limited myself to 30 grams of carbs a day, and lost 5 pounds the first week. I still hadn't read Dr. Atkins' Diet Revolution, *but I cut myself down to 15 grams of carbs daily. Then I lost ten pounds a week. Finally, I bought the book so I could follow the program exactly. I was breathing normally for the first time in my life.*

Then in 1981, I got divorced and went to work as a chef at a resort that focused on macrobiotic food. With its reliance on organic vegetables, grains, and soy products, a macrobiotic diet seemed to be a healthy way to eat. Before I knew it, though, I had gained 10 pounds, and then 20. When I noticed my weight gain, I went back to a controlled-carb lifestyle and lost a few pounds. But I seesawed back and forth for years afterward. In 1991, I suffered a severe asthma attack. I was in intensive care for four days. The only way to control my breathing was through steroids, which increased my appetite. Four years later, my weight was up to 280 pounds. By 2000, I was waking up in the night short of breath and with heart palpitations. I thought I was going to die.

Getting remarried in 2000 gave me the impetus to buy Dr. Atkins' New Diet Revolution. *On April 1, 2000, I announced to my listeners that*

I was going back to doing Atkins. (Before starting, I went to see my doctor to get my lipids, blood sugar, and blood pressure checked.) Three days later, my cravings vanished. I lost 30 pounds in the first 45 days on Induction. I remained in the Induction phase for almost a year, and had my lab tests repeated several times. As the weight fell off, I felt like a jerk for letting myself slide.

I was so happy when I read the July 7, 2002, article in the New York Times Magazine *confirming that Dr. Atkins' controlled-carbohydrate program was a healthy lifestyle, despite its allowance of natural fats and eschewing of excessive consumption of fruits and grains. Finally, someone else was explaining why low-fat dieting hasn't worked for countless people! I had some new ammunition for the naysayers around me, friends and family alike, who'd been telling me that eating the Atkins way would come back to haunt me.*

I have since gone through another painful divorce. I also changed jobs and moved. These kinds of stresses commonly cause people to overeat and eat the wrong kinds of foods. But I managed to control the stress through exercise, refusing to revert to the old, sick me. My two-year-old twins, one boy and one girl, are going to need me for the next 20 or 30 years. I have every intention of being here for them.

Note: Your individual results may vary from those reported here.

Chapter 5

WARNING: PREDIABETES!

As the term implies, there can be no clearer warning of impending Type 2 diabetes than the fourth stage of the six-step progression: prediabetes—or, more technically, insulin resistance with hyperinsulinism and impaired glucose tolerance. For many years, before it was given official recognition, doctors called this stage a variety of names, such as the insulin resistance syndrome, subclinical diabetes, borderline diabetes, or mild diabetes.

In 2002 and 2003, the American Diabetes Association revised its guidelines for the diagnosis and treatment of diabetes.[1] Among other things, the new guidelines formally defined prediabetes. You have prediabetes if you have one or both of these blood sugar problems:

- Impaired fasting blood sugar (also known as impaired fasting glucose, or IFG). To measure your fasting blood sugar (FBS) level, a blood sample is taken in the morning after you have fasted for a minimum of eight hours. Normally, your blood sugar at that point would be less than 100 mg/dL. If it's between 100 mg/dL (5.6 mmol/L) and 125 mg/dL (7.0 mmol/L), you may have impaired fasting blood sugar. If it's higher than that, you may have diabetes. A single high blood sugar reading on the fasting blood sugar test isn't necessarily a definite indication that you have prediabetes. If the elevation is found on a second test on another day, however, this is a reliable indication.

- Impaired glucose tolerance (IGT). This condition is defined by an abnormal rise in blood sugar after consumption of a specifically defined amount of carbohydrate. People who have IGT don't produce insulin quickly enough after a meal to clear away the blood sugar, so they become hyperglycemic an hour or two after meals (this is known as *postprandial* hyperglycemia). IGT has two components—the blood sugar rise just discussed, and the slow initial response in insulin production. To diagnose IGT, doctors use the 2-hour oral glucose tolerance test. After a fast of 8 to 12 hours, your fasting blood sugar is measured. You then drink a sugary liquid and your blood sugar is tested at the 1- and 2-hour marks. Normally, your blood sugar would go up no higher than 140 mg/dL 2 hours after having the drink. If your blood sugar goes above 140 mg/dL(7.8 mmol/L) but stays below 200 mg/dL(11.1 mmol/L), you have impaired glucose tolerance.[2] We'll go into the details of the very useful 5-hour oral glucose tolerance test in Chapter 6, Diagnosis: Diabetes.

These blood sugar cutoff points for prediabetes are based on a large body of research showing that damage to the tiny blood vessels of the eyes and kidneys starts to happen at these levels—in other words, the damage to your body from hyperglycemia has already begun.

Clearly, if you have prediabetes, you already have a serious medical condition. And you will almost certainly develop Type 2 diabetes within ten years if you are overweight unless you take action now.[3] Prediabetes should be your wake-up call to take charge of your health.

When Justine M. came to see me, she related the following history. In 1996, at age 52, five feet one inch tall, and weighing 237 pounds, her laboratory results were close to normal, with a fasting blood sugar (FBS) of 92. By 1997, her weight had climbed to 248 and her FBS had climbed to 109. A year later she had put on another 10 pounds and her glycated hemoglobin (A1C) had climbed to a diabetic level of 8.3. She was referred to me three years later, at which time she weighed 306 pounds. Her girth at her navel was 60 inches and her BMI was 58! Justine was taking two medicines for blood sugar and one for blood pressure. Now, two years later, after following Atkins, she weighs 191 pounds, her waist is down to 41 inches, and she is medication-free. Her labs look like this: FBS: 102; c-peptide: 2.2; A1C: 5.7; cholesterol: 159; triglycerides: 42; HDL: 57; and LDL: 93. She looks great, feels great, and, as a bonus, her medication costs have plummeted.   —MARY VERNON

SCREENING: TOO LITTLE, TOO LATE

As Dr. Atkins knew from observing patients over the years, the standard blood sugar tests do not detect the presence of insulin and glucose changes early enough. Also, the fasting blood sugar test is not foolproof. By now you realize that this process can be diagnosed and treated at an earlier stage if your doctor knows how to test for it.

Today the American Diabetes Association guidelines call for routine fasting blood sugar tests on everyone over age 45. If the test is normal, it should be repeated at three-year intervals. If you have other risk factors for diabetes, the guidelines call for testing to start earlier and to be repeated as appropriate.[4] Unfortunately, the screening guidelines often aren't always followed, which is why about a third of diabetes cases in the United States go undetected. If everyone with just a single risk factor for diabetes were screened, nearly 100 percent of all cases would be found.[5]

Here's the problem: Some doctors are not following the current testing guidelines, but even if they were, many people would still not be diagnosed early, as early as possible. We have a diagnostic test that Dr. Atkins believed was imprecise and used too late in the game. No wonder so many people are slipping through the cracks!

THE PREVALENCE OF PREDIABETES

Just about everyone who develops Type 2 diabetes has prediabetes first. According to the National Institutes of Health, at least 20.1 million people in the United States ages 40 to 74 had prediabetes during the years 1988–1994.[6] That works out to 21.1 percent of the population. But today many people much younger than age 40—even children and teens—have prediabetes. That means the total number of people with this condition is probably considerably larger—perhaps as many as one in three Americans.

THE PREDICTIVE POWER OF PREDIABETES

There's strong evidence that having prediabetes is almost as dangerous to your health as having diabetes itself. By the time your blood sugar falls into the prediabetes range, your risk of heart disease and of dying goes way up.[7,8] Recently, researchers found that many people hospitalized for heart attacks have undiagnosed prediabetes or diabetes. A recent study in Sweden, for instance, looked at 181 patients admitted to the hospital for heart attack. During their hospital stays, 31 percent were found to have diabetes and 35 percent to have prediabetes—but not one of them knew it. This was no fluke. Three months after discharge, the blood sugar tests were repeated and the results were consistent. The authors noted that perhaps the true prevalence of diabetes in patients admitted for heart attacks could be as high as 45 percent.[9]

The results of this study reinforce what Dr. Atkins said all along: It is absolutely imperative that early screening and treatment become standard practice to avoid heart attacks in those who have not yet even been diagnosed with prediabetes. We are committed to giving you the tools to prevent getting even this far. Undiagnosed prediabetes almost guarantees that the silent damage will continue until it reveals itself in an acute cardiovascular event. Let's try to make sure that doesn't happen to you.

HOP, SKIP, AND A JUMP TO DIABETES

If you have prediabetes and don't do anything about it, what are your odds of progressing onward to full-blown Type 2 diabetes? Dr. Atkins was convinced it was almost a guarantee. A study of a large group of people in Holland showed that over a six-year period, 64.5 percent of those who had both impaired fasting glucose and impaired glucose tolerance became diabetic. That compares with only 4.5 percent of those who had normal glucose levels at the start of the study. To put it another way, the people with IFG and IGT had roughly ten times the risk of developing diabetes as the people with normal blood sugar.[10]

In his practice, Dr. Atkins frequently encountered this situation. Many of his patients came to him only after they had progressed to full-blown Type 2 diabetes, which could have been avoided had they started on a controlled-carb program the moment they received a diagnosis of the metabolic syndrome. One good example of this is Ruth T. Several years before Dr. Atkins first saw her, her doctor had told her she had the metabolic syndrome and advised her to lose weight. She failed at every diet she tried, however, and by the time she came to see Dr. Atkins, she had become diabetic. It was only when she started following his dietary approach that she had any success with weight loss and improving her blood sugar and lipids. If only she had taken the controlled-carb route sooner! She could easily have avoided the unseen damage from years of high blood sugar.

At 39, Janet M. came to me complaining of fatigue. She generally felt terrible and had begun to lose weight. Her initial blood sugar was 326, indi-

COULD IT BE TYPE 1 DIABETES?

If you've been given a diagnosis of prediabetes, you'll also know that you have a good chance of progressing along the continuum to diabetes—unless you're able to *immediately* make the appropriate lifestyle changes. So, if you suddenly start having symptoms such as excessive thirst and hunger and frequent urination, it's natural to assume that you've tipped over into Type 2 diabetes. That may well be the case, but it's also possible that you have a late-developing case of Type 1 diabetes. Although this form of the disease usually strikes people under age 25, it can occur at any age. When it happens to older people, it's generally known as latent autoimmune diabetes in adults (LADA). This is a serious condition that needs to be diagnosed and treated quickly to avoid dangerous complications. See your doctor at once if you suddenly notice symptoms of diabetes.

cating diabetes, with a glycated hemoglobin (A1C) higher than 16 and a nondetectable c-peptide, indicating that she was not producing insulin and therefore had late-onset Type 1 diabetes. Her cholesterol was 217, triglycerides 179, HDL 46, and LDL 135. As she wanted to use as little medication as possible, she chose to begin to control her carbohydrates, took about ten units of long-acting (NPH) insulin twice a day, and carefully checked her blood sugars. When her blood work was rechecked three months later, her fasting blood sugar was normal at 96, her A1C was normal at 5.3, and her lipids had improved. Her cholesterol was now 165, her triglycerides 47, her HDL 62, and LDL 93. She had also regained the 15 pounds she had lost as a result of her severe Type 1 diabetes.

—MARY VERNON

DO YOU HAVE PREDIABETES?

Do the following statements describe you? Your answers will determine if you have prediabetes.

1. I am overweight and my excess fat tends to be in the abdomen.   True ❑   False ❑
2. I don't get much exercise.   True ❑   False ❑
3. I have two or more signs of the metabolic syndrome (see Chapter 4).   True ❑   False ❑
4. My doctor has told me I have the metabolic syndrome.   True ❑   False ❑
5. My doctor says my fasting blood sugar is above 100 mg/dL but below 125 mg/dL.   True ❑   False ❑
6. I have taken an oral glucose tolerance test and my blood sugar was above 140 mg/dL but below 200 mg/dL.   True ❑   False ❑

If you answered true to any of the first four statements, you may well have prediabetes. If you answered true to the fifth or sixth statement, you almost certainly already have prediabetes and need to take immediate action to prevent Type 2 diabetes. Please read on for more information to discuss with your doctor.

Chapter 6

DIAGNOSIS: DIABETES

It is a sad day when we have to tell a patient that he or she has Type 2 diabetes. As upsetting as this news is to patients, it is made worse by the knowledge that the situation could have been prevented. That's why we wrote this book. It is our hope that by reading it, you will never need to have this unpleasant conversation with your physician—or if you've already had that conversation, that *Atkins Diabetes Revolution* can deliver new hope.

If you've already been diagnosed, you have likely been told to follow a low-calorie, low-fat diet, take prescription medications, and engage in regular exercise. With the exception of exercise, that's a bleak prospect—years of denying yourself food when you're hungry and popping pills that are expensive and often have unpleasant—or even dangerous—side effects. Fortunately, there's another option. Dr. Atkins' teachings can introduce you to a way of eating to control your diabetes that is easy to stick with for the long term. These teachings can also show you the way to a future without drugs—or, at the very least, lower doses of those drugs. You'll still have to exercise, but we have tips for you on how to make it an enjoyable part of your life. (See Chapters 22 and 23.)

DIABETES BY THE NUMBERS

You officially have Type 2 diabetes when your fasting blood sugar (FBS) is 126 mg/dL or higher on two separate blood tests, or when your blood sugar is above 200 mg/dL two hours after a meal or at the two-hour point in a glucose tolerance test. At this point, you would be at the fifth stage of the progression—significantly elevated blood sugar, insulin resistance, and high insulin production. If that's where you are, let's hope you can still avoid the sixth and final stage, Type 2 diabetes with low or virtually no insulin production. It's no fun having to take oral antidiabetic medications or, worse, to give yourself daily doses of insulin. Don't put this book down until you've learned how to take immediate steps to avoid these consequences.

WARNING SIGNS OF DIABETES

A shocking number of people have progressed to Type 2 diabetes and don't even realize it. Following is a list of common symptoms that patients with diabetes may experience. You must see your doctor as soon as possible to evaluate any of the following symptoms:

- Extreme thirst
- Extreme hunger
- Frequent urination
- Weight loss without trying
- Unusual fatigue
- Blurry vision
- Irritability
- Tingling or numbness in hands or feet
- Frequent skin, bladder, or gum infections
- Slow healing of cuts and bruises

THE MOST IMPORTANT TOOL

The hallmark of Dr. Atkins' approach was his focus on the role of insulin and glucose function. He believed that it goes to the very heart (pardon the pun) of maintaining optimal health, preventing disease, and even treating chronic illness. Because insulin is a basic and fundamental hormone, whose job it is to regulate how your cells use energy, any disruption in this hormone's function will interfere with your health. And in today's sedentary, "carb-o-holic" society, insulin function is disrupted in an extremely large percentage of people.

That is why in his practice, regardless of the patient's weight and reason for coming to see him, Dr. Atkins almost without exception performed a five-hour glucose and insulin tolerance test (GTT). This is not a standard test, as it is time-consuming and expensive. Nevertheless, he believed the GTT is the best way to find out how your body reacts to carbohydrates. A *single* test such as fasting blood sugar is like a snapshot; the GTT is like making a movie of your metabolism.

It is through observing the results of thousands of patients and correlating the results with their reported symptoms that Dr. Atkins came to fully understand the importance of controlled-carbohydrate nutrition in the prevention of diabetes and heart disease and in the treatment of the other chronic health problems that plague us today. By observing the changes in blood sugar and insulin levels that occur during the test, he learned just how early on we can diagnose those at risk for developing the metabolic syndrome. He also learned how, with proper education and intervention, we can not only prevent the metabolic syndrome, but also stop the progression to prediabetes and Type 2 diabetes.

If after reading this far you think that you might have the metabolic syndrome or prediabetes, you need to be your own patient advocate and have a serious discussion with your doctor about performing the full five-hour glucose tolerance test.

DISCUSSING THE GTT WITH YOUR DOCTOR

If your doctor tells you you don't need the glucose tolerance test, what should you say? We suggest that you ask your doctor to order the test anyway. Offer to pay the bill ahead of time. Call your insurance carrier and obtain a letter indicating the company will cover the cost (if it will). You could also offer to pay a deposit and ask for the bill to be filed with your insurance carrier. Most physicians will agree to order the test if the cost doesn't directly affect them. Some insurance plans will charge a physician for ordering a test not considered "medically necessary." In that case, your only choice is to pay the bill yourself. You may be able to negotiate a discount for cash payment.

PREPARING FOR THE GTT

For the results of your oral glucose tolerance test to be accurate, you will need to start preparing a few days in advance. The test is only accurate if you've been eating 150 or more grams of carbohydrate a day for several days running. Of course, if you're following the standard American diet, you're eating that much and more and you won't have to change your diet to prepare for the test. If you've been following a low-carbohydrate eating plan, however, you'll have to go off it and eat at least 150 grams of carbs each day for four days. Is that a reason to eat a whole bunch of jelly doughnuts? No way. Use those carb grams on the best possible foods, such as whole grain breads, fruit, potatoes, legumes, and starchy veggies. Spread the carbs evenly across your meals, and eat them with foods that contain protein and fat.

Before the test, you must fast for 12 hours. It's okay to drink as much water as you want during this time. You'll also be able to drink water during the test, but you won't be able to eat (or smoke). Some prescription medications, such as thiazide diuretics, beta-blockers, oral contraceptives, steroids, and some psychotropic medications, can affect the results of your test. Be sure to tell your doctor about all your medications in advance and discuss whether any will affect the test.

DOING THE GTT

As we just discussed, if you are currently restricting carbs, to ensure an accurate result on the glucose tolerance test, you'll have to prepare a few days in advance by eating more carbs. The GTT has three components: It measures blood sugar levels, insulin levels, and the presence or absence of sugar in the urine. The first blood sample, taken before you drink the glucose solution, measures what's called your *baseline* fasting blood sugar and insulin. A urine specimen is also tested for the presence of glucose. (If glucose is found in the baseline urine sample, your doctor should check your fasting blood sugar before proceeding with the test.) It is then up to your doctor's discretion whether to give you the glucose drink or proceed instead with a postprandial test—see page 71 for more on that. Assuming it is okay to proceed, you then drink a measured amount of a very sugary solution to test your body's response over the next five hours.

Here are the measurements Dr. Atkins would take during the glucose tolerance test:

Time	Blood Sugar	Blood Insulin	Urine Glucose
Fasting (start)	x	x	x
½ hour	x		
1 hour	x	x	x
2 hours	x	x	x
3 hours	x		x
4 hours	x		
5 hours	x		

Dr. Atkins would ask his patients to keep a journal noting any symptoms they experienced after drinking the glucose solution and the time the symptoms occur. Some people will feel fine during the test; most people do not. It is useful to be able to correlate symptoms with abnormal results on the test. He also found that charting symptoms can be an eye-opener for patients, helping them understand that the migraine headaches or intense irritability they may have experienced in the past can be related to an unstable blood sugar pattern.

During the test, if the blood sugar goes too high early on, the patient may feel sleepy or nauseated, or have difficulty concentrating. Later, as the blood sugar drops too low or too fast, the patient may experience irritability, shakiness, palpitations, headache, anxiety, and numerous other symptoms. The more symptoms the patient has, the more carb intolerant he or she is, even if the blood sugar and insulin numbers are not yet way out of line. How you feel during the test is your window into your body and this silent illness. Your symptoms provide you with valuable information about the ups and downs in your insulin and blood sugar and how much stress these vacillations put on your body.

Linda K. was obese and had severe and frequent migraine headaches. When Dr. Atkins gave her the GTT, her insulin was mildly elevated at the start of the test and went up very high as the test continued. Although her blood sugar levels didn't rise above the normal levels, she reported typical symptoms. At the half-hour mark, for instance, she was lightheaded and had a headache. By the two-hour point, she still had those symptoms—but in addition she was now nauseated and jittery. By the fourth hour of the test, she had all the previous symptoms, plus irritability. The symptoms correlated with her rising insulin levels. When she started following the Atkins Nutritional Approach, she lost weight but, even better, her insulin normalized and she was free of her migraines as long as she continued to follow her individualized controlled-carb plan.

WHAT THE GTT REVEALS

Back in Chapter 2, we explained the stages of insulin/blood sugar abnormalities that culminate in Type 2 diabetes. They're important enough to bear repeating.

The first four stages are milestones on the road to diabetes:

1. Insulin resistance of cells
2. Insulin resistance with hyperinsulinism (the production of large amounts of insulin)

3. Insulin resistance with hyperinsulinism and reactive hypo-glycemia (low blood sugar)
4. Insulin resistance and hyperinsulinism with impaired glu-cose tolerance (prediabetes)
5. Type 2 diabetes with insulin resistance and high insulin pro-duction
6. Type 2 diabetes with low or virtually no insulin produc-tion

The GTT is valuable because it reveals the *earliest* signs of hyperin-sulinism, stage 2 on the six-stage continuum to diabetes. Insulin levels can be higher than normal even before the blood sugar becomes un-stable enough to cause many symptoms.

The case of Joe B. illustrates this point very clearly. Joe was 52 years old when he first came to see Dr. Atkins. At five feet seven inches, weighing 208 pounds, and with high blood pressure, he showed the classic signs of the metabolic syndrome. His fasting blood sugar was 87 mg/dL, and during the GTT, his blood sugar rose to 158 at the end of the first hour. His insulin, however, soared sky-high. At the one-hour point, it reached 347 µIU/mL, which indicates hyperinsulinism with insulin resistance. Had Joe been given only the standard FBS test as part of an annual checkup, or even if he had taken the usual two-hour GTT, both of which check only blood sugar levels, his hyperin-sulinism would have gone unnoticed until things got much worse.

Unless someone who is at stage 2 makes dietary modifications, in-sulin resistance and high insulin production will continue and reac-tive hypoglycemia (stage 3), with all its unpleasant symptoms, will surely follow. Dr. Atkins diagnosed hypoglycemia from the glucose tolerance test when the blood sugar dropped 60 points or more from one hour to the next or there was more than a 100-point change be-tween the highest and lowest reading during the test. As the six stages make clear, hypoglycemia is not the opposite of diabetes. Rather, it's on the continuum that leads inexorably to diabetes.

The following chart and its comments parallel Dr. Atkins' thoughts regarding optimal blood sugar levels. As you can see, there is a differ-ence between what are considered normal ranges and what he consid-ered optimal.

GLUCOSE TOLERANCE TEST—GLUCOSE AND INSULIN VALUES

TIME	NORMAL GLUCOSE VALUES	NORMAL INSULIN VALUES	WHAT THE RESULTS MEAN
Fasting	<126 mg/dL	<10 μIU/mL	Normal glucose results are 70–90; 111 or over is impaired; 126 or over is diabetic. Insulin levels above 10 show insulin resistance.
½ hour	<200 mg/dL	40–70 μIU/mL	A truly normal glucose response will not exceed 150.
1 hour	<200 mg/dL	50–90 μIU/mL	Some want to lower the threshold on glucose to <180 to identify early stages of diabetes. Insulin >80 shows insulin resistance, or a level 5 times that of the fasting level (i.e., a fasting of 11 followed by a 1 hour >55).
2 hours	<140 mg/dL	6–50 μIU/mL	A truly normal glucose response is 110 or lower. Insulin >60 is IR [insulin resistance].
3 hours	<120 mg/dL		
4 hours	<120 mg/dL		

This chart provided with permission from INCIID, the InterNational Council on Infertility Information Dissemination, Inc. (www.inciid.org). Use of materials provided by INCIID is voluntary, and reliance on such materials should only be undertaken after consultation with a physician.

WHAT THE INSULIN NUMBERS MEAN

When your blood is drawn at the various intervals during the glucose tolerance test, the amount of insulin in your blood should be checked along with your blood sugar levels.

Insulin is measured in micro International Units per milliliter, or µIU/mL. According to the preceding chart, a normal fasting insulin level (also called fasting serum insulin) would be 10 µIU/mL or lower. Half an hour into a glucose tolerance test, normal insulin would rise to between 40 and 70 µIU/mL. (Note: Although the preceding chart lists a half-hour insulin level, Dr. Atkins felt he could obtain the information he needed by measuring the one- and two-hour levels.) According to the chart, at the one-hour mark, normal insulin would be between 50 and 90 µIU/mL. People with insulin resistance, however, will have insulin levels that are at least five times their fasting level. If you start out with a fasting blood insulin of 11, for instance, you have insulin resistance if your insulin level is 55 µIU/mL or more one hour after swallowing the glucose drink—even though that's still in the normal range. According to the chart, no matter what your starting blood insulin, a level of 80 µIU/mL or more at the one-hour mark indicates insulin resistance.

By the two-hour point in the test, insulin levels usually begin to drop down again, falling into the 6- to 50-µIU/mL range. If your insulin level is still at 60 µIU/mL or more at this point, you have insulin resistance. Insulin level is a bit tricky to measure, and results will vary among testing labs. (The lab at which your tests are analyzed will report the normal range for *their* labs.)

Once you have reached stage 3, progression to stage 4 is inevitable if you make no lifestyle changes. In stage 4, the blood sugar rises to a higher than normal level as insulin resistance and high insulin production continue to worsen. This is where the GTT is especially valuable as compared with standard screening recommendations from the American Diabetes Association.

As part of a typical annual physical exam, your health care provider will probably check only your fasting blood sugar (FBS). Insulin levels are not routinely checked. At stage 4, however, it is likely that your FBS is still within the normal range. Getting the A-OK on your blood sugar gives you a false sense of security, allowing you to continue with the illusion that any extra pounds are purely a cosmetic problem. You won't be able to see the effect of that fat storage on your body chemistry with the FBS test alone.

The FBS test doesn't measure what happens to your blood sugar after a typical high-carb meal. Your real concern at this point should be excessive insulin and the silent damage that comes from high blood sugar. You are now making more fat and storing it in your body; at the same time, this storage process is clogging your arteries. Your blood pressure may be creeping up while endothelial dysfunction worsens. Also at this point many of you are finding it increasingly more difficult to control carbohydrate cravings.

If your doctor recognizes your risk of diabetes and wants to investigate further, he or she is likely to order a two-hour glucose tolerance test that will *not* include insulin measurements. The test will measure fasting and two-hour blood sugar levels, following an oral glucose challenge. If your blood sugar reading at the second hour falls between 140 mg/dL and 200 mg/dL, you have impaired glucose tolerance, or prediabetes. That's useful knowledge, but it's incomplete. Because your insulin levels weren't checked, you won't know how much insulin you are making, and therefore you don't know how severe your metabolic abnormality really is. Your insulin numbers could be quite high, but because the two-hour test looks only at blood sugar, it misses this important finding.

Prediabetes is also diagnosed when fasting blood sugar is between 100 mg/dL and 125 mg/dL—above normal but not yet in the diabetic range. But the FBS test can be misleading at this stage in the progression. Based on the FBS, you can *look* like you have prediabetes, but in reality you already *have* Type 2 diabetes.

This was the case with Susan F., a 53-year-old woman who had fasting blood sugar of 117 mg/dL, which is below the cutoff point of 126 mg/dL for diabetes. Her primary-care doctor had diagnosed her with hypoglycemia several years before and now told her she had prediabetes. She came to Dr. Atkins because, at five feet one inch and 260 pounds, weight loss was a priority for her. He was almost certain Susan had progressed beyond prediabetes, and the glucose tolerance test proved him right. Her blood sugar jumped to diabetic levels, and her insulin levels were among the highest he had ever seen. Her high insulin levels kept her from losing much weight at first, but after five months she was losing slowly but steadily and many of her other health issues were improving as well.

Another patient, Patricia G., could have avoided her diagnosis of diabetes had she only come to see Dr. Atkins earlier. When he first saw Patricia, she was five feet three inches and weighed 268 pounds. She had been diagnosed with the metabolic syndrome and was taking drugs to treat her high blood pressure and high blood lipids. Because there was a history of diabetes in her family, Dr. Atkins strongly suspected she had already moved well beyond the metabolic syndrome to diabetes, even though her fasting blood sugar was 111 mg/dL, still in the prediabetes range. The GTT showed he was right—she did indeed have Type 2 diabetes, and had probably had it for several years. She did extremely well once she started controlling her carbs. Over the next 11 months, she lost more than 20 pounds, her blood sugar came down, and so did her blood pressure and blood lipids.

As you can see, another virtue of the GTT is that it can detect "hidden" diabetes, as happened in this unusual case: Bernadette S. was a very large woman, standing six feet one inch and weighing 363 pounds. Someone who is that severely overweight (BMI of nearly 50) is almost certainly diabetic, yet because her fasting blood sugar was normal, her regular doctor never investigated any further. Dr. Atkins did and found that Bernadette's GTT results clearly showed she had Type 2 diabetes. After five months of following the Atkins program, Bernadette had lost nearly 30 pounds. Her fasting blood sugar was normal, and her glycated hemoglobin (A1C)—see Chapter 7 for more details on this—was 5.1, an excellent reading that indicated her blood sugar had been at normal levels for the past three months.

The GTT is also useful for revealing the subtle changes that happen as you begin to creep up to the higher ranges of normal glucose or insulin values. Even a slight shift toward the high end of normal can be cause for concern, especially if you are also gaining weight, craving carbs, or have a family history of diabetes. Your blood sugar doesn't suddenly change from normal to abnormal; rather, it's like a watercolor in which one color imperceptibly shades into another.

During his many years in clinical practice, Dr. Atkins learned to recognize these subtle changes and to use them as a tool in diagnosing blood sugar abnormalities, educating patients, and preventing illness. A test in the normal range does not necessarily mean that an individual is at his or her metabolic healthiest. When he reviewed the results of a GTT, in addition to looking at the values for each hour, Dr. Atkins looked at the pattern of change in blood sugar and insulin values, and also observed how the patient felt at various points over the course of the test.

Although there are normally accepted values that are used to analyze the results of the GTT (as indicated on the chart on page 66), Dr. Atkins did not see matters in such a black-and-white fashion. When seeing someone at risk for blood sugar problems, he certainly would have agreed with the commentary on the chart, but if a patient's blood sugar rose much above 150 mg/dL after the glucose drink, Dr. Atkins would be alerted to the possibility of that patient's having insulin/glucose metabolism abnormalities. The closer the blood sugar got to 200, the more concerned he would get. He also always took into consideration the symptoms the patient reported during the test.

The more symptoms the patient has, the more carb intolerant he or she is, even if the blood sugar and insulin numbers are not yet way out of line. The important point to remember is this: How you feel during the test reflects how much your body is stressed by the ups and downs in your insulin and blood sugar.

THE END GAME

If excessive demand for insulin caused by eating high-carb foods continues over a long period, the insulin-producing beta cells in the pancreas can become exhausted. They can no longer make enough insulin—or they may even stop making insulin altogether. This is stage 6 of Type 2 diabetes, and it now typically requires administering insulin to yourself for the rest of your life. Still, even when the disease has progressed this far, you can improve your situation. If you stop overloading your pancreas with carbohydrates, you may be able to restore some insulin production. By learning to control your carbs and making other lifestyle changes, you may be able to go off insulin completely or at least keep your dose to a minimum and avoid complications, such as hypoglycemic episodes, that often accompany insulin administration.

OTHER BLOOD TESTS

In addition to the GTT, Dr. Atkins would typically order:

- a *lipid panel* consisting of total cholesterol, triglycerides, HDL, and LDL;
- routine chemistry tests (also known as a *comprehensive chemistry panel*), including those for liver function, kidney function, uric acid, and electrolytes;
- CBC (complete blood count);
- thyroid function, including TSH, free T3, and free T4.

As a cardiologist, he also screened for markers of cardiovascular risk, such as C-reactive protein (hs-CRP), homocysteine, lipoprotein(a), and fibrinogen. These tests are crucial for patients who have elevated lipids, hypertension, known heart disease, diabetes, or a strong family history of heart disease. We'll discuss these risk factors in more detail in Chapter 9, The Cardiac Connection.

ARE YOU MAKING INSULIN?

If you have been newly diagnosed with diabetes, stressing the system with a glucose tolerance test may not be appropriate. The key question is discovering how much insulin your pancreas is still producing. Does your pancreas produce high, normal, or low amounts of insulin? The answer is extremely important, as it can influence the kind of treatment you are given.

Instead of the GTT, Dr. Atkins would have these patients do a two-hour postprandial (after a meal) test. This is a way of determining how high your insulin and blood sugar go two hours after you eat a high-carb meal. To do the two-hour postprandial test, you fast for 12 hours (water is allowed) before the test. A blood sample is drawn for blood sugar and insulin. You then eat a standard high-carb breakfast as recommended by the American Diabetes Association: six ounces of orange juice, a bowl of plain oatmeal, two slices of toast, decaf coffee or tea sweetened with a teaspoon of sugar. Two hours after you finish the meal, blood is drawn again to measure sugar and insulin.

If the two-hour insulin level has at least doubled from the baseline level, your pancreas is still clearly producing insulin. That's excellent news, because it means the ABSCP alone should be effective for managing your blood sugar. If the two-hour insulin level hasn't doubled, this suggests that your insulin production is low. Don't despair. You may well need medication or even supplemental insulin at this point, but the ABSCP will still be extremely helpful to you. Many of Dr. Atkins' patients started the program needing diabetes medications and were able to reduce the doses or even stop taking the drugs completely. (We'll discuss drug treatment for Type 2 diabetes in detail in the next chapter.)

THE C-PEPTIDE TEST

Another, somewhat indirect way to check your insulin production is a blood test for c-peptide. This protein is a normal by-product of insulin production, so your level of c-peptide is an indication of how much insulin your pancreas is making. Because the normal ranges may vary among laboratories, you should compare your results with the normal results reported by the lab you use. The higher above the norm your c-peptide level goes, the more hyperinsulinemic you are.

Krystal M. was only 19 years old when she first came to see me, but she already had a well-advanced case of the metabolic syndrome. At 5 feet 8¾ inches tall, she weighed 288 pounds. Her c-peptide blood level was 9.8 ng/mL (more than twice the normal range), her triglycerides were 180, her total cholesterol was 182, her HDL was 33, her fasting blood sugar was 95, and her A1C was 5.6. In addition, she required two medications that made it difficult to manage her weight. Nine months after beginning her controlled-carb program, Krystal had lost 40 pounds and 5¼ inches from her waist. Her lab values improved: her c-peptide was normal at 3.6 ng/mL, her triglycerides were 161, her total cholesterol had dropped to

161, her HDL was 35, her LDL was 113, her fasting blood sugar had dropped to 78, and her A1C was 4.6. At the two-year point, Krystal weighed 186, and she had lost 15¼ inches at her waist. Her lipid lab values had also continued to improve, with triglycerides of 109, total cholesterol of 143, HDL of 56, and LDL of 65.   —MARY VERNON

While the c-peptide test does reflect insulin production in the body, unlike the GTT performed by Dr. Atkins, it does not measure the glucose response to the insulin that is present.

DIET OR DRUGS?

If you are diagnosed with Type 2 diabetes, the chances are good that your doctor will immediately prescribe at least one drug to control your blood sugar. If you're not already taking medications for high blood pressure and high blood lipids, chances are good you'll be prescribed those drugs as well. And then your doctor will probably hand you a booklet that describes the American Diabetes Association (ADA) diet for people with Type 2 diabetes. You'll be urged to follow this low-fat, high-carb approach—in fact, your health insurance company may even pay for you to attend classes that teach you all about this "healthy" diet.

In Dr. Atkins' opinion, nothing could be better designed to turn you into a perpetual patient destined to face increasingly severe health problems as time goes by. If you have diabetes, your body can't process carbohydrates normally. Does it make any sense at all to prescribe a diet that is 55 percent or more carbohydrate? Of course not. The logical treatment is a low-carbohydrate regimen that uses protein and fat to stabilize your blood sugar and preserves your pancreatic function.

Dr. Atkins battled the medical establishment on this issue for decades. In the few years before his death, he was heartened to find that mainstream research was increasingly bearing out his ideas, and that some of his colleagues had spoken out on the folly of high-carb diets for those with blood sugar abnormalities. Dr. Gerald Reaven, who first defined syndrome X (now called the metabolic syndrome), is one of them. In an important article written for heart doctors in 2001, he plainly stated that "in the absence of associated weight loss, the usually recommended low-fat, high-carbohydrate diet makes the manifestations of syndrome X worse." [1]

In the end, only you can decide what's best for your health—in concert with your physician. You can choose to use the Atkins approach, or you can choose the ADA approach. If, despite everything you've read so far in this book, you make the ADA choice, be aware that your odds of doing well on it are low.

That's not just our opinion—it's the result of an important study that appeared in that most mainstream of medical publications, the *Journal of the American Medical Association,* in January 2004. Researchers from the U.S. Centers for Disease Control and Prevention and the NIH's National Institute of Diabetes and Digestive and Kidney Diseases looked at 12 years' worth of diabetes data from national cross-sectional surveys. What they found is that only about a third of all adults with Type 2 diabetes were meeting treatment goals for their blood sugar, their blood pressure, or their blood lipids. How many were meeting their treatment goals for all three risk factors? A mere 7 percent. [2]

Could there be a more clear illustration of the fact that putting people with Type 2 diabetes on the ADA diet and bombarding them with drugs is a complete failure? Their inability to meet treatment goals is putting these patients at greater risk for the multiple complications of diabetes, not to mention other health problems and side effects from the arsenal of prescription drugs.

There are several possible reasons for these appalling statistics. The main one, of course, is simply that people with diabetes should not be eating a high-carb diet. A second reason is that many people undoubtedly find it impossible to comply with the ADA dietary guidelines—this diet seems designed to cause hunger and cravings in patients with this metabolic pattern. The third possibility is that many people mistakenly believe that their diabetes medications allow them to eat anything they want without ill effect. That leads to the disastrous result of greater fat storage, higher blood sugar and blood pressure, lipid problems, and increased risk of suffering a heart attack or stroke. And that's just for starters. Farther down the road are kidney disease, blindness, amputations, and other unpleasant—even deadly—complications.

We sincerely hope that the rising tide of evidence in favor of the low-carb approach to treating diabetes will soon become an unstoppable tidal wave that will prove to the medical establishment that providing these diagnostic and treatment tools will benefit their patients.

ARE YOU AN UNDIAGNOSED DIABETIC?

If you think you might have an undiagnosed case of diabetes, take this self-test and share the results with your physician.

Do you experience the following symptoms?

- **Extreme thirst**
- **Extreme hunger**
- **Frequent urination**
- **Weight loss without trying**
- **Unusual fatigue**
- **Blurry vision**
- **Irritability**
- **Tingling or numbness in hands or feet**
- **Frequent skin, bladder, or gum infections**
- **Slow healing of cuts and bruises**

Chapter 7

MANAGING YOUR DIABETES

All too many patients arrived on the doorstep of Dr. Atkins' office only after they had received a diagnosis of diabetes. When you're told you have a serious disease, it's usually pretty terrifying. And that fear often drives people to consider alternatives to what their mainstream doctors advise. That's where Dr. Atkins usually came in. Perhaps the patient had heard a success story about someone who had used his approach, or maybe they had read one of his books and felt it was talking to them. Very often, they felt that medicine had failed them, and they just wanted to get their health back.

Dr. Atkins had two goals for his patients with diabetes. First, by teaching these patients the Atkins Blood Sugar Control Program (ABSCP), he helped them get their blood sugar under control. Second, he worked with them to cut back on the amount of medication they took each day. Success comes when a patient has good blood sugar numbers and needs no drugs at all, or is down to the least possible number of drugs taken in the smallest possible doses. Most of Dr. Atkins' patients were able to achieve that success within a year. Many were also well along to achieving their weight-loss goals.

TRACKING YOUR BLOOD SUGAR

If you have diabetes, your primary goal is to bring your fasting blood sugar below 126 mg/dL—and preferably to 100 mg/dL or less. Once you start following the ABSCP, this may happen with surprising speed, but for many people some time may be required to return the insulin/glucose metabolism to normal functioning. After all, it took a long time to get to this stage of diabetes. You can't expect to reverse years of high blood sugar overnight.

You'll monitor your progress by using a home blood sugar meter. A number of high-quality meters are now available at pharmacies or medical supply stores. Work with your doctor or pharmacist to choose the one that's right for you and learn how to use it correctly.

When you start following the ABSCP, your meter becomes a useful tool for monitoring your progress. Check your blood sugar first thing in the morning before eating or drinking anything other than water and keep a record of the numbers. (If you're taking insulin, you'll probably need to test your blood sugar several times a day—first thing in the morning, just before meals, and at bedtime.) As you change your way of eating and start exercising more, you should see your blood sugar numbers improve. Once you've got your blood sugar normalized and your glycated hemoglobin (A1C) number is coming down (see page 78), you don't need to check your blood sugar quite so often. Every other day is fine at that point, unless your doctor instructs you otherwise. As your blood sugar continues to improve, you can move to checking it just twice a week. Continue to keep a record—we think you'll be very pleased with the results.

Important note: Talk to your doctor about what to do if your blood sugar goes up to a higher level or drops to a lower level than is usual for you. You will probably be told to call him or her if your blood sugar rises beyond a particular level—be sure you and your doctor are in agreement as to what that level should be. Illness, infection, surgery, or high levels of stress can make your blood sugar go higher than is normal for you. Call your physician if you don't feel well or have new symptoms that you can't explain.

THE A1C TEST

A blood test called the glycated hemoglobin (A1C) is extremely important for tracking your blood sugar over time. This test measures the amount of sugar that has become bound to a protein molecule called hemoglobin, which is found in your red blood cells. The A1C is sometimes called the blood test with a memory, because it gives a pretty good picture of what your blood sugar has been doing over a three-month period. Once a person has been diagnosed with diabetes, the A1C is the standard method used to assess "glycemic control," or how close your blood sugars are to the normal range. A normal A1C result in a healthy person without diabetes would be in the 4 to 6 percent range. When diabetes is first diagnosed, a person's A1C will probably be above that range, possibly even as high as 15 percent. The higher the A1C, the greater the risk for diabetes-related complications such as kidney disease, eye disease, and nerve damage.

The standard therapeutic goal for people with diabetes, as set by the American Diabetes Association (ADA) and other professional organizations, is an A1C of 7 percent or less. Dr. Atkins' goal for his patients was 6 percent or less. Almost all his patients achieved significantly lower A1C numbers within a few months of controlling their carbohydrates and exercising more. His recommendation was to have the A1C test done every three months until good control, meaning A1C below 7, was achieved, then two or three times per year unless there is weight gain or a worsening of blood sugar control.

THE SCOOP ON ANTIDIABETIC DRUGS

If you are diagnosed with Type 2 diabetes, in addition to the high-carb ADA diet, your doctor will almost certainly put you on one or more prescription drugs to control your blood sugar. You may also be prescribed drugs to control your blood pressure and blood lipids.

Dr. Atkins believed that drugs for treating blood sugar abnormalities and diabetes should be avoided if at all possible. If your diabetes is far advanced, however, drugs may indeed be necessary. In serious cases, he had no hesitation in prescribing drugs, but there were only two blood sugar medications he used: metformin (Glucophage) and, if necessary, insulin.

Why did Dr. Atkins avoid all the other drugs that are often prescribed for controlling blood sugar? Let us explain. Some of the drugs prescribed for Type 2 diabetes stimulate the pancreas to release more insulin; others make your cells more sensitive to insulin. The fact is this: No drug works as well as controlling your carbs and getting more exercise. And most drugs for diabetes end up actually making your situation worse. Why? Because with the exception of metformin, every drug for diabetes makes it almost impossible to lose weight and may well make you gain weight. In addition, some diabetes drugs make you retain water, which can only worsen blood pressure (creating the scenario for, yes, more medications). Dr. Atkins felt that almost all diabetes drugs get you into a futile cycle that leads to larger doses of more drugs, rather than actually improving your health.

As a result, the only drug (other than insulin when necessary) Dr. Atkins usually prescribed for blood sugar abnormalities was metformin (Glucophage). This is the only diabetes drug that doesn't cause weight gain. Metformin is helpful for people who have dangerously high blood sugar that needs to be lowered quickly—more quickly than dietary change and exercise alone can accomplish. It's also helpful for those who are very metabolically resistant to the effects of dietary change and exercise. For these patients, taking metformin can be very helpful, and Dr. Atkins didn't hesitate to prescribe it—along with the Atkins Blood Sugar Control Program, of course. As the combination starts to work, the metformin dose can often be gradually reduced and eventually stopped. There are, of course, some who may need to remain on it indefinitely.

Often, Dr. Atkins' patients came to him already taking two oral diabetes drugs—usually metformin in combination with another drug such as glyburide (Glucovance), which is an insulin-stimulating drug. In most instances, he would switch the patient to metformin alone. As the ABSCP begins to lower blood sugar, the insulin-stimulating drugs can lower blood sugar *too much*, causing a dangerous hypoglycemic reaction. **An important precaution:** If you take any of these medications and are about to start following the ABSCP, speak with your doctor first. You need to plan a strategy for lowering your medications as your new dietary approach starts to work. It is, of course, still necessary for you to continue to monitor blood sugar readings at home.

THE INSULIN DECISION

If you have progressed to stage 6 of Type 2 diabetes, the beta cells in your pancreas are now producing less insulin than you need. In fact, after years of a high-carb diet and high blood sugar, your beta cells may not be making much insulin at all. You need insulin to survive, however, so at this point you will probably have to start administering this powerful hormone to yourself, often several times a day. Your insulin dose, the type of insulin you use, and when you administer it depend on a number of factors. Every person who needs to use insulin is different, and you'll have to work closely with your doctor to design an individualized program that works for you.

Because taking insulin can cause dangerous episodes of hypoglycemia, and because it almost invariably causes weight gain, Dr. Atkins always aimed to help patients who were using it to discontinue it or reduce their dose. Fortunately, many of his patients were able to do exactly that by following the ABSCP. In fact, there were situations where the patient was able to discontinue the use of insulin immediately. (See the case of Glenda Carter on page 151 for an example of someone who was able to stop using insulin as a result of the ABSCP.) Let us say at once, however, that this is not always the case. Stopping or changing your dose of insulin must be handled on an individual basis, working with your doctor and closely monitoring your blood sugar. This is a complex process that needs to be handled carefully—*never try to adjust your insulin dosage without discussion with your physician.*

When you start controlling your carbs and bringing your blood sugar under control, you break a vicious, long-standing cycle in your body. When your blood sugar finally stabilizes, the beta cells in your pancreas may very well be able to resume their normal response. Insulin production will often improve—in fact, it may even return to normal levels.

WHAT YOUR FUTURE HOLDS

Often when people are first diagnosed with Type 2 diabetes, they go home with dark and gloomy images of a lifetime administration of insulin, wounds that won't heal, or even amputations. Those images are worst-case scenarios, but they are real possibilities—especially if you continue to eat in the way that led you to gain weight and become diabetic in the first place. In case your blood sugar has been too high and your mind foggy, let us remind you: The diet that brought you here is the one that includes large amounts of nutrient-empty carbohydrates.

Continuing on that diet could even cause your doctor to prescribe insulin unnecessarily. In our experience, many people are put on insulin even when they continue to produce high amounts of it themselves. That's because their blood sugar is so high that their doctors assume they are no longer producing enough insulin. One reason blood sugar might be so high is that their diets may be chock-full of the high-carb foods that cause blood sugar to skyrocket.

Unfortunately, most doctors simply assume that their patient needs insulin without investigating any further (e.g., performing the two-hour postprandial test discussed in Chapter 6). They prescribe a powerful hormone that you may have to take for the rest of your life without any real understanding of whether you truly need it. Dr. Atkins could never understand why the postprandial test is so often skipped. Whenever he considered prescribing insulin for a patient, he would order a two-hour postprandial test that let him compare the fasting blood sugar and fasting insulin levels with the levels reached two hours after a high-carb meal. This is how he would find out how much insulin was being produced and what the patient's glucose response was.

One of the downsides of prescribing the powerful hormone insulin is that in *the absence of carbohydrate restriction* it will often cause weight gain. With the exception of metformin, the other drugs used to stimulate insulin production and increase insulin sensitivity are also problematic when it comes to weight management, which makes every other aspect of managing diabetes more difficult. Remember Larry H., a patient we discussed back in Chapter 3? When Dr. Atkins first saw Larry, he had been taking glipizide (Glucotrol) for a year. Not surprisingly, he had gained weight over that period and was now carrying 255 pounds on a five-foot-nine-inch frame. Aside from making him gain weight, the glipizide wasn't doing much for Larry. His fasting blood sugar was just over 200 mg/dL and his glycated hemoglobin (A1C) was 7.3 percent. Dr. Atkins immediately switched Larry from glipizide to metformin. Within four weeks, he began losing weight and his fasting blood sugar was down to 130 mg/dL, a definite improvement, but Larry remains a work in progress.

Of course, some patients most certainly do need insulin and always will. In those cases, the ABSCP can still be very helpful. By controlling the carbohydrates in the diet, people who must take insulin can gain better control over their blood sugar, have a chance to decrease their insulin doses, manage their weight more successfully, and avoid the dangerous hypoglycemic episodes that plague so many diabetics who use insulin.

Your future doesn't have to be a downward spiral of multiplying drugs, insulin administration, and poor health. Even if you have gone so far down the diabetes road that you must use insulin, it is still possible to slow or even halt the progression to more serious illness.

The next two chapters will discuss high blood pressure and heart disease—two very common complications of diabetes. But, as you'll learn in later chapters, you have the power to limit the complications of diabetes and to optimize your health

COMMON DRUGS FOR TYPE 2 DIABETES

Although Dr. Atkins used very few of the following medications, we think it is important that you understand how they work and their potential side effects.

Drugs for treating Type 2 diabetes fall into these main groups:

SULFONYLUREAS. These drugs stimulate your pancreas to release more insulin. They include chlorpropamide (Diabinase), tolazamide (Tolinase), glipizide (Glucotrol), tolbutamide (Orinase), glimepiride

(Amaryl), glyburide (DiaBeta, Micronase), glibenclamide, and gliclazide.

Side effects include weight gain, fluid retention, and a slightly increased risk of a cardiac event such as a heart attack.

MEGLITINIDES. These drugs stimulate your beta cells to produce insulin. They include repaglinide (Prandin), nateglinide (Starlix), and mitiglinide.

Side effects include diarrhea, headache, and a slightly increased risk of a cardiac event such as a heart attack.

BIGUANIDES. The only drug now available in this group is metformin (Glucophage). Although the mechanism of action is not fully understood, metformin probably works by making your cells more sensitive to insulin and reducing glucose production in your liver. Metformin doesn't cause weight gain or fluid retention.

Side effects include nausea, diarrhea, and a metallic taste in the mouth. (Our experience has been that most people can adjust to any gastrointestinal side effects by starting with a lower dose and gradually increasing to the prescribed amount.) People with heart failure or kidney disease should not take this drug.

THIAZOLIDINEDIONES. Also known as TZDs or glitazones, these include rosiglitazone (Avandia) and pioglitazone (Actos). These drugs improve your sensitivity to insulin. They are usually prescribed in combination with other diabetes drugs.

Side effects include weight gain, fluid retention, anemia, and liver problems. These drugs can be very risky for people with heart failure.

COMBINATION THERAPY. The combination of metformin and glyburide (Glucovance) is often used to increase insulin sensitivity and to help your pancreas release more insulin.

Side effects include diarrhea and hypoglycemia.

INSULIN. If your diabetes has progressed and you can no longer produce much or any insulin, you may need to administer additional insulin. Insulin use is complex; miscalculated doses can lead to hypoglycemic episodes. If you are on insulin and using the ABSCP, it is essential that you plan ahead and work with your doctor to adjust your dosage as your blood sugar begins to stabilize naturally.

Side effects: Insulin usually causes weight gain.

WHAT'S YOUR DIABETES IQ?

The more you know about managing diabetes, the easier it will be for you to follow the ABSCP and avoid complications. Check your diabetes knowledge with this quiz.

1. Call your doctor if:
   a. Your blood sugar meter needs a new battery.
   b. Your blood sugar reading is normal.
   c. Your blood sugar reading is unusually high or low for you.
   d. You forget to check your blood sugar.
2. Check your A1C knowledge:
   a. A1C is a blood test.   True ❏ False ❏
   b. Target A1C is 7 percent or higher.   True ❏ False ❏
   c. A1C measures your blood sugar for
      that day.   True ❏ False ❏
   d. A1C gives a picture of your blood sugar
      over two to three months.   True ❏ False ❏
3. Which of the following diabetes drugs *don't* cause weight gain?
   a. Sulfonylureas such as chlorpropamide (Diabinase), tolaza-mide (Tolinase), glipizide (Glucotrol), tolbutamide (Orinase)
   b. Metformin (Glucophage)
   c. Meglitinides such as repaglinide (Prandin) and nateglinide (Starlix)
   d. Thiazolidinediones such as rosiglitazone (Avandia) and pio-glitazone (Actos)
4. Insulin may be needed if:
   a. Your blood sugar drops too low.
   b. The beta cells in your pancreas make too much insulin.
   c. Your cholesterol is too high.
   d. The beta cells in your pancreas don't make enough insulin.

Answers

1. c. 2. a. True; b. False; c. False; d. True. 3. b. 4. d.

Chapter 8

TWIN PEAKS: HIGH BLOOD PRESSURE AND HIGH BLOOD SUGAR

They are like two sides of the same coin: If you have high blood pressure, you're very likely also to have high blood sugar—and vice versa. This is because they are both evidence of the same underlying metabolic imbalance. Correct this imbalance and both will likely improve.

BLOOD PRESSURE BASICS

Let's start by taking a look at what blood pressure is and why it matters. Your blood pressure is a measure of the force your bloodstream exerts against the walls of your arteries as your heart beats and rests. It's measured in two numbers: the systolic pressure, when your heart contracts and pumps the blood, and the diastolic pressure, when your heart relaxes between beats. When discussing blood pressure, the systolic number is always given first, followed by the diastolic number, as in 127 over 84 (usually written as 127/84).

When those numbers are too high, you have high blood pressure, also known as *hypertension.* Hypertension is linked to increased risk for heart attack, congestive heart failure, stroke, and kidney damage. Today about 50 million Americans—one in four adults—have high blood pressure.[1] Hypertension is sometimes called the silent killer,

HYPERTENSION GUIDELINES

In the United States, the official guidelines for diagnosing hypertension are set by the National High Blood Pressure Education Program, part of the National Heart, Lung, and Blood Institute. The guidelines were updated in 2003. Here's how your blood pressure measures up according to the new guidelines:

- Normal: below 120 systolic and below 80 diastolic
- Prehypertension: 120–139 systolic and 80–89 diastolic
- Hypertension Stage 1: 140–159 systolic and 90–99 diastolic
- Hypertension Stage 2: 160 and above systolic and 100 and above diastolic [2]

because it doesn't really have any symptoms. Many people who have it don't know it.

Under the old guidelines, which date back to 1997, what's now defined as prehypertension was called *high normal*. With this change in the guidelines (published in 2003), about 22 percent of American adults, or about 45 million people, are now classified as having prehypertension. [3] The new guidelines are based on evidence that damage to the arteries occurs at blood pressure levels that physicians previously deemed acceptable. These studies have also shown that prehypertension is very likely to progress to hypertension as well as to additional health problems, unless changes are taken to correct the underlying cause. Controlling insulin levels and weight with the ABSCP addresses the underlying causes of high blood pressure. [4, 5]

Just as conventional medicine has recently begun to understand the importance of screening for glucose abnormalities by defining prediabetes, it is recategorizing blood pressure values to allow for earlier identification and treatment of this potentially devastating disease. The root of the blood pressure problem in some people is the same metabolic imbalance we have discussed in previous chapters: high-carbohydrate intake, leading to excessive fat storage, leading to inflammation at the cellular level. You may recall the discussion in Chapter 4 regarding endothelial dysfunction and its relationship to insulin/blood sugar abnormalities. Because endothelial cells line all blood vessels, all blood vessels are at risk for damage. This is why we are committed to helping you identify where you are on the blood sugar imbalance continuum—and to halting its progression.

At first glance the new guidelines seem like a good thing. No one was more of an advocate of early identification of health risks and intervention than Dr. Atkins. If these revisions led to lifestyle changes, in the form of exercise and dietary recommendations that could impact the underlying cause, we would be well on our way to truly addressing the epidemics of obesity and diabetes. Our fear is that, instead, these new guidelines and recommendations could lead millions of Americans not to better health but to the pharmacy—and to the "Band-Aid" solution of pharmaceuticals that are both expensive and potentially dangerous. (See Appendix 6, Drugs for Hypertension, on page 475.)

In this sense, the new guidelines are a bonanza for the companies that make blood pressure drugs. Most people with high blood pressure

GETTING AN ACCURATE BLOOD PRESSURE READING

Your blood pressure normally varies quite a bit—as much as 20 points or more—over the course of a day. A single reading showing high blood pressure doesn't necessarily mean you have hypertension. If your doctor suspects hypertension, your blood pressure reading may be repeated during the course of the office visit to be sure the stress of the visit itself isn't raising your pressure. You may be asked to monitor your blood pressure yourself at home for a few days or to return to the office for another reading. On occasion, you may be asked to wear a monitor that records your blood pressure over 24 hours.

Different blood pressure cuffs should be used for children and people of various sizes. The standard blood pressure cuff may be too small for people with large arms, for instance, giving an inaccurate reading.[6]

need at least two and often three drugs to bring it down, and they must take the drugs indefinitely.[7,8] Moreover, assuaged by a false sense of security, people on these drugs may not realize that, although their blood pressure may improve, the underlying condition silently progresses.

THE BLOOD PRESSURE–BLOOD SUGAR CONNECTION

High blood pressure often goes hand in hand with obesity, high blood sugar, the metabolic syndrome, prediabetes, and diabetes because in many cases they share the same metabolic root cause. If you have any one of those conditions, there's a good chance you're hypertensive, too. People with hypertension are almost 2.5 times more likely to develop diabetes than those with normal blood pressure.[9] In a study of almost 70,000 individuals, 30 percent of men over 40 years of age with a systolic blood pressure of between 140 and 159 mm/Hg had impaired fasting glucose, or prediabetes.[10]

Although very common, the combination of high blood pressure and high blood sugar is quite dangerous. If you have both, you are at much greater risk for blood vessel injury, leading to stroke, heart attack, kidney failure, blindness, and amputations. But don't get discouraged. Research has shown that even small improvements in blood pressure and blood sugar—along with weight loss—can improve your chances of avoiding those dire outcomes.[11] It's worth noting that none of these studies restricted carbohydrates. We see much better results in patients using the Atkins program.

The increased risks in people with diabetes begin at blood pressure readings of 120/70 and above—in other words, as soon as you reach the prehypertension level. That's why most experts agree that people with blood sugar abnormalities should aim for a target blood pressure of less than 130/80—and preferably lower.[12] Let us remind you that the Atkins Blood Sugar Control Program is designed to address the underlying metabolic abnormalities that are largely responsible for high blood pressure. Once patients have been following the program for a few months, it is not unusual to find blood pressure readings that reflect optimal health—that is, 120/70 or lower—often without medication. This is no Band-Aid!

When 71-year-old Dorothy W. came in for her annual physical, she was five feet tall and weighed 151 pounds. She had been taking three medications to control her blood pressure, but it was still 196/84, meaning she would need yet another drug. She would also need a medication for her lipids, as her lab results showed the following: fasting blood sugar: 122; glycated hemoglobin (A1C): 5.8; total cholesterol: 282; triglycerides: 485; HDL: 38. Her LDL cholesterol could not be evaluated due to her extremely high triglycerides.

Dorothy was interested in decreasing her medications, so under my supervision, she began the Atkins Nutritional Approach, with frequent follow-up visits. After three months, during which I tapered her medications, Dorothy's triglycerides had dropped to 86; her total cholesterol was now 209, with HDL of 86 and LDL of 57. Seven months later, she was able to eliminate one of her blood pressure medications. She is now down to 123 pounds, takes a very small dose of one medication, and her blood pressure is 120/70. Her fasting blood sugar is 112; c-peptide: 2.3; A1C: 5.1; total cholesterol: 197; triglycerides: 39; HDL: 74; and LDL: 115.   —MARY VERNON

THE NONDRUG APPROACH TO HYPERTENSION

What can you do to lower your blood pressure without drugs? You've probably already guessed the single most important step you can take: Control carbs! When you control both the quantity and quality of the carbs you eat, you directly address the metabolic abnormality that drives blood vessel damage—damage that is the basis for the long list of complications we've just discussed. When you control carbs, fat is no longer stored. Rather, the proper level of carb intake allows the body to burn excess body fat for energy.

Other very important lifestyle steps to lower your blood pressure include:

- Be more physically active. Lack of exercise, especially in combination with obesity, makes you more likely to develop high blood pressure. Adding exercise brings your blood pressure down— and helps your blood sugar levels and insulin resistance as well, which in turn helps bring your blood pressure down even further. Before starting an exercise program, read Chapter 22 and check with your physician.

• Limit alcoholic beverages. If your blood pressure is elevated and you drink alcohol, stop drinking altogether and observe the impact on your blood pressure. If your blood sugar is abnormal and/or you are overweight, you probably should not be consuming alcohol at all. (We'll discuss this more in Chapter 19.)

• Stop smoking or using other forms of nicotine.

DIET AND BLOOD PRESSURE

As soon as you start the Atkins Blood Sugar Control Program (ABSCP) and eliminate worthless carbs from your diet, you start to normalize your metabolism. This helps to lower your blood pressure in two ways. First, because your primary source of carbohydrates is now leafy green vegetables and other low-glycemic vegetables (those that have a limited effect on blood sugar), you're naturally getting a lot more potassium, magnesium, and calcium. These minerals have been found to be effective for lowering your blood pressure.[13]

Second, controlling your carbs will stop the abnormal salt and water retention caused by your former high-carb way of eating—fluid retention that can raise blood pressure. You may assume this has something to do with the salt content of foods. Although in salt-sensitive people, salt in the diet does lead to fluid retention, by no means is everyone with high blood pressure salt sensitive. In Dr. Atkins' experience, and according to some research, a high-carbohydrate diet and high insulin levels are more likely to cause fluid retention than salt does.[14] We find that on the ABSCP, salt restriction is rarely needed. Some people may actually need some supplemental salt (a cup of bouillon will do the trick) to prevent nausea or weakness when they burn fat rapidly. When you control your carbs, your body soon self-regulates to a more normal salt and water balance. Others who have studied this type of dietary approach concur with this advice.[15] Also, on the ABSCP, you will probably find that your taste buds become much more sensitive to the taste of salt (and to sugar). So, instead of salting your food before tasting it, let your newly sensitive taste buds be your guide.

EXERCISE AND BLOOD PRESSURE

Exercise is an integral part of the ABSCP and crucial for lowering blood pressure and blood sugar. In fact, a recent meta-analysis of 54 major studies on the value of exercise for high blood pressure showed without question that regular exercise can lower your systolic blood pressure by nearly 4 points and your diastolic pressure by nearly 3 points. Best of all, you get the benefit no matter how old you are, how much you weigh, or how high your blood pressure is.[16] Understand that exercise alone will not fix all the problems caused by excessive carbohydrate intake. It must be done in concert with controlled-carb nutrition to get the full benefit. (See Chapters 22 and 23 for more information on the value of exercise.)

STRESS AND BLOOD PRESSURE

The word *hypertension* sounds as if it should have something to do with stress. It is true that any stressful situation will make your blood pressure go up. However, that rise is normally temporary. Blood pressure usually returns to normal when the situation is over, even if it takes days or weeks. Whenever you're under stress, your body produces extra batches of the stress hormones, such as cortisol and epinephrine. These "fight-or-flight" hormones ready your body for action by raising your blood pressure, blood sugar, and heart rate; by making you more alert; and by stimulating your body to draw energy from stored fat and muscle. These hormones raise your blood sugar—so that there will be plenty of glucose available for immediate energy needs during the crisis. The aftermath of this hormonal outpouring? Carbohydrate cravings. Ever found yourself finishing off a giant bag of chips when you're on a deadline for work or school?[17, 18]

(continued)

Under normal circumstances, when the crisis is over, a complex series of feedback loops tells your body to turn off the stress hormones. But when stress is continual—as it often is in modern life—the stress switch gets stuck in the "on" position. When hormone levels remain elevated, the body is in a state of chronic biochemical stress, resulting in insulin resistance, increased hunger, cravings for carbohydrates and other comfort foods, elevated blood pressure, and weight gain. This stress-related weight gain, which usually ends up around your waist, is linked with the metabolic syndrome.[19, 20]

The solution? Find healthy ways to cope with stress. They include:

- Stabilize your insulin/blood sugar metabolism by implementing the ABSCP.
- Start or step up your exercise regimen, according to the guidelines in Chapters 22 and 23.
- Establish a regular schedule for eating, exercising, and sleeping.
- Implement relaxation techniques such as meditation and yoga.
- Reach out to friends and family for support.
- Avoid sleep deprivation. When you're short on sleep, you produce more stress hormones; getting more sleep can help flip off the switch.[21, 22]

DRAWBACKS OF DRUGS

Current guidelines recommend starting drug treatment for people with diabetes as soon as their blood pressure reaches the prehypertension level of 130/90.[23] If a patient's systolic blood pressure is in the 130–139 range, or diastolic blood pressure is in the 80–89 range, and if after a maximum of three months lifestyle changes have not improved the blood pressure, then medication(s) should be prescribed. This usually means taking two and sometimes three different drugs in combination. (For a list of pharmaceuticals used for hypertension, as well as other conditions, see pages 94–96.)

While drugs for hypertension are effective, they often have unpleasant side effects, such as dry cough, fatigue, and erectile dysfunction. They can also cause *orthostatic hypotension*—blood pressure that's too low when you're standing up—in people with diabetes. That's bad enough, but if you have blood sugar abnormalities, some blood pressure drugs, particularly beta-blockers (Inderal, Lopressor, Corgard), as well as thiazide diuretics (drugs that make you urinate more), could raise your blood sugar even more and tip you over into diabetes.[24, 25] The combination of a beta-blocker and a thiazide diuretic can make you six times more likely to become diabetic. There's also some evidence suggesting that for people with blood sugar problems, treating hypertension with a thiazide diuretic alone or with a combination of a beta-blocker and a thiazide diuretic may actually *increase* the risk of having a heart attack.[26, 27]

We have seen all too many patients who have ended up in worse health as a result of taking drugs for high blood pressure. In the case of Allison C., for instance, her doctor failed to realize that her high blood pressure was a sign of the metabolic syndrome. He didn't investigate any further, which means he never discovered that Allison already had high blood sugar. Instead, he treated her high blood pressure as an isolated problem and prescribed a thiazide diuretic. Sure enough, the drug raised her blood sugar to the point that she became diabetic. When she came to Dr. Atkins, he put her on the ABSCP and stopped her medications. Her blood pressure came down right along with her blood sugar.

All of that said, there is a place for blood pressure medication. Lowering your blood pressure the natural way through weight loss, exercise, and other lifestyle changes takes time. The risks of uncontrolled high blood pressure are serious. While you should avoid some antihypertensive drugs if you have high blood sugar, others such as ACE inhibitors, calcium channel blockers, and angiotensin receptor blockers (ARBs) don't negatively impact blood sugar and may be safe for you. Discuss the use of hypertension medications with your doctor and weigh the pros and cons carefully. Remember that your doctor is probably following recommended guidelines that advise beginning treatment with thiazide diuretics.

DRUGS FOR HYPERTENSION

Doctors now have a truly impressive array of pharmaceuticals from which to choose when it comes to treating high blood pressure. Here's a rundown of the current arsenal. (Note: Every time you combine two drugs, as is often the case when treating hypertension, you increase the risk of side effects and adverse reactions; when you combine even more drugs, the odds of a negative interaction go up considerably.)

Diuretics

The first drug most hypertension patients are prescribed is a diuretic—a drug that makes you excrete more water and salt. Why do these drugs help? If you are eating a high-carb diet, high insulin levels can make you retain both salt and water, which raises your blood pressure.[28] Diuretics reverse this, but of course they don't solve the underlying condition that is causing your hypertension. Diuretics fall into three categories:

- Thiazides. One of the most commonly used drugs, especially when first beginning drug treatment of hypertension, thiazides cause a moderate amount of water, salt, and mineral loss. These drugs can worsen glucose metabolism to the point of causing Type 2 diabetes and/or gout.
- Loop diuretics. Loop diuretics cause greater salt and water loss than thiazides—so much so that these drugs are usually given with a potassium supplement and may cause severe dehydration.
- Spironolactone. This commonly used diuretic is potassium-sparing—you retain more potassium in your body instead of excreting it, which helps prevent dangerous electrolyte imbalance. It must be used cautiously in combination with other drugs to avoid excessive potassium retention.

Beta-Blockers

Another group of medications commonly used to treat high blood pressure are the beta-blockers. These drugs work by blocking a receptor that regulates your heart rate and blood vessel tightness. This keeps your heart from speeding up and relaxes the blood vessels, but there's a major downside: The very same receptor that's found in the cells of your heart and blood vessels is also present in fat cells.[29] Beta-blockers block your body's ability to move stored fat out of fat cells. For many patients, this results in weight gain, which only worsens high blood pressure. If you take insulin, you could be at risk for life-threatening problems from beta-blockers, because they prevent your body's normal response to low blood sugar. The combination of insulin and a beta-blocker can cause dangerously low blood sugar that is very difficult to raise.[30–32]

Calcium Channel Blockers

Calcium channel blockers (amlodipine, bepridil, and others) are also used to treat hypertension. These drugs relax your blood vessels, but when used alone they may not bring your blood pressure down enough. Constipation is a major side effect.

ACE Inhibitors

Angiotensin-converting enzyme inhibitors (ACE inhibitors) are popular among patients with diabetes because they don't have any effect on insulin, blood sugar, or weight, and because they have been shown to slow the progression of kidney damage. However, these drugs often cause a persistent dry cough, which means some patients with asthma and other respiratory problems can't take them.

Angiotensin Receptor Blockers

Closely related to ACE inhibitors is a newer group of drugs called angiotensin receptor blockers, or ARBs. People who can't take ACE inhibitors can usually take ARBs. Like the ACE inhibitors, ARBs help protect the kidneys in patients with diabetes. If you take either of these types of drugs, you need to have your kidney function monitored regularly, because they can impair kidney function in people with decreased blood flow to the kidneys.[33, 34]

Before Dr. Atkins even considered prescribing powerful pharmaceuticals, he would ask his patients to follow the ABSCP until he could evaluate their response. The dietary changes alone are often enough to bring blood pressure down significantly. But multivitamin and mineral supplements and exercise are major parts of the program as well, and these, too, play a crucial role in lowering blood pressure. For patients who require more help to bring down their blood pressure, Dr. Atkins would prescribe additional supplements, targeted to their individual needs.

He found that people with high blood pressure usually respond well to a combination of several different supplements, including magnesium, the amino acid taurine, essential fatty acids, and coenzyme Q_{10}. (We'll discuss these supplements and others for heart health in Chapter 21.)

When a patient's blood pressure was only mildly elevated or if it had responded well to a controlled-carb approach and exercise, Dr. Atkins would use lower supplement doses. Of course, if a patient's blood pressure was so high that he or she was already taking drugs, or that it posed an immediate risk, he used medications and larger supplement doses until the ABSCP had taken effect. In many cases, his patients found their blood pressure came down to normal or near normal levels within a few months, if not sooner. For those patients who still needed medication for hypertension, he was able to keep the doses to a minimum and was often able to get them down to just one drug.

Remember, if you're already taking blood pressure drugs and start following the Atkins approach, you'll probably need to lower your dosages as the benefits of controlling carbohydrates kick in. Establish *in advance* with your doctor a plan about which medications to taper as your blood pressure improves.

Jeff T., a university professor, had severe metabolic syndrome and hypertension. He took three drugs daily for hypertension alone. He decided to begin the Atkins Nutritional Approach, but because of his demanding schedule, he didn't wait to come in for an appointment and medication plan. After three days of doing Atkins on his own, he was forced to discontinue all his medications. Unfortunately, this required a hospital stay because his blood pressure dropped so low. He laughed and told me, "Well, Doc, it really works!" It does work but this is a good example of why it is so important to work closely with your doctor to plan a strategy in advance, so medications can be safely tapered. —MARY VERNON

As your blood pressure improves, so will your heart health—but there's more to improving your cardiac health than blood pressure alone. That's what we'll discuss in the next chapter.

WHAT'S YOUR BLOOD PRESSURE IQ?

1. Systolic pressure is the pressure:
   a. when your heart beats
   b. when your heart relaxes between beats
   c. when your heart stops
2. Normal blood pressure is less than 120/80. What are the readings for the stages of hypertension?
   a. prehypertension
   b. stage 1 hypertension
   c. stage 2 hypertension
3. The main symptom of prehypertension is:
   a. headache
   b. dizziness
   c. tiredness
   d. nausea
   e. none
4. High blood pressure increases your risk of:
   a. heart disease
   b. stroke

(continued)

c. kidney disease
d. eye disease
e. all of the above

Answers

1. a. 2. prehypertension is 120/80 to 139/89; stage 1 hypertension is 140/90 to 159/99; stage 2 hypertension is 160/100 and higher. 3. e. 4. e.

A SPARKLING ACHIEVEMENT

Barbara Woodruff had the metabolic syndrome, but despite taking several medications for hypertension, she was not able to control her blood pressure. Now that she has dropped 70 pounds, significantly lowered her blood pressure, and felt her energy skyrocket, she can pursue her hobby as a fireworks technician.

NAME: **Barbara Woodruff**
AGE: **62**
HEIGHT: **5 feet 1½ inches**
WEIGHT BEFORE:
  216 pounds
WEIGHT AFTER:
  145 pounds

People look at me and think I'm just a little gray-haired grandmother who does needlework and has semiretired to Florida. Little do they know that at 62, I am so filled with energy because of my adherence to the Atkins Nutritional Approach that I spend much of my free time shooting off fireworks!

Yes, you read that right. I'm a pyrotechnics expert. I shoot off fireworks both by computers and by hand. I even choreograph shows to music. It's a hobby I simply love. I wouldn't be able to do it if it hadn't been for Dr. Atkins. I adopted the Atkins lifestyle on April 1, 2001, and lost 70 pounds in less than one year. That was great, but even better was that I

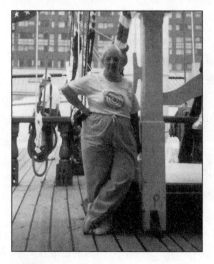

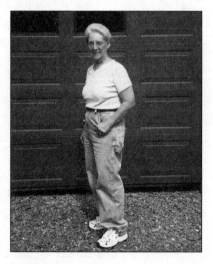

BEFORE   **AFTER**

*significantly lowered my blood pressure while my energy level skyrock-
eted. I was working once on a fireworks job with a 23-year-old guy and
literally wore him out. He quit at the end of the day!*

*If I had not gotten control of my blood pressure (today I take only one
blood pressure medication, instead of three), I would not be allowed near
the fireworks. If I had a heart attack or a stroke out on the field (the area
where fireworks are shot off), who knows what could happen? No one
would be able to help me because even firefighters can't be within a certain boundary around the fireworks.*

*In my "real job," I work at Disney World. It's work that requires me to
be on my feet for most of the day, and I would not have had the stamina to
keep up if it wasn't for my Atkins lifestyle. I'm trying to get on the Disney
World pyrotechnics team (my dream job), but for now I am working in
the shops on Main Street. One of them is the fudge shop. People always
ask me, "Don't you want to eat everything?" I can honestly say, "No, I
don't." Doing Atkins has permanently taken away my sugar cravings. If a
slight urge for something sweet trickles in, I eat an Atkins Endulge bar
and that takes care of it.*

*I can always tell when I've slipped up a bit and had too many carbo-
hydrates, usually around the holidays. When I eat something high-carb,
my heart starts racing and my face gets flushed. When I've gone up to 150
pounds from my normal weight of 145, I can tell because I start huffing
and puffing as I walk through the tunnels underneath Disney, which are
used by employees to get around quickly. Then I go right back to Induction and in a week, the weight is gone and I feel great again.*

*As with many women, my weight problem started after I had chil-
dren. The pounds crept on after each pregnancy. At age 42, I became a
single parent, and the stress resulted in my putting on even more weight.
Then I had a hysterectomy, began hormone replacement therapy, and
ballooned up 20 pounds almost overnight. A few years later, I developed
high blood pressure.*

*When I reached 216 pounds, I said, "That's it." In the early 1990s, I
had tried doing Atkins and lost 15 pounds. But it was hard to stay on it
with people pestering me that it defied the government recommendations
in the form of the food guide pyramid. Also, it was difficult to know which
foods were high in carbohydrate, because the labeling on products was
quite poor back then.*

This time around, no one, not even my doctor, was going to stop me. I lost about 12 pounds during the first week. About eight weeks later, I had my blood pressure checked and it had already dropped. By January 1, 2002, I had lost 70 pounds and felt terrific. Now, my blood pressure has gone from 160/90 to 145/85.

It's so easy to maintain this lifestyle today because there are so many delicious low-carb products in stores. Even restaurants are making it easy by offering low-carb meals. I work out along with a daily exercise program on local television.

I recently studied for, and got, a Florida commercial driver's license, as well as certification to haul hazardous materials. I love driving an 18-wheeler! I've also taken up counted cross-stitching as a hobby. I guess the latter is a more typical "grandmotherly" activity. I bet you've never met someone whose grandchildren watch a fireworks show and can say, "My Nana did that!" I'm thrilled to say that mine can.

Note: Your individual results may vary from those reported here. As stated previously, Atkins recommends initial laboratory evaluation and subsequent follow-up in conjunction with your health care provider.

Chapter 9

THE CARDIAC CONNECTION

Are you ready for the most alarming statistic you will find in this book? About 75 percent of people who have diabetes will die of heart disease.[1]

The deteriorated state of health—now known as the metabolic syndrome—that brought you to your diabetes diagnosis eventually leads to the formation of artery-narrowing plaques that cause reduced blood flow to your heart. In the worst cases, this progresses to arterial blockage, causing a heart attack. Half of those who do not survive their heart attack will die within the first hour; many will not make it to the hospital.[2] Even if you do survive that heart attack, your heart muscle will never be the same.

PROTECTING YOUR HEART

Heart disease and diabetes are a deadly duo. In fact, if you have diabetes, your risk of having a first heart attack is about as high as the risk of someone without diabetes who's already had a heart attack.[3] In other words, the moment you officially become a diabetes patient, you are automatically at risk for heart disease, even if you've never had any heart problems. During the decades in which you gradually developed diabetes, your blood vessels were suffering the kind of damage that often leads to a heart attack.

Because you can control what goes in your mouth, you have a unique opportunity right now to choose the alternative path to better health. Heart disease and diabetes aren't inevitable—there's plenty you can do to minimize your risk. In addition to getting your blood sugar and blood pressure under control, you also need to look at your

RESEARCH REPORT: A HIGHER RISK OF HEART DISEASE

Wherever you are on the road to diabetes, your risk of heart disease is already substantially higher than that of people not on the diabetes continuum. How much higher? According to results from the 118,000 women in the Nurses' Health Study, it's almost four times as high. The researchers in charge of this long-running study observed the women over a 20-year period. At the start, about 1,500 already had diabetes and 394 had a history of a heart attack. Over the next two decades, nearly 6,000 more developed diabetes and 2,500 women were newly diagnosed with coronary heart disease. The study found that women with both diabetes and prior heart disease were 20 times more likely to die from any cardiovascular disease such as a stroke and 25 times more likely to die from coronary heart disease.[4]

The risk doesn't apply just to women. Middle-aged men with high blood sugar levels, even if they don't have diabetes, are at greater risk of death not just from heart disease but also from all causes. We know this from a revealing analysis of three long-term studies conducted in Europe. Over a 20-year period, the health of some 17,000 men was carefully followed. The researchers found that among all three groups, the men who fell into the top 20 percent of the normal blood sugar range had an overall risk of death 1.6 times higher than the men whose blood sugar was in the lower 80 percent of the normal range. The men whose blood sugars were in the upper 2.5 percent of the normal fasting and normal two-hour glucose ranges were about 1.8 times as likely to die from heart disease as the men with low-normal blood sugar.[5]

blood lipids—the cholesterol and fats in your blood. And instead of relying on the standard pharmaceutical approach of cholesterol-lowering drugs to manage high blood lipids, wouldn't you rather target the underlying reason for this condition? That's what you'll do on the Atkins Blood Sugar Control Program (ASBCP).

Here's an example of how well the program works—even for people who have suffered years of health problems related to their blood sugar. When 73-year-old Muriel R., whom you met in Chapter 4, first came to see Dr. Atkins, she had been a Type 2 diabetic for 30 years. She was on numerous medications to control her blood sugar and lipids—and they weren't working. Her blood sugar was high, her total cholesterol was 318, and her triglycerides were almost off the chart at 1,455.

A SILENT KILLER

The classic symptoms of a heart attack include a crushing sensation in the chest, chest pain (angina), pain radiating into the left arm or up into the jaw, and shortness of breath. However, it's important to realize that women and people with diabetes may not experience these symptoms. For them, symptoms are more likely to include nausea and vomiting, tiredness, sweating, and collapse. Doctors call these silent heart attacks. They are actually more dangerous than the more obvious sort, because life-saving, heart-preserving intervention may be delayed or never even administered.

The message: Don't wait until you're facing a crisis. If you have the metabolic syndrome, prediabetes, or diabetes, discuss with your physician a course of action should you experience any of these symptoms. It is in these emergency situations that standard American medicine shines—but you must recognize the signs and get help quickly.

Heart attacks are not the only problem. Obesity alone can overwork your heart to the point where its ability to pump blood efficiently is severely compromised.[6] This problem, heart failure, can also be caused by hypertension and the leftover scarring caused by a heart attack. Among people with heart failure, 20 to 40 percent have diabetes.[7]

After just three months on the ABSCP, she had lost only five pounds, but her risk factors for a heart attack had dropped considerably. Her blood sugar was down, her total cholesterol had fallen to 202, and her triglycerides had plummeted to 101! Muriel is a classic example of how it's never too late to improve your health.

UNDERSTANDING BLOOD LIPIDS

Throughout this book, we talk a lot about your blood lipids: LDL cholesterol, HDL cholesterol, and triglycerides. Now that we're talking about your heart health, it's time to take a closer look at them.

People with the metabolic syndrome, prediabetes, or Type 2 diabetes almost always have low HDL cholesterol, high triglycerides, and normal or only somewhat elevated levels of LDL cholesterol. As more and more research shows, the combination of low HDL and high triglycerides is practically a formula for a heart attack.[8–10] Whether or not you need to lose weight, if you have problems with your lipids, controlling your carbs will help. A high-carb diet is often associated with bad lipids, and controlling your carbs can help lower your triglycerides, raise your HDL, lower your LDL, and shift your overall cholesterol production toward less dangerous forms.

IS LDL CHOLESTEROL BAD?

High levels of LDL cholesterol in your blood are associated with a greater risk of vascular disease such as heart disease and stroke from clogged arteries—that's why it's often called the "bad" cholesterol. Calling LDL cholesterol "bad," however, is a simplistic approach that's more useful for selling cholesterol-lowering drugs than it is for helping you to avoid blocked arteries. When you look closely at LDL cholesterol, the picture is more complex.

Types of LDL can be divided into subfractions based on the size of the cholesterol particles. Very low density lipoprotein (VLDL) particles are fairly large; intermediate-density lipoprotein (IDL) particles are smaller, and low-density lipoprotein (LDL) particles are the smallest of all. The smaller the particle, the more potentially athero-genic (damaging to the arteries) it is.[11] In people with the metabolic syndrome, prediabetes, and diabetes, the particles tend to be mostly small, dense LDL cholesterol, rather than the bigger, lighter, "fluffier, less dangerous" particles.

The reason for this is a lot more complex than we have space to dis-cuss here. Suffice it to say that high insulin levels shift your production of cholesterol away from the larger, lighter particles and toward the smaller, denser particles. Lower your insulin by controlling your carbs, and you help move your cholesterol production back in a healthier di-rection—think of it as loosening or "fluffing up" these particles of cholesterol.[12]

Why are we explaining this in such detail? After you've been follow-ing the ABSCP for a few months, your LDL cholesterol number will probably be the same or might even go up a bit, even as your HDL cholesterol rises and your triglycerides drop. For most people, the LDL increase is modest and temporary and not at all harmful, and it's more than offset by the improved HDL/triglyceride ratio. In almost all peo-ple following the ABSCP properly, LDL numbers drop back to normal levels in three to six months. If your LDL did go up, see your physician to discuss further evaluation, as discussed below. Ask him or her to pay attention to other positive changes in your blood lipids. He or she is likely to respond to a rise in your LDL—or even to no drop in your LDL—by reaching for the prescription pad and writing out an order for a statin drug.

Before you take a drug to lower your LDL cholesterol, ask your doc-tor to investigate your LDL further to find out the proportions of dense and light particles. Even if your total LDL number has gone up, there's a good chance that your switch to a controlled-carb approach has raised the proportion of lighter, fluffier particles and shifted you toward what doctors call Pattern A. Recent studies have confirmed that the Atkins Nutritional Approach can shift your LDL to the favor-able, "fluffy" type.[13, 14]

You can also ask your doctor to do a blood test for a type of lipid called *lipoprotein little a* and written lipoprotein(a), or lp(a) for short. This is another form of blood lipid that has been shown to be an inde-pendent risk factor for heart disease.[15] Even if your LDL cholesterol is normal, your lp(a) number could be high. Most doctors believe that your lp(a) number is inherited and can't be changed by diet or anything else, but Dr. Atkins reported seeing some cases where it went down when the patient went on a controlled-carb program and lowered his or her insulin levels.

An example of such improvement resulting from dietary changes also occurred in one of my patients. Maureen Y., a 28-year-old woman who weighed only 100 pounds, lowered her lipoprotein(a) from a dangerously high 64 mg/dL to a safer level of 36 mg/dL, simply by controlling her intake of carbohydrates. The process took about six months—and her other blood lipids, which had been on the high side, improved as well. All this happened without weight loss, which was not appropriate in her case. —MARY VERNON

Research in this area is still emerging; however, there's not enough information yet to say that lowering your insulin can also lower your lp(a) number.

WHY IS HDL CHOLESTEROL GOOD?

Offsetting the LDL cholesterol is HDL cholesterol, the "good" or "protective" cholesterol. HDL cholesterol clears unused cholesterol from your bloodstream and carries it back to your liver. The higher your HDL level, the more cholesterol is being removed from your bloodstream before it has a chance to oxidize and damage your blood vessels; this explains the current thinking about why high HDL levels are protective of your heart and arteries.[16]

Like LDL, HDL comes in different particle sizes, or subfractions. People with the metabolic syndrome not only have low HDL levels, but their type of HDL tends to be small, dense particles, just as is the case with LDL. These particles, called HDL_3, aren't as efficient as the large, fluffy variety (called HDL_2) at transporting stored lipids to your liver. The more you have of the lighter, larger HDL_2 particles, the lower your risk of heart disease. And as with LDL cholesterol, high insulin levels shift your cholesterol production away from HDL_2 particles and toward smaller, denser particles called HDL$_3$. Lower your insulin level by following the controlled-carb approach, and you help shift your HDL production toward the more desirable, lighter HDL$_2$ particles.[17, 18]

The fat globules in your blood known as triglycerides are sometimes called triacylglycerol. High levels of triglycerides are undesirable. Dr. Atkins felt the optimum number should be under 100. Here's where controlling your carbs really pays off, because high levels of carbs in the diet translate directly into high triglycerides in the blood.[19, 20] Just about everyone who follows the controlled-carbohydrate approach finds that his or her high triglyceride levels drop considerably. We have seen triglycerides that were literally off the chart drop to less than 100 within a few months of the patient's starting to control carbohydrates. The combination of lowering triglycerides and raising HDL markedly improves your cardiac risk.[21, 22]

STATIN DRUGS AND LDL CHOLESTEROL

Because people with diabetes often have normal or only slightly elevated LDL cholesterol levels, there's been some question as to whether these patients should still try to lower their levels to the low-normal range. Some researchers say yes and believe all patients with diabetes should take statin drugs, even if their LDL is normal.

But we say: Not so fast. Some studies of statin drugs show that modest lowering of LDL, even if it's not on the high side, may help some people with diabetes lower their risk of heart disease. What they don't prove is that you need statin drugs to do this, although of course the patients in the studies were treated with statins. The drugs weren't compared with a controlled-carbohydrate program. Dietary changes that control carbohydrates are a very effective way to improve your lipid profile. So why take an expensive drug that can cause muscle pain and weakness, liver problems, and a possible increased risk of heart failure, when you can accomplish the same thing with the ABSCP? Most patients who follow the Atkins program correctly manage to bring their blood lipids to normal or near-normal levels within three to six months without the use of drugs.

Some of you who have a strong hereditary tendency toward extremely high cholesterol and triglycerides may not want to disagree with your physician on the issue of cholesterol-lowering drugs. Even if that is the case, taking the drugs shouldn't prevent you from following the ABSCP. Many will be pleasantly surprised by the results you will experience in your lipid values and other blood work—results that you didn't get from taking the drugs alone. Once your doctor sees these results, he or she may be willing to discuss making an adjustment in your medication.

A SECOND LOOK AT STATIN DRUGS

A popular group of drugs used to treat lipid abnormalities, statins (see the sidebar on page 111) are often prescribed for patients with the metabolic syndrome, prediabetes, and diabetes. In fact, if you have high cholesterol, your doctor may feel the only treatment option is to suggest these drugs to you. That's because doctors today are strongly pressured to follow the recommendations of the National Cholesterol Education Program (NCEP), which advise them to use these medications.[23] A large body of research shows that statins lower cholesterol, however, Dr. Atkins rarely needed to use them. Ask your doctor to give you the opportunity to try lowering your cardiovascular risk factors without medication.

Statins were initially thought to exert their cholesterol-lowering effect by blocking production of an enzyme your body uses to make cholesterol. Recent research, however, suggests that much of their effect may not be related to cholesterol lowering at all. Instead, statins seem to work by decreasing inflammation, especially in the endothelial cells that form the lining of your blood vessels.

However they work, these drugs require careful monitoring and have the potential for serious side effects. Because they block the synthesis of a compound called coenzyme Q_{10} (CoQ_{10} or ubiquinone), used in your cells for energy metabolism, statins can cause liver and muscle damage—including damage to the heart muscle.[24] Muscle damage can be so severe that one statin drug (Baychol) was voluntarily withdrawn from the market after some deaths occurred. Liver injury can occur as well. The manufacturers of statin drugs recommend blood tests every three to six months to monitor for evidence of liver damage.[25]

If there were no other way to improve your lipids, we would agree that the significant health risks of statins were worth it. But here's why we don't agree. With regards to lowering risk factors, the same effect that is achieved by the drugs can be achieved by following the Atkins controlled-carb approach. That's because decreasing insulin concentrations in the body can theoretically lower your production of an enzyme called HMG Co-A reductase—the same enzyme targeted by statin drugs—simply and naturally. And what's the most effective tool for bringing insulin down to normal levels? Controlling your carbohydrate intake.[26]

What about the statins' ability to reduce inflammation in the blood vessel lining? The controlled-carb approach can help there, too. High levels of insulin increase inflammation—and controlling insulin levels by controlling dietary carbohydrates can help control inflammation all over the body.[27, 28] Also, controlling carbs helps rid the body of excess fat, the secretions of which contribute to the inflammation of the cells that line blood vessel walls.[29] Add in the beneficial effect of essential oils from both diet and supplements, which further decrease inflammation, and you've got an effective, natural way to impact inflammation without statins or any other drugs.

TARGETING BLOOD LIPIDS

In 2001, the third Adult Treatment Panel (ATP III) of the NCEP issued new guidelines for the evaluation and treatment of high blood cholesterol.[30] The panel significantly lowered the thresholds for high cholesterol. This had the effect of substantially increasing the number of Americans who would be candidates for drug treatment—from an estimated 15 million adults under the old 1993 guidelines to an estimated 36 million under the new guidelines.[31] At the same time, the panel issued new low-fat, high-carb dietary recommendations. The panel's findings were a dream come true for drug manufacturers. The dietary recommendations are practically guaranteed not to work, unless the patient loses weight, meaning more patients will "need"

COMMON STATIN DRUGS

Generic ingredient: atorvastatin
Brand name: Lipitor

Generic ingredient: fluvastatin
Brand name: Lescol

Generic ingredient: lovastatin
Brand name: Mevacor

Generic ingredients: lovastatin and niacin
Brand name: Advicor

Generic ingredient: pravastatin
Brand name: Pravachol

Generic ingredient: Simvastatin
Brand name: Zocor

statin drugs.[32] Combined with the more aggressive approach to lowering cholesterol, the new guidelines guarantee the drug companies huge profits for years to come.

These guidelines were developed from statistical data on patients who ate the typical high-carb American diet. The guidelines do not take into account the total lipid picture, which includes other cardiovascular risk factors such as homocysteine, lipoprotein(a), fibrinogen, and C-reactive protein. As you already know, in the presence of high glucose and insulin, your cells immediately stop burning fat and prepare to store fat instead. To manage these risk factors effectively, the problem must be corrected where it starts. By controlling carbohydrates, you can prevent the hormonal fat storage effect of excessive insulin, which results in increased cardiovascular risk factors. These include high triglycerides, low HDL, and small, dense, dangerous

RESEARCH REPORT: CHOLESTEROL AND CONTROLLING CARBS

Two highly significant recent studies have shown that controlling carbohydrates can have a powerful impact on blood lipids. In the first study, 12 healthy, normal-weight men followed a very low carbohydrate diet for six weeks. At the end of that time, their HDL cholesterol was up and their triglycerides were down. Perhaps more important, among the men who had mostly small, dense LDL particles at the start of the study, LDL size went up, moving these men toward a better cholesterol profile.[33] A similar study of 10 healthy, normal-weight women also showed excellent results. Their triglycerides went down and HDL went up. The beneficial effects of a low-carb approach in women were even stronger than they were in men. Three of the women with small particles at baseline had particles change to the large, fluffier type.[34]

lipoprotein particles. Standard guidelines focus simply on the total and LDL cholesterol values.[35]

Whether or not the ATP III guidelines make sense, they're the ones that set the lipid standards for physicians all over the country. Check the following chart to see what these guidelines are.

ATP III GUIDELINES

LDL CHOLESTEROL

Optimal	less than 100 mg/dL
Near optimal/above optimal	100–129 mg/dL
Borderline high	130–159 mg/dL
High	160–189 mg/dL
Very high	190 mg/dL or more

HDL CHOLESTEROL

Low	less than 40 mg/dL
High	60 mg/dL or more

TOTAL CHOLESTEROL	
Desirable	less than 200 mg/dL
Borderline high	200–239 mg/dL
High	240 mg/dL or more

TRIGLYCERIDES	
Normal	less than 150 mg/dL
Borderline high	150–199 mg/dL
High	200–499 mg/dL
Very high	500 mg/dL or more

Source: National Cholesterol Education Program.

WHEN TLC IS BAD FOR YOU

The latest dietary recommendations from the NCEP are known as TLC, or Therapeutic Lifestyle Changes. The current version of this low-fat, low-cholesterol diet isn't very different from the diet that NCEP has been promoting for years. This diet calls for keeping total fat to 25 to 35 percent of daily calories and limiting dietary cholesterol to less than 200 mg a day, and it recommends getting 50 to 60 percent of total calories from carbohydrates. This approach may lower your LDL cholesterol somewhat—but at the expense of also lowering your HDL cholesterol. Not only that, the TLC diet may also shift your HDL production to smaller, denser particles that aren't as good at clearing LDL cholesterol from your blood. And of course, eating all those carbs will probably raise your triglycerides.

THE BETTER WAY TO BETTER BLOOD LIPIDS

The Atkins approach improves all aspects of your blood lipids naturally—not by blasting your body with drugs and judging the results by the numbers on only one blood test. Controlling your carbs is the first step. Your triglycerides will drop as your insulin-glucose metabolism improves. Even before you lose the first ten pounds, you may see an immediate improvement in triglyceride levels. HDL will begin to rise—although in our experience it takes between three and six months to get HDL to its best level—after glucose metabolism is normalized. At the same time, levels of tiny LDL particles will decrease, and LDL will shift toward those larger, fluffier particles that aren't as dangerous to your arteries. As you follow the program, your lipid profile will almost certainly continue to improve.

One of Dr. Atkins' patients, 68-year-old Claudia W., had the lowest HDL he had ever seen—at only 20 mg/dL. She started following the ABSCP and three months later her HDL had risen to 70 mg/dL. In fact, she was now unusual in a much healthier way, because her HDL number was higher than that of her triglycerides.

Although the dietary changes of the ABSCP are a very effective way to elevate your HDL, exercise and supplements provide additional improvement. Is that because of the exercise itself or because exercise helps you lose weight? It's hard to tell, because in just about every study that has looked at the effect of exercise on HDL, the subjects lost weight. It's hard to separate the two effects, but it doesn't really matter. After all, losing weight also raises your HDL level, along with all its other benefits. And exercise is undeniably good for every aspect of your health.

THE DANGEROUS CHEMISTRY OF ABDOMINAL FAT

In case you thought it was all about your cholesterol, we're about to disabuse you of that misconception. Cholesterol is only part of the heart disease story. Did you know that it is quite possible to have cholesterol numbers that fall within the normal range and still have a heart attack?

Remember, a heart attack is caused when blood flow to the arteries of the heart is blocked, usually by a blood clot. The biochemical imbalance driving the metabolic syndrome causes an increased tendency toward blood clotting. In part, this is because the abdominal fat that is such a telltale sign of the metabolic syndrome secretes chemicals that raise the level of clotting factors in your blood and make your platelets "stickier" and more likely to form a clot. The inflammatory response that occurs in the metabolic syndrome—partly due to those same secreted chemicals—damages the endothelial cells that line your blood vessels.[36] This is a recipe for blood clot formation, arterial blockage, and deep venous thrombosis. If you have ever wondered why our society is plagued by stroke, heart attacks, and blood clots in the lung (pulmonary embolus), now you know.

Here's the good news! Dr. Atkins observed in his practice that when people with abdominal obesity and the metabolic syndrome, prediabetes, or diabetes start following the Atkins approach, they generally lose proportionally more weight in the abdominal area. In many cases, even when total weight loss is fairly modest, the effect is powerful if the weight comes from fat stored in the abdominal area: HDL cholesterol goes up and triglycerides go down more than the weight loss alone would normally accomplish. Other dangerous substances in your blood, such as clotting factors, also can go down, because you have less of the fat that makes them. Add in some exercise, which also seems to target abdominal fat, and the effect on your lipids and inflammatory and clotting factors is even greater. Losing even small amounts of visceral fat may be enough to bring your metabolic syndrome under control and improve your heart health.

OTHER RISK FACTORS

So much attention gets paid to cholesterol as a risk factor for heart disease that other important risk factors tend to be ignored, especially if your cholesterol is in the normal range. Let's look at three additional independent risk factors Dr. Atkins considered to be more important than total cholesterol level.

Homocysteine

A normal by-product of metabolizing the amino acid *methionine,* high levels of homocysteine in your blood are an independent risk factor for heart disease from clogged arteries. This automatically raises the risk of death from heart disease for the estimated 25 percent of the population that has a genetic tendency toward high homocysteine levels. And if you have the genetic tendency and also have diabetes, your risk is about 2.5 times greater.[37] A recent study in Finland found that even moderately elevated homocysteine is an independent risk factor for fatal heart attacks in people with Type 2 diabetes, even when other risk factors such as smoking and high blood sugar were taken into account. The study found that the elevated risk began at homocysteine levels of 15 μmmol/L or higher—or not that much higher than the upper end of normal.[38]

Whether or not they have the genetic tendency to high homocysteine, people with insulin resistance or diabetes seem more likely to have high homocysteine levels than do people with normal glucose tolerance; also, people with diabetes and high homocysteine are more likely to have complications such as kidney disease.[39] Dr. Atkins would treat his patients who had high homocysteine levels with the dietary changes of the ABSCP and also with additional supplements of vitamins B_6, B_{12}, and folic acid. Although the normal range for homocysteine is 5.2 mmol/L to 12.9 mmol/L, his goal for his patients was a homocysteine level of 8 mmol/L or less. Most of them were able to achieve this goal.

C-reactive protein (CRP)

An elevated level of this protein, produced in your liver, is a sensitive marker of inflammation. Because inflammation is believed to be one of the underlying processes that causes your arteries to clog, high CRP levels in general turn out to be a good warning sign of heart disease. In the Physicians' Health Study, for instance, the men who had higher levels of CRP when the study began were much more likely to have a heart attack over the next ten years than the men who had normal CRP levels—even though they seemed equally healthy based on other measurements, such as their cholesterol.[40] Results for women in the Nurses' Health Study were similar.[41]

People with abdominal obesity, impaired glucose tolerance, and Type 2 diabetes generally have elevated CRP levels.[42] Other factors, such as an acute illness or the use of some hormones, can also elevate CRP.) But again, there's reason to be optimistic. A recent study of overweight women with high levels of inflammation (according to blood markers such as CRP) showed that when they lost just 10 percent of their body weight through a diet and exercise program, the markers fell back to much healthier levels. In fact, their levels were very close to those of normal-weight women.[43] And despite some claims to the contrary, following a low-carbohydrate approach does not raise CRP levels.[44]

Fibrinogen

This is a protein in your blood that plays a crucial role in the complex process of blood clotting. When your fibrinogen levels are high, your blood may clot too easily—and a clot that blocks an artery can cause a heart attack or stroke. People with the metabolic syndrome, prediabetes, or diabetes can all have elevated fibrinogen levels, as well as an increase in other chemicals that increase blood clotting.[45] This tendency to clot may be related to the inflammatory process that is part of the metabolic syndrome. (As with CRP, other factors, such as the use of certain birth-control medications and hormone imbalances, can increase fibrinogen levels.) This is one of the reasons many doctors recommend low-dose aspirin as a way to lower your risk of heart disease. Dr. Atkins found that aspirin, with its risk of gastrointestinal bleeding, wasn't necessary for most of his patients. Instead, he prescribed fatty acid supplements to decrease platelet stickiness and for their anti-inflammatory effects.

TAKE HEART!

As this chapter makes clear, first, if you have the metabolic syndrome, prediabetes, or diabetes, you have an increased risk of heart disease. Second, and most important, no matter where you are on the diabetes continuum, heart disease is not inevitable. By following the

ABSCP you'll begin to correct the underlying metabolic problems that threaten your heart health. And once you start controlling your carbohydrate intake and normalizing your metabolism, the risk to your heart drops—safely, naturally, and without the use of drugs.

WHAT'S YOUR HEART RISK?

Use the self-quiz below to assess your risk of cardiovascular disease.

1. I am:
   a. male [1]
   b. female [0]
2. My age is:
   a. under 40 [0]
   b. 41 to 44 [0]
   c. 45 to 49 [1]
   d. 50 to 54 [2]
   e. 55 to 60 [3]
   f. 61 or older [4]
3. I smoke or use other forms of tobacco:
   a. yes [2]
   b. no [0]
4. I have prediabetes or diabetes:
   a. yes [4]
   b. no [0]
5. My blood pressure is:
   a. normal (less than 120/80) [0]
   b. prehypertensive (130/90) [1]
   c. hypertensive (140/90 or higher) [3]
6. My triglycerides are:
   a. desirable (150 mg/dL or less) [0]
   b. high (151 mg/dL or more) [1]
7. My HDL cholesterol is (according to ATP III guidelines):
   a. low (40 mg/dL or less) [2]

b. borderline low (50 mg/dL or less) [1]
c. high (60 mg/dL or more) [0]

To determine your risk of developing heart disease, add up the numbers in square brackets for each of your answers.

Scoring
0 to 6: lowest risk
7 to 10: moderate risk
11 and above: high risk

A NEW LEASE ON LIFE

Joe McCoy had a heart attack at age 44. While he was on a prescribed low-fat diet, his blood sugar and blood pressure careened out of control. Today, thanks to Atkins, it's on a smooth ride.

NAME: Joe McCoy
AGE: 53
HEIGHT: 5 feet 10 inches
WEIGHT BEFORE: 278 pounds
WEIGHT NOW: 196 pounds

TOTAL CHOLESTEROL BEFORE: 880
TOTAL CHOLESTEROL AFTER: 168
BLOOD PRESSURE BEFORE: 200/130
BLOOD PRESSURE AFTER: 145/78
TRIGLYCERIDES BEFORE: 6,600
TRIGLYCERIDES AFTER: 273

My father was a doctor and, I realize now, he was ahead of his time when it came to diet and nutrition. My brother, sisters, and I were raised on a diet of protein and vegetables. I never ate bread or dessert at home, except for the occasional birthday cake, until I was out on my own. In high school, I also played lots of sports, including football, and being overweight was never an issue.

I started to gain weight after I got married, mostly due to my wife Karen's home cooking and unbelievably delicious challah bread. It took about 15 years, though, before I reached the point where I really needed to lose weight. In 1995, I had a heart attack and my doctor put me on a low-fat diet. I had been hypoglycemic prior to this time and I believe this low-fat regimen plunged me into full-blown Type 2 diabetes by 1999. My glycated hemoglobin (A1C) was an abysmal 13. My blood sugar numbers ranged between a scary 500 and 600. I also developed a case of peripheral neuropathy, a common side effect of diabetes that causes numbness and soreness in the feet and hands. I was in so much pain, you wouldn't wish it on your worst enemy. One of my friends suggested I see Dr. Mary Vernon, who practices in Lawrence, Kansas, where I live. I didn't know then that she used the Atkins Nutritional Approach.

In her office, Dr. Vernon took one look at me and said, "You certainly have the body type that will benefit from carbohydrate restriction." As she wrote my menu she told me to stop taking Glucovance. I wasn't surprised that she said I needed to lose weight, but I couldn't believe my ears when she told me to stop taking my diabetes medication. I was feeling so lousy, though, I just jumped right in and did what I was told. It took a month for me to lose ten pounds. Within three months my blood sugar, cholesterol, and triglycerides all improved. As did my kidney function. Five months later, I contracted pneumonia in both lungs and spent three weeks in the hospital. I know that I probably would have died if I had not made such a remarkable improvement in my health from doing Atkins. I resumed the program after I recovered and after six more months, I was down to 220 pounds. By then I needed a whole new wardrobe. I probably should have invested in a pair of suspenders because I was having trouble keeping my pants up!

I have been hovering around 200 pounds since February 2003, and I still keep my grams of Net Carbs at around 20 per day. Still, I'd like to lose another 15 pounds. I continue to test my blood sugar every day and take a very small amount, about one-quarter to a half tablet, of Glucovance, which keeps my blood sugar around 110. My A1C reading is 5.3, which is quite good. My triglycerides are still a little high and I'd like to improve that number, too. I'm told my heart is also in excellent shape. The pain from the neuropathy is not nearly as bad as it once was and one of the nerves has regenerated in my right hand—I'm hoping that more of them will do the same. I can't really exercise or return to work as an auto mechanic because of this problem, but I'm telling you, I have an energy that wasn't there before going on the program.

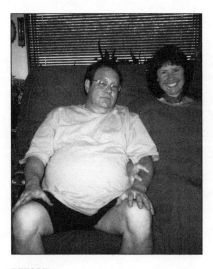

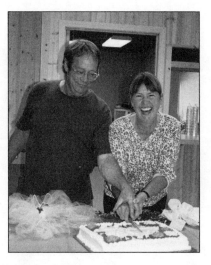

BEFORE   **AFTER**

When I was fat and sick with diabetes, I prayed and prayed that I would live to see the birth of my grandchildren. Now, our only son and his wife are due to have their first baby soon, right around our 25th anniversary. It's easy to understand why my wife and I recommend Atkins every chance we get.

Note: Your individual results may vary from those reported here.

Part Two

Taking Charge of Your Health

Chapter 10

THE ATKINS BLOOD SUGAR CONTROL PROGRAM

Now that you have a better understanding of the progression of this epidemic disease and all the health risks associated with it, you are probably more than ready to get started on your new path. We couldn't be happier about that. The sooner you start dealing with your metabolic imbalance, the better.

Before telling you about the right way to eat for your condition, let us briefly introduce you to the wrong way to eat if you have insulin-blood sugar abnormalities. If you have seen your physician and have received a diagnosis of either the metabolic syndrome, prediabetes, or diabetes, he or she has likely prescribed a diet endorsed by groups such as the American Diabetes Association (ADA) and the American Heart Association (AHA). By now you won't be surprised when we tell you that Dr. Atkins would recommend another approach.

His 40 years of experience treating patients with the metabolic syndrome, prediabetes, and Type 2 diabetes made it clear to him that these low-fat, high-carb diets are likely to make you feel worse—and your blood sugar, blood pressure, and blood lipid measurements will probably get worse, too. You may have discovered this for yourself. Perhaps you have followed your doctor's advice, only to find that you actually gained weight—meaning fat—and your blood sugar, blood lipids, and blood pressure numbers worsened instead of improving.

Sometimes, the lack of improvement in your blood tests might lead your dietary counselor to believe that you didn't follow his or her recommendations, even though you did. Your doctor may tell you that you have no choice but to resort to medications.

Health care practitioners who really understand carbohydrate metabolism know that this sequence of events—from diagnosis to dietary changes that don't work to medication—is about as predictable as the sun rising each morning. Indeed, recent research is now confirming Dr. Atkins' years of clinical experience. (See Scientific Studies That Validate the Atkins Nutritional Approach, page 448, for a comprehensive list of recent work in this area.) What *is* a surprise is that much of the medical establishment persists in this outdated thinking when rapidly accumulating evidence points to the fact that these programs don't work for the vast majority of people.

Whether you have the metabolic syndrome, prediabetes, or diabetes, if you want to do all you can to prevent your condition from getting worse (and who in their right mind wouldn't?), these dietary recommendations could hinder you. They are simply too high in carbohydrates for many people. You have learned in the first few chapters of this book about what eating excessive carbs do to your body. Let's take another look, step-by-step:

1. Eating a carb-heavy diet causes a rapid rise in blood sugar. To control this elevation, the body produces insulin to transport the blood sugar to the cells.
2. As the cells become more and more resistant to the insulin, the pancreas increases its output of insulin.
3. As the effect of the excessive insulin kicks in, blood sugar drops too fast and too low, making you feel irritable, jittery, and hungry.
4. When blood sugar takes a dramatic dive, your body releases stress hormones such as epinephrine and cortisol.
5. The side effects of this response can cause a variety of unpleasant yet common symptoms: mood and energy swings, palpitations, food cravings, difficulty concentrating, irritability, headaches, and even high blood pressure.

This cycle is more common in overweight individuals, but it can occur even if you are slim, especially if you eat the standard American diet (or SAD), which is high in refined carbohydrates. Eating excessive amounts of carbs or even frequently eating refined carbs triggers the fat-storage mechanism. Remember, insulin promotes the storage of fat. Your body burns sugar (derived from carbohydrates) for energy and stores the excess sugar as fat for future use. Fat can be stored anywhere in the body, including around the belly, in the liver, around your internal organs, and even in the walls of the blood vessels. Triglycerides are one form in which fat is transported in your bloodstream. Other lipoproteins also transport fat—and insulin is involved in regulating their production. So when you put the wrong kind or amount of carbohydrates in your mouth, insulin goes up—and so do the fats in your bloodstream. Now let's talk about your new lifestyle—the diet, exercise, and supplement program that's going to turn your health around.

THE ATKINS WAY

The Atkins Blood Sugar Control Program (ABSCP) is designed to help you control your individual metabolism through food and other lifestyle choices. We stress the word *individual* because, with ABSCP, one size doesn't fit all. For many of you, this program will be the very tool that prevents further blood sugar stress (such as hypoglycemia), and takes diabetes off your road map altogether. For those of you who have later stages of blood sugar stress (prediabetes) or full-blown diabetes, it will help you to control your blood sugar and even normalize it, which means you may be able to minimize or even stop the use of some prescription medications.

As Dr. Atkins routinely observed in his patients, the ABSCP increases patients' energy, decreases aches and pains, improves numerous other symptoms, and enhances the overall quality of life. Likewise, published studies of people with diabetes and the metabolic syndrome document improvements in blood sugar and blood lipid values on a controlled-carbohydrate program. This dietary approach provides the tools you need to take control of your metabolism.

Because the ABSCP is based on the famed Atkins Nutritional Approach (ANA), let's start with an overview of this safe, effective, controlled-carbohydrate approach to rebalancing the metabolism, managing weight, and improving health. Later we'll look at how the ABSCP differs from the ANA.

If you're overweight or if you have only a slightly impaired insulin/glucose mechanism, the ANA alone will probably help you lose weight as well as lower and stabilize your blood sugar and insulin levels. At the same time, you'll improve your health in other important ways, because weight loss and normalizing blood sugar help improve lipids, lower blood pressure, and reduce the inflammation markers associated with heart disease. As your blood sugar stabilizes, you'll have more energy, and you'll probably find that your mood and mental sharpness improve as well.

Some of you undoubtedly are already familiar with the ANA as a weight-loss program. For those of you who are not acquainted with it, a brief review of the four phases is in the next section. When people are on the ANA, their body fat slowly, steadily, and safely vanishes; most of them do not experience food cravings after the first few days. You progress toward your goal of improved health without feeling deprived. And this is not a temporary fix; learning how to do Atkins provides you with a tool for lifelong control of your weight and metabolism. A brief review of the ANA follows.

THE FOUR PHASES OF THE ATKINS NUTRITIONAL APPROACH

Phase 1: Induction. To kick-start weight loss, limit your carbohydrate intake to 20 grams of Net Carbs a day. (The simple way to calculate Net Carbs in a whole food is to subtract the grams of fiber from the total number of carbohydrate grams in the portion. Net Carbs are the only carbohydrates that have an appreciable impact on your blood sugar.) During this phase, which lasts a minimum of two weeks, you satisfy your appetite with foods high in protein and natural fats, along with carbohydrates in the form of 3 cups of salad greens (dressed with olive oil and vinegar, lemon juice, or your favorite controlled-carb dressing). Alternatively, you can have 2 cups of salad and a cup of fresh, nonstarchy cooked veggies, such as broccoli or zucchini. You can also eat 3 to 4 ounces of aged cheese, a handful of olives, and half an avocado each day.

Phase 2: Ongoing Weight Loss (OWL). When you move on to OWL, you deliberately slow your weight loss as you continue to eat protein and natural fats, along with salad greens and nutrient-dense and fiber-rich vegetables. As you continue to lose weight, you gradually add back nutrient-rich carbohydrates. Each week, you increase your daily carb count by just 5 grams of Net Carbs by eating more vegetables, nuts and seeds, and even berries. After incorporating these foods, some people can even reintroduce small portions of legumes (beans) and fruits other than berries—until weight loss stalls. At that point, drop back 5 grams of Net Carbs and you should have discovered your Critical Carbohydrate Level for Losing (CCLL)—the amount of Net Carbs you can eat while continuing to lose weight. To continue your steady progress, keep your carb intake at or below your CCLL.

Phase 3: Pre-Maintenance. When you are within five to ten pounds of your goal weight, you'll want to slow down your rate of weight loss even more, so that your new, improved eating habits become in-grained. (Expect it to take at least two months to trim the last ten pounds.) You can now broaden your food choices to include moderate portions of starchy vegetables such as sweet potatoes and peas and even some unrefined whole grains. Each week, simply add another 10 daily grams of Net Carbs to your program—or treat yourself to an extra 20 to 30 grams of high-quality carbs twice a week—until weight loss stops. Then drop back down 5 or 10 grams, and you will have found your revised CCLL. Continue at this level until you reach your goal weight. When you have maintained your goal weight for one month or more, you will have achieved your Atkins Carbohydrate Equilibrium, or ACE, the number of grams of Net Carbs you can eat without gaining or losing weight, and you are now officially in the Lifetime Maintenance phase.

Phase 4: Lifetime Maintenance. Now that you've achieved your goal weight, you can continue to enjoy a wide range of delicious foods. Of course, you still need to keep an eye on your total carb intake. Remember, this program is not simply about the quantity of carbs, but their quality as well. Accept the fact that junk food is a thing of the past;

instead, spend your carb allowance on nutrient-rich and fiber-rich foods. Understand that you may or may not be able to add back whole grains, such as oats, brown rice, wild rice, and barley, and higher-carb fruits (like bananas) and vegetables (like potatoes). Your ACE will depend upon your age, gender, activity level, hormonal status, and any metabolic issues you have. Most people can raise their ACE if they exercise regularly.

For more details on weight loss and the science behind controlled-carb intake for weight control, good health, and disease prevention, read *Dr. Atkins' New Diet Revolution, Atkins for Life,* and *The Atkins Essentials* or visit www.atkins.com.[1-3] To track your carbohydrate intake easily, we recommend using *Dr. Atkins' New Carbohydrate Gram Counter.*[4]

THE NEXT STEP

When it comes to weight loss, the ANA works for just about everyone. And because slimming down almost automatically ameliorates many health problems—including blood sugar abnormalities—losing even a moderate amount of weight might well be enough for you to start feeling a lot better.

But if your health picture now includes the metabolic syndrome, prediabetes, or diabetes, you may well need to take a next step beyond the ANA. Why? Because you must work on reversing health problems that have developed over months or even years. That's where the Atkins Blood Sugar Control Program comes in. As in the ANA, weight loss is a crucial component of the program, but now there are also other very important goals. In fact, some of you may be at normal weight or only slightly overweight but still have blood sugar abnormalities, high blood pressure, high blood lipids, and other markers of metabolic imbalance.

The ABSCP concentrates on getting your metabolism back into balance by normalizing your insulin/blood sugar levels and blood lipids, reducing other markers associated with impending heart disease, and lowering your blood pressure. As your metabolism improves, you will almost certainly lose weight (if you need to).

A LITTLE CAN DO A LOT

The loss of stored fat and an improved ability to burn fat are very important steps on the road to improved health. However, weight loss may be secondary to the other improvements on the ABSCP. In fact, it is possible to improve your blood sugar, lipids, and blood pressure numbers without losing all—or even very much—of your excess fat. Your journey back to health begins with improvements that will happen before the pounds begin to fall away. Until these occur, your weight loss may well be slow or even nonexistent—and that's just fine. More important than seeing the numbers on the scale move down is stabilizing your metabolism. For now, your lab values (your blood sugar number, for instance) are more important than how much extra fat you have. When you start following the ABSCP, these lab values can be positively improved early on, even before significant weight is lost. When those numbers improve, it means you can reduce the dose or even stop taking some or all of the medications you might be on.

A 75-year-old patient with diabetes named Jim H. came in to see Dr. Atkins; at the time he was taking nine different drugs to control his blood sugar, blood pressure, blood lipids, and some other ailments. After six months on the ABSCP, Jim was down to just three drugs (and lower doses of those), and his blood sugar was under control. Jim had lost just five pounds in that time.

I had a patient who likewise did not lose a lot of weight, but the weight she did drop made a tremendous difference in her health. At age 37, Maureen J. had the lab results of someone twice her age. Weighing 197 pounds and five feet six inches tall, she had a total cholesterol of 327; her triglycerides were 298; her HDL, 53; and her LDL, 214. Moreover, her blood pressure was creeping up to 138/80. I put her on the Induction phase of the Atkins Nutritional Approach for two weeks and she then moved to 25 and later 30 grams of carbohydrates a day. After six weeks, although she had only lost ten pounds, Maureen's improvement was remarkable: Her total cholesterol was down to 199, her triglycerides, to 121; her HDL was 46 and her LDL was down to 172. Her waist was also two inches smaller.   —MARY VERNON

Remember, long before your lab values become abnormal, the gradual shift from good health to increased risk and finally to outright illness has been set in motion. Years before tests reveal that you have a problem, damage to the blood vessels in your heart, eyes, nerves, kidneys, and brain may have been silently accumulating. Although some of these changes may be permanent, the good news is that you can impact your metabolism *immediately* by simply changing the food you eat. This will give your body every chance to repair itself.

On the other hand, if you do need to lose weight, don't take this as license to settle for only minimal weight loss as your final goal. We're not going to let you off the hook that easily. You owe it to yourself to ultimately take off those extra pounds, which increase your risk for a litany of diseases and contribute to the insulin/blood sugar abnormalities. Fat is not only a sign of the problem; excess fat also contributes to the problem.

It is important to understand that we are talking about a *permanent* lifestyle change. If you have a tendency toward the metabolic syndrome or diabetes, you can manage this with careful attention to your diet—but your blood sugar problems don't ever go away. If you return to your old way of eating, the old symptoms and risk factors will come roaring back. To get your blood sugar under control and keep it there, you'll almost certainly need to follow the basic principles of the ABSCP for a lifetime.

THE ATKINS BLOOD SUGAR CONTROL PROGRAM

The ABSCP is fundamentally very simple: Control carbohydrates—meaning both quantity and quality—to control blood sugar, insulin levels, and your metabolism. As with the ANA, you can eat satisfying portions of a wide variety of nutritious, delicious foods, and you never have to go hungry. The difference is that in addition to careful carbo-

SEE YOUR DOCTOR

Dr. Atkins designed the ABSCP to help the specific health issues caused by the metabolic syndrome, prediabetes, and Type 2 diabetes. But before you begin to follow this program, you must have a complete medical examination and discuss the results with your doctor.

The ABSCP is safe and effective, but you may have special medical problems, such as advanced kidney disease, which may mean this program is not right for you—unless it is prescribed and monitored by a physician trained in this type of metabolic management. You also need to know your baseline lab results for important markers such as insulin/blood sugar, blood lipids, and blood pressure *before* you begin the program. Finally, if you take prescription medications, you need to plan ahead for possible changes in the doses as your metabolism normalizes.

hydrate control, your diet will be rich in foods that have been shown to help control not only blood sugar but also lipid levels, high blood pressure, and the many other health problems that go along with the metabolic syndrome, prediabetes, and diabetes. Two of the reasons that the Atkins Blood Sugar Control Program is so easy to follow are that those foods can be found in any supermarket and that they just happen to taste great.

SETTING REALISTIC GOALS

In the earlier chapters of this book we explained exactly what happens to your body when your insulin and blood sugar levels rise. With that information in mind, now let's look at your objectives as you start following the ABSCP.

Metabolic Improvement

You want to return your metabolism to its optimum function to be healthy and energetic, to feel great, and to take as few medicines as

FINDING A NUTRITIONALLY ORIENTED PHYSICIAN

As an increasing number of physicians become aware of the science supporting the Atkins approach and see how much their patients benefit, many are recommending Atkins to their patients. Even though the subjects of controlled-carbohydrate nutrition and ketogenic diets are not commonly taught in medical school, your own physician might have experience in monitoring and supervising them. If your physician does not have specific training or is uncomfortable with Atkins, he or she may be able to refer you to a provider who is. If your doctor is unable to make such a referral, you can contact one of the following organizations, which have a focus on nutrition. Understand that not all their members are familiar with controlled-carbohydrate nutrition. (See page 139 for questions you might ask to ascertain an individual physician's expertise and level of comfort with the Atkins approach.)

American College for Advancement in Medicine: www.acam.org
American Society of Bariatric Physicians: www.aspb.org

possible. That's the aim of the ABSCP. For years you've been experiencing the metabolic abnormalities we've discussed. It may take some time to turn all this around. You'll have to do your part: It is up to you to learn how to manage your metabolism with carbohydrate control, to include exercise in your daily routine, and to take the necessary supplements to support your body's return toward normal. This book, based on Dr. Atkins' clinical experience, will provide the road map, but you must stay the course.

Stabilized Insulin and Blood Sugar

The Atkins Blood Sugar Control Program is designed to improve blood sugar levels. By this we don't mean simply using drugs to drive your fasting blood sugar below the magic number of 100 mg/dL.

Rather, Dr. Atkins designed the ABSCP to treat the underlying prob-lem—the whole person, not just your blood sugar number. The goal is to teach you a way to keep your insulin/blood sugar steady at a health-ier level.

Improved Blood Lipids

A common initial finding related to insulin and blood sugar imbal-ance is disturbed lipid levels, particularly high triglycerides and low HDL, which are recognized as serious risk factors for heart disease. Even if your blood lipid numbers are within the normal range, you may still be at increased risk, because high blood sugar shifts these lipid particles toward a smaller, denser, more dangerous form. (For more on this, review Chapter 9, The Cardiac Connection.) Control-ling your carbs moves you toward a more desirable lipid profile.

Lowered Blood Pressure

High insulin and blood sugar levels go hand in hand with high blood pressure. Getting your insulin/blood sugar levels under control by controlling your carbs will simultaneously help tackle the cause of hy-pertension. (Review Chapter 8, Twin Peaks: High Blood Pressure and High Blood Sugar.) Exercise and weight loss (if necessary) will bring down your blood pressure even more.

Reduced Medication Needs

The average adult with Type 2 diabetes takes several different prescrip-tion drugs to treat various aspects of the disease. All those drugs may succeed in temporarily producing test results that *appear to* indicate improved health, but the reality is that most of them are doing noth-ing to solve the underlying problem. In addition, all those drugs may actually create a downward spiral of worsening health. Reducing med-ications with your doctor's help means fewer chemicals for your liver to process and less chance of a dangerous drug interaction. You may think these interactions are rare; they're not. According to a study published in the *New England Journal of Medicine,* about 25 percent of all prescriptions lead to some adverse event.[5] Here's something else you probably didn't know. In a study published in the *Journal of the American Medical Association,* reporting on adverse drug reactions in the United States in 1994, it was found that about 100,000 hospitalized patients died as a result of a drug interaction—making legally prescribed and administered drugs somewhere between the fourth and sixth leading cause of death for that year.[6]

Weight Loss

Why have we saved this important goal for last? Because until you get your blood sugar under control, and perhaps until you can reduce or eliminate some of the drugs you are now taking, you may find it difficult to lose weight. Most of Dr. Atkins' patients with the metabolic syndrome, prediabetes, or diabetes did gradually lose weight once they began the program. Although the loss can be agonizingly slow at first, it almost always picks up once patients get their insulin and blood sugar normalized and reduce their medications. For those of you with the metabolic syndrome who are not presently taking medications, of course, weight loss could happen quickly. Whether or not you are taking medications, if you already have prediabetes or Type 2 diabetes, the weight-loss process will likely take a while to begin and may initially go slowly.

In the short run, there is much benefit to be gained from even small amounts of fat loss. Remember that even a small change in the amount of stored fat has been shown to favorably impact the risk factors for heart attack and stroke.[7] In the long run, once your insulin/blood sugar metabolism normalizes, you will find it easier to decrease your fat stores.

A good example of metabolic improvement with minimal weight loss is Pia S., a 48-year-old, who came to see me with a fasting blood sugar of 370. At the time of her first visit, she weighed 217 pounds. Two weeks after starting the ABSCP she had lost only 3 pounds but her blood sugar was down to 268. One month later, her blood sugar dropped to 198 although her weight stayed the same. After six months, her blood sugar was down to 150, her glycated hemoglobin (A1C) went from 12.5 to 7.6, her cholesterol from 242 to 156, her triglycerides from 118 to 63, her LDL from 161 to 93, and her CRP from 12.9 to 5.5. In addition, her 24-hour urine test for microalbumin (a test to measure kidney function, which I monitor every three months) went from 482.9 to 390.6. Although she lost only 10 pounds, her waist went from 45 inches to 42. At eight months, her fasting blood sugars were down to 120, and she weighed 202 pounds.

—MARY VERNON

The basic principles of the Atkins Blood Sugar Control Program are straightforward and scientifically sound. But can you put theory

WHAT IS KETOSIS?

One of the most frequent misconceptions concerning both the ANA and ABSCP is about the body's normal production of ketones. To understand why following the ABSCP is safe for your kidneys and the rest of your body, you'll have to understand a bit about your metabolism. When you initially cut back on carbohydrates the Atkins way, your body starts primarily burning fat for energy, a process that's known as lipolysis. Your body breaks down fat into chemicals called ketones, which are used by your muscles and other cells for energy. Most of the cells in your body can "burn" both glucose and ketones for energy production, so your stored fat can be used for energy. That's how you lose fat when you control carbohydrates. When your body burns fat very rapidly, some of the ketones escape into your breath and urine. The process is entirely normal; in fact, our bodies use ketones for energy when we are asleep. When you produce more ketones than you can burn, and extra ketones are excreted, then you are said to be in ketosis, more accurately called benign dietary ketosis. Remember, you can be making and burning ketones without them showing in your urine, meaning you are still burning fat even without "spilling" ketones. (Occasionally, ketones turn up in the urine even without a change in your weight.)

Benign dietary ketosis is a perfectly safe bodily function. Did you know that even on an overnight fast, a normal individual may produce ketones? Humans are adapted to live for long periods of time this way—

that's how we are able to survive periods of famine. It's worth noting that a 30-day fast (drinking water but eating no food) raises ketones to ten times the levels experienced by individuals who are restricting carbohydrate intake.

All too often, benign dietary ketosis is confused with the dangerous metabolic state called "ketoacidosis," which may occur in Type 1 diabetics with very high blood sugar or in severe alcoholics after a binge.

into practice and still enjoy good food without a lot of fuss? Absolutely. You'll learn how in the next chapter.

HOW TO TEST FOR KETONES

The presence of ketones in your urine indicates that you are now burning fat for energy—a perfectly normal bodily response to controlling your carbohydrate intake. To determine if ketones are present, you can use lipolysis test strips (also called ketosis testing strips). You can buy these in any pharmacy.

If you want to know if you're in ketosis, test your urine before your evening meal or before bedtime. Simply follow the instructions on the package. Understand that the color the test strip turns varies by individual—in some people the strip turns dark purple, in others it turns only pale pink. And in some people the strip never turns color. That doesn't necessarily mean you're not following the program correctly. Even if you're making and burning ketones, and therefore still burning fat, you might not be making enough ketones to "spill" over into your urine. Don't panic. As long as your blood sugar level, weight, and blood pressure are improving, and your appetite is under control, the presence of urinary ketones is irrelevant. And if you've reached the point of eating 50 grams or more of Net Carbs, you probably won't be spilling ketones anymore, even though you will probably still be losing weight. Again, this is perfectly normal.

DOES YOUR DOCTOR UNDERSTAND THE ABSCP?

We strongly suggest that you work closely with your doctor as you follow the Atkins Blood Sugar Control Program. To see if your physician understands the controlled-carb approach and is experienced in managing patients who decide to follow it, ask these questions as a basis for a dialogue:

1. What dietary approach do you usually recommend?
2. What experience do you have in following patients on a controlled-carb diet?
3. Have you worked with patients following the Atkins approach?
4. Do you use nutritional supplements for blood sugar, blood pressure, or lipid disorders?

Chapter 11

TAKE ACTION

You now have a good knowledge base about insulin/blood sugar problems, the metabolic syndrome, and diabetes. We've also explained how and why the Atkins Blood Sugar Control Program (ABSCP) can help you turn your health around. It's finally time to tell you how to put the plan into action—and get you on your way to a healthier life.

FIRST THINGS FIRST

As we said in the previous chapter, before you start the ABSCP, it's important to visit your doctor to assess your current state of health. In particular, you need to know if you have any special medical problems that will require monitoring and you need your baseline lab results.

Know Your Numbers

You'll be measuring your success *not so much by weight loss* as by improvements in your blood sugar, your blood pressure, and your blood lipids. When your goal is metabolic control, you use your lab values and body measurements, such as your waist-to-hip ratio, as a way to gauge results. When you visit your doctor for a complete checkup, he or she will order tests to reveal your baseline numbers. When you repeat the tests after following the ABSCP for even three months, you may be pleasantly surprised to find evidence of your metabolic improvement. (Note that once you are controlling carbohydrates, there is no need to repeat the GTT.) After six months, you're likely to be even happier. As you see from the chart that follows, routine blood chemistries and lipids are monitored fairly soon. These time frames are simply guidelines. Your physician will determine timing individualized to your situation. Dr. Atkins recommended the following tests, which may vary from those your physician usually recommends:

THE IMPORTANT TESTS					
LAB TEST	START (BASE-LINE)	4–6 WEEKS	3 MONTHS	EVERY 3 MONTHS UNTIL NORMAL	ANNUALLY IF NORMAL
GTT with insulin*	x				
Chemistries and lipids**		x	x	x	x
CV risk factors†		x			

* See page 63.   ** See page 71.   † See Chapter 9.

If these numbers begin to change for the worse or get stuck at undesirable levels, it will be a clear indication that you need to drop back to a lower level of carbohydrate intake.

GETTING WITH THE PROGRAM

The basic phases of the ABSCP parallel those of the Atkins Nutritional Approach (ANA), as you learned in Chapter 10. However, because your primary goal is normalizing insulin/blood sugar, the time you spend in each phase of the program, and when you decide to move on to the next phase, will be based on your lab values, not just on your weight loss.

It All Begins with Induction

Start by lowering your daily Net Carb intake to the Induction level of 20 grams a day, primarily in the form of vegetables. This will start to get your metabolism under control rapidly. Judge your progress at first by your blood sugar numbers. Once they normalize, continue at the 20-gram level until slow, steady weight loss begins. Many patients with diabetes stay at this level for weeks or even months—and a few even must stay at that level indefinitely. (Net Carbs are explained on page 128.)

Moving On to the Ongoing Weight-Loss Phase

One difference between the ANA and the ABSCP is that moving on to this phase should not occur until your metabolism is fairly well under control. Once it is, you can slowly start to add more carbs to your diet. If either your blood sugar or blood pressure rises or weight loss stops, you've gone too far, too fast. Your body wasn't yet ready to expand your carbohydrate budget.

Find Your ACE

When you are following the ANA, the Atkins Carbohydrate Equilibrium (ACE) is the number of grams of Net Carbs you can eat in one day and maintain your goal weight. However, if you've already developed the metabolic syndrome, prediabetes, or diabetes, your ACE number will also be the amount of carbohydrates that keeps your blood sugar at an acceptable level, improves your blood lipids, and keeps your blood pressure down. If you're overweight but have not yet demonstrated blood sugar problems, your Critical Carbohydrate Level for Losing (CCLL) will probably be higher (see Chapter 10) than it would be for someone who shows blood sugar dysfunction. This will also likely be the case with your ACE when you have achieved your goal weight.

How will you know what the right number is for you? Start by following the Induction phase described above. When your lab values have shown improvement, start adding carbs back into your daily diet in 5-gram increments. On the ANA, you can typically increase carbs week by week. On the ABSCP, however, you should proceed more slowly, adding in carbs as you observe the status of your weight, blood sugar (if possible), and blood pressure closely. You'll know you've passed your ACE if:

- You start to regain weight.
- Your fasting blood sugar goes up.
- Your blood pressure goes up.
- Your cravings or hunger increase.

If any of these signs of diminished metabolic control occur, cut back on your carb consumption until they improve. When they do, you've discovered your ACE. For some of you, that number will be only 20 grams a day; others may be able to go up as high as 40 or even 60 grams a day. As you continue to follow the program, lose weight, and taper off some of the prescription medications that may be slowing or preventing weight loss, you might be able to moderately raise your carb intake. But don't forget that if you're reading this book, you are very likely highly sensitive to the effects of carbohydrates in your diet. Because of that, your long-term ACE, even after you lose weight and normalize your blood sugar, may well remain at no more than 60 grams a day and possibly less.

Use the Atkins Glycemic Ranking (AGR)

If you have the metabolic syndrome, prediabetes, or Type 2 diabetes, you need to keep your carbohydrate intake at a level that keeps your blood sugar and blood lipids in a normal range. But quality counts as much as quantity when it comes to carbs. You need to choose your carbohydrates carefully and select those that will have the least impact on your blood sugar. You'll learn exactly what that means in Chapter 16, but in simple terms, use your carb grams on low-carb veggies and controlled portions of nuts. Most of you will also be able to enjoy some low-glycemic fruit; some of you will also be able to eat legumes, other vegetables, and occasional servings of whole grains.

To get an understanding of how the AGR is organized, we are including the fruit portion below. (Other portions begin on page 468.) When you are still in the earlier phases, you discover whether you can eat a fruit from column 1, such as strawberries, before attempting to introduce those in column 2. Likewise, fruits in column 2 are introduced before those in column 3. Even when you are maintaining your goal weight, you will still primarily choose from foods in column 1. Understand that the AGR is a general guideline, but you may find that you can eat certain foods in a column but not necessarily others. Also, some people are never able to move beyond foods in the first two columns or even in the first column.

1. EAT REGULARLY	2. EAT IN MODERATION	3. EAT SPARINGLY
Apple	Apricots, canned in juice	Banana
Blackberries	Apricots, dried	Cranberry cocktail,
Blueberries	Apricots, fresh	no added sugar
Cherries	Grapes, green and red	Cranberry juice, no
Cranberries	Grapefruit juice,	added sugar
Grapefruit	no added sugar	Fruit cocktail, canned
Orange	Kiwifruit	in juice
Peach	Mango	Grape juice
Pear	Melon, cantaloupe	Orange Juice
Plum	Melon, Crenshaw	Prunes
Pomegranate	Melon, honeydew	Raisins
Raspberries	Nectarine	
Strawberries	Papaya	
Tangerine	Pineapple, fresh	
	Watermelon	

Control Carbohydrate Portions

When you follow the ABSCP, you should feel hungry only as mealtime approaches because you're limiting your intake of carbohydrates. By restricting carbs and adding good fats, protein, and fiber to your diet, you feel satisfied without eating large portions. (You'll learn a lot more about these dietary components in later chapters.) When you eat this way, your food is absorbed slowly throughout the day, providing a steady stream of nutrition to your cells without blood sugar peaks and valleys. We promise you that once you understand the roles of all the dietary components for maintaining good health, you'll be able to follow the ABSCP without needing to feel hungry or deprived.

Although most of you don't have to count calories when you do Atkins, it is important to keep track of your carbohydrate grams. That means keeping track of your portions, because the carbs can add up fast and you may need always to limit your intake to 60 grams a day or less. (Remember, the more you exercise, the more liberal your program can be.) To help you understand how your carbohydrate portions fit into satisfying meals, we've included a month's worth of meal plans in Chapter 26.

Eat Regular Meals

Skipping meals or eating on an irregular schedule can cause your blood sugar to drop. These drops in blood sugar and the body's hormonal response create excess hunger and carbohydrate cravings, along with energy and mood swings that can disrupt your day and even cause weight gain.

To start, eat at least three meals and one snack, spaced evenly throughout the day. Each meal or snack should contain protein and fat. Always eat your carbohydrates as part of a meal or a snack that also includes protein or fat; eating carbs alone can result in a blood sugar spike. Because you will experience diminished hunger and enhanced satiety, be sure to eat as much at each meal as you need to feel comfortable but not stuffed. However, if you prefer, you can have five or six small low-carb, high-nutrient "feedings" throughout the day. With experience and a little experimentation, you'll find the eating schedule that works best for you. And once your blood sugar is more stable, you will likely feel less need for snacking.

No matter which meal schedule you choose, it's important to balance your nutrients over the course of the day. If you save up all your carbohydrates for just one meal, for instance, you'll get a big blood sugar spike. Instead, spread out your carbs—and everything else— over the day. You'll keep your blood sugar steadier and get better over- all nutrition. As long as you eat regularly, stick to your daily Net Carb limit, combine protein and fat in every snack or meal, and spread out your carbohydrates as evenly as you can over the day; it's okay to do whatever works best for you.

Eat the Right Foods

Many common foods have been shown to be particularly helpful for people with impaired glucose tolerance and diabetes. Not coinciden- tally, those foods are also low in carbohydrates and low on the Atkins Glycemic Ranking. Here are the top foods for you:

- Vegetables high in antioxidants and rich in vitamins, minerals, and fiber—such as broccoli, cauliflower, and other members of the cabbage family; and kale, collards, and other dark leafy greens, including salad greens.

SNACK STRATEGY

When you follow the ABSCP, between-meal snacks become an impor- tant part of your strategy for maintaining stable blood sugar. Instead of eating junk food such as doughnuts, however, you now snack the low- carb way. That means you eat a snack that contains protein and fat (a baked chicken leg or a piece of cheese, for example) and, for some of you, a small amount of carbohydrate (a handful of blueberries, say) along with some protein and/or fat. By substituting high-quality protein and fat for low-quality carbs, you satisfy between-meal hunger without sending your blood sugar off into a wild swing. By eating carbohydrates with protein and/or fat instead of alone, you slow the entry of glucose into your bloodstream. That helps keep your blood sugar, your energy, your appetite, and your mood on an even keel.

- Fish, particularly oily cold-water fish such as tuna, salmon, mackerel, and sardines.
- Foods high in calcium but low in carbs, such as cheese, tofu (bean curd), and dark leafy greens.
- High-fiber whole grains, such as barley, bulgur, and brown and wild rice. But remember, since one size doesn't fit all, some of you may not be able to include these higher-carb foods on a regular basis or even at all.

We'll explain in detail what makes these foods and others so valuable in later chapters.

Eat Healthy Fats

The low-fat message has been so persistent for so many decades that you may have trouble believing that eating *more* fat could actually help you control your blood sugar. Chapter 12 explains why dietary fat is not only good for you, it's essential. For now, let's just say that it's crucial to get a balance of healthy fats from eggs, cheese, meats, poultry, olive oil, flaxseed oil, peanut oil, nuts, avocados, and fatty cold-water fish like salmon, tuna, and sardines. The ABSCP automatically guides you toward foods that have a favorable fat balance.

Count Calories If Necessary

The basic principles of the ABSCP help the vast majority of people overcome the metabolic syndrome, prediabetes, and diabetes simply by controlling carbohydrate intake. For a small number of people, however, controlling carbs isn't quite enough. Their bodies are so resistant to insulin that they also have to cut back on total dietary intake to reverse their insulin resistance. The culprit could also be a prescription drug; many medications make it more difficult to lose weight, probably by increasing insulin resistance.

Caloric restriction needn't mean starvation or even going hungry, however. It does mean keeping carbohydrates to a minimum, reducing portions somewhat, and being aware of the calorie content of your foods. As a general rule of thumb, a woman who needs to restrict calories should cut back to between 1,200 and 1,800 calories a day, a man to between 1,500 and 2,000 calories.

An important note about restricting calories: There are 9 calories in a gram of fat and only 4 calories in a gram of carbohydrate or protein. This might lead you into the trap of thinking you should eat more low-fat foods and fewer high-fat foods. Don't do it. Your body needs those grams of fat and protein to keep your blood sugar stable and provide you with essential nutrients. It also needs them because they are what make you feel satisfied. If you cut the fat, you'll be cutting calories but virtually guaranteeing hunger and poor nutrition. What happens then? You experience cravings for carbohydrates—and if you give in to those cravings, your blood sugar and insulin levels will skyrocket.

If you must cut calories, do it the Atkins way. Continue to eat moderate amounts of good dietary fat and protein, but decrease your portion sizes, keep your carbohydrates down, and make sure that your primary source of carbs is fresh vegetables. Eat protein, fat, and fiber at every meal. Restricting portion size will speed weight loss and help improve insulin resistance. Once you have things under control, you may well be able to eat larger portions. We recommend the reduced-calorie option only when the natural appetite-control aspect of the ANA/ABSCP, in conjunction with exercise and supplements, does not produce the initial improvement needed in an individual case. Some patients are so far down the diabetes path that, at the start, they need every tool available to pull them back from the brink of metabolic disaster.

Get Moving

Exercise is so essential for controlling blood sugar and improving insulin resistance that it's not an option. It's mandatory. Following the dietary aspects of the program will do a lot to improve your health, but the addition of moderate daily exercise will improve your health a lot more—and a lot faster. It's also easy. To make a noticeable difference all it takes is a daily walk or some other moderate daily exercise for a minimum of just half an hour. Any exercise is better than none. No excuses. Even if you're very out of condition or have health problems that limit your activity, the information in Chapters 22 and 23 will help you incorporate exercise into your life in a safe and enjoyable way.

PRESCRIPTION DRUGS AND THE ABSCP

As you reduce your carb intake, your need for insulin (if you take it) and other prescription medications will almost certainly decrease or even vanish. You may be able to work with your doctor to decrease your medications gradually as you control your carb intake and thus take back control of your metabolism. When you have reduced or eliminated medications (especially the ones for blood sugar control) and your fasting blood sugar levels have stabilized in the normal range (below 100 mg/dL), you can experiment a bit with your ACE. You may be able to eat a few more carbs without gaining weight or making your blood sugar go up.

If you take any drugs—prescription or over-the-counter—discuss your decision to follow the controlled-carb approach with your doctor before you start. Work with him or her to monitor your condition regularly and lower your doses in a systematic way that will avoid sudden changes and possible over- or undermedication.

We hope we've convinced you that the ABSCP will help you restore your own health by solving underlying metabolic imbalances. The program requires a permanent change in the way you eat and the amount of exercise you get. Is that difficult? Thousands of Dr. Atkins' patients say just the opposite. Once they were under way on the program, they felt so much better that making the long-term commitment to the Atkins approach was a very easy choice. It will be for you too.

TRACK YOUR PROGRESS

Before you start following the Atkins Blood Sugar Control Program, visit your doctor for the tests listed below. (Refer to Chapters 6, 8, and 9 for explanations of these tests and what they mean.)

Record your starting numbers and then track the changes as you repeat the tests over the next year. We've suggested intervals, but items such as blood pressure and waist-to-hip ratio and lipids can be monitored more frequently.

STARTING VALUES	3 MONTHS	6 MONTHS	1 YEAR
Weight	_____	_____	_____
BMI	_____	_____	_____
Waist-to-hip ratio	_____	_____	_____
Fasting blood sugar	_____	_____	_____
A1C	_____	_____	_____
Blood pressure	_____	_____	_____
Total cholesterol	_____	_____	_____
LDL cholesterol	_____	_____	_____
HDL cholesterol	_____	_____	_____
Triglycerides	_____	_____	_____
Lipoprotein(a)	_____	_____	_____
C-reactive protein	_____	_____	_____
Homocysteine	_____	_____	_____
Fibrinogen	_____	_____	_____

A LUCKY HOSTESS

Glenda Carter used to be the pharmaceutical industry's dream, taking prescription drugs for diabetes, high cholesterol, high blood pressure, and arthritis. But a fortuitous reservation at her bed-and-breakfast helped her become medication-free and 56 pounds slimmer.

I've had a perennial weight problem since I was 13 years old. Over the years, I have probably lost a cumulative 1,000 pounds and gained back 1,000 pounds. By the time I was 37, I was already hav-

NAME: Glenda Carter

AGE: 53

HEIGHT: 5 feet 3 inches

WEIGHT BEFORE: 245 pounds

WEIGHT NOW: 189 pounds

BLOOD PRESSURE BEFORE: 165/110

BLOOD PRESSURE AFTER: 100/60

TOTAL CHOLESTEROL BEFORE: 220

TOTAL CHOLESTEROL AFTER: 144

HDL BEFORE: 48

HDL AFTER: 52

LDL BEFORE: 137

LDL AFTER: 113

TRIGLYCERIDES BEFORE: 313

TRIGLYCERIDES AFTER: 128

ing troubles with my blood pressure. And at 44, I was diagnosed as a diabetic. My doctor put me on a low-fat diet, and I really did stick to it most of the time, but I didn't lose any weight. I used to feel shame when I went in for an office visit because I thought they believed I was cheating on their diet and lying about it. I began to go in for appointments only to get my prescriptions refilled. I was taking insulin for diabetes, Cozzar and Lozol for high blood pressure, Lipitor for cholesterol, Vioxx for arthritis. My drugs cost between $600 and $700 per month. As a former nurse and mental health therapist, I can tell you I was not a happy camper.

Everything changed for me in August 2003. My husband, Bob, and I run a bed-and-breakfast near Jasper, Alberta, in the Canadian Rockies. A lady from Virginia called to make a reservation with us. I asked, as I routinely do, if she had any dietary restrictions. She said she followed the Atkins program. I had heard about Atkins in the seventies and even tried it for a while, but found it too restrictive. She talked my ear off and told me that she was absolutely sure it would work for me.

The very next day, my husband and I went on the program together using Dr. Atkins' New Diet Revolution *and the Internet for guidance. We vowed that we would do the program correctly without breaking any*

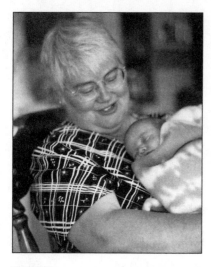

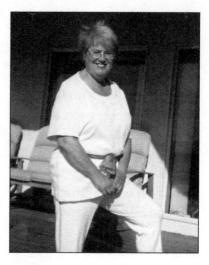

BEFORE   **AFTER**

rules. Within 32 hours, I had to stop taking my insulin. My blood sugar had dropped to 48. I just couldn't believe it. My doctor was away for three weeks. When she returned I went to see her. She was happily stunned by my improved numbers but was very wary. "Glenda, this is going to wreck your kidneys." She agreed to support me in continuing the program if I would have the following tests every four weeks: A1C, lipids, ALT, AST (both routine liver chemistries), creatinine for kidneys, fasting glucose, and potassium. After four months of great results, she no longer needed any proof. Now, she is a believer.

Bob and I both keep our carb level at a maximum of 20 to 30 grams per day. I have never felt so good in my life and I am taking no medications whatsoever. I don't miss the bread or pasta at all. For breakfast twice a week, I have eggs and sausage; the other days, I'll have homemade flaxseed muffins or flaxseed porridge with strawberries, whipped cream, and cinnamon. Lunch might be canned salmon salad made with mayonnaise, onion, and celery rolled in lettuce leaves. If Bob and I are working outdoors, we sometimes have a "party tray," formerly forbidden things like sliced pork sausage, olives, cheese, and dips with veggies. A typical dinner might be baked chicken legs and a spinach salad with avocado and goat cheese. You need to think outside the box for variety. I've discovered a recipe for faux mashed potatoes using puréed cauliflower, cream cheese, and sour cream. The beauty of being a diabetic is that because I test my blood sugar every day I can try adding new things to my food plan and see how my levels are affected. For instance, butternut squash was too high in carbs for me, but spaghetti squash worked just fine. I stuff it with meat sauce, top it with Cheddar, and bake it. It's just delicious.

Two months after I started Atkins, I bought a Bow-Flex machine and started using it. I also continued curling—it's like shuffleboard on ice— three times per week in the winter. I used to need a two-hour nap every day. Now when I want to take a break, I read instead because I have so much energy. The arthritis is gone from my spine, knees, hands, and feet. Only two fingers are still gnarled and I am confident they will improve, too.

In December, four months after we'd started the program, I had to shop for a dress for a Christmas party. I went to the big-ladies store where I've shopped for 25 years. I had worn a size 44, or a 3X or 4X. Everything I tried on that day hung on me. "Glenda, you can shop at a regular store," I said to myself, amazed, and didn't even know where to go. In a department store, I bought a size 16 glittery silver-and-black dress and bought new bras for the first time that didn't look like horse halters! By the end of six months, I had lost 56 pounds. Bob, who is six feet two inches, went from 275 pounds to 220 pounds in the same time period. His waist measurement dropped from 44 to 36 inches, and he wants to reach his goal of 190 pounds.

I've started an Atkins section on a bulletin board for B&B owners across Canada. Fifteen have joined it and many are diabetic. My doctor even suggested that I start an Atkins group. Hinton is a small town, population around 10,000, yet 16 people signed up in less than 24 hours. When I walked into a restaurant recently, one of the waiters said, "Hi, Mrs. Low Carb," so I know word is getting around. I would like to lose about 30 more pounds to reach a very achievable goal of 160. Rather than focus on a timetable, I rejoice that I am medicine free, eating nutrient-rich foods, and looking better than ever before in my whole adult life. Doing Atkins helped my body heal itself.

Note: Your individual results may vary from those reported here. As stated previously, Atkins recommends initial laboratory evaluation and subsequent follow-up in conjunction with your health care provider.

Chapter 12

THE IMPORTANCE OF GOOD FATS

Dietary fat is one of the most important tools you have for controlling your insulin and blood sugar. That might seem impossible, given the simplistic antifat message that has been relentlessly hammered into our collective consciousness for so long. The reality is that most fats—in fact, all natural fats—are fine when carb intake is controlled. In fact, natural fats are absolutely necessary for good health, and are actually helpful for preventing and treating diabetes.

CHEMISTRY 101: DIETARY FATS

Fats are oily, organic compounds that don't dissolve in water—think of the way oil floats on top of water—but do dissolve in other oils. Fatty acids (the chemist's way of describing fats) are long chains of carbon and hydrogen atoms with some oxygen atoms stuck on at one end. (Technically speaking, it's the oxygen at the end that makes the molecule an acid.) How many hydrogen atoms the chain contains, and where those atoms are located on the chain, determines what sort of fat it is.

The natural fats we regularly eat fall into three basic categories:

- *Saturated fats.* Almost all of these fats are solid at room temperature; butter, lard, and suet are good examples. They are solid because the carbon-and-hydrogen chain contains as many atoms as it possibly can. This is why it's called "saturated." Although we tend to think of saturated fats as animal fats, a few vegetable oils, such as coconut oil and palm oil, are also highly saturated. Unlike saturated animal fats, they stay liquid at room temperature.
- *Monounsaturated fats (MUFA).* Liquid at room temperature, monounsaturated fats include olive oil and the oils found in nuts and seeds; avocados also contain monounsaturated fat. These fats are monounsaturated because a single carbon atom somewhere in the chain has a double bond, meaning that the chain is missing a hydrogen atom.
- *Polyunsaturated fats (PUFA).* Polyunsaturated fats are also liquid at room temperature. Canola oil and safflower oil are polyunsaturated fats, as is flaxseed oil. The oil found in fatty fish is also polyunsaturated. These fats are polyunsaturated because more than one carbon atom along the chain has a double bond, so more hydrogen atoms are missing. The number of double bonds and where they are in the chain determines the type of polyunsaturated fat.

THE ESSENTIALS

Just as your body absolutely must have vitamins every day, and just as you can get those vitamins only from food or from supplements, your body also needs certain dietary fats. These essential fatty acids, as nutritionists call them, are basically two types of polyunsaturated fats: omega-3 fatty acids (also called alpha linolenic acids or n-3 fatty acids) and omega-6 fatty acids (also called gamma linoleic acids or n-6 fatty acids). These fatty acids support a range of crucial bodily functions. You need them to make cell membranes, to make the oxygen-transporting hemoglobin in your red blood cells, and to make eicosanoids and prostaglandins—natural chemicals that play a crucial role in regulating many body functions such as inflammation.

Omega-3 fatty acids are found in eggs, fish, vegetable oils, nuts and seeds, and dark green leafy vegetables. The main dietary sources of omega-6 fatty acids are vegetable oils, such as soybean oil, canola oil, and safflower oil. In the modern diet, the balance of these fats is sadly off-kilter. Because omega-6 fatty acids are found in the cheap, highly processed vegetable oils that are used in so many prepared and processed foods, the average American now eats about 16 times as much omega-6 fatty acids as omega-3s, instead of a more natural ratio of about one to one.[1] When you get rid of the processed, high-carb foods in your diet, you shift your intake of essential fatty acids away from these lopsided proportions and back toward a more desirable ratio. To be on the safe side, consider taking a balanced essential fatty acid supplement. (For more on essential fatty acid supplements, see Chapter 20.)

Omega-9 fatty acids aren't essential, but we recommend getting plenty of them in your diet. Good dietary sources of omega-9s are extra-virgin olive oil, sesame oil, peanuts, all tree nuts, and avocados. There are also some omega-9 fatty acids in poultry and pork.

A QUICK COURSE IN CHOLESTEROL

We've talked a lot about cholesterol already, and we'll be talking about it even more in the chapters that follow. It's time to get down to some details about this controversial yet vital substance.

- Cholesterol is a waxy chemical compound manufactured by your body—it's not really a fat at all, and your body doesn't burn it for energy as it does with fats.
- Cholesterol is essential for a wide variety of crucial functions, including manufacturing the hormones testosterone, estrogen, and progesterone, making cell walls and brain tissue, and producing vitamin D in your body.
- Your body manufactures most of its own cholesterol. However, a

small amount comes from the cholesterol you digest, found in animal foods like meat, dairy products, and egg yolks.

- Your body makes cholesterol as it needs it, mostly in your liver, at the rate of about 800 mg to 1,500 mg a day. The average American also eats about 300 mg to 450 mg or more of cholesterol daily, but of that amount, no more than half—and perhaps only as little as 10 percent—is actually absorbed by your body.

To move waxy cholesterol through your watery bloodstream, your body turns it into lipoproteins—complexes of cholesterol and protein. There are several kinds of lipoproteins, but the two most important are low-density lipoprotein, or LDL cholesterol, and high-density lipoprotein, or HDL cholesterol. Just to remind you, LDL cholesterol carries fat and cholesterol *from* your liver, where most of your cholesterol is manufactured, to the parts of your body that need it. HDL cholesterol carries unused cholesterol *back* to your liver, where about half of it then gets recycled again into LDL cholesterol; some is excreted in the bile acids used in digestion, and some is recycled for other purposes. While it is true that high levels of LDL cholesterol can be bad, and that low levels of HDL are also undesirable, the story is a lot more complex: See Chapter 9, The Cardiac Connection.

CHOLESTEROL BY THE NUMBERS

According to the latest recommendations from the National Cholesterol Education Program (NCEP III), here's what your blood lipids should be:

- Total cholesterol (HDL and LDL combined): less than 200 mg/dL
- LDL cholesterol: less than 100 to 130 mg/dL
- HDL cholesterol: 40 mg/dL or more for a man; 50 mg/dL or more for a woman
- Triglycerides: less than 150 mg/dL

GOOD FATS AND BAD FATS

If you have a rudimentary understanding of fats, you've probably picked up the standard take on the subject. That is, saturated fat is bad and mono- and polyunsaturated fats are good. That popular oversimplification is very misleading. For one thing, all naturally occurring fats are actually mixtures of different kinds of fatty acids. The fat found in beef, for instance, contains a mixture of saturated and mono-unsaturated fats—in fact, there's actually more *unsaturated* fat (whether from monos or polys) in beef than saturated. Beef fat is solid at room temperature, however, so it's misleadingly lumped into the saturated fat category.

The standard dietary advice comes down especially hard on saturated fats. That's because a diet high in saturated fats and cholesterol from animal foods is often linked with heart disease. But that link is tenuous at best. The much-touted connection between saturated fat and cholesterol in the diet and high cholesterol levels and heart disease is a lot less solid than you might think. Respected science writer Gary Taubes pointed this out in a watershed article published in the *New York Times Magazine* in July 2002, entitled "What If It's All Been a Big Fat Lie?" One significant problem with most studies that claim saturated fat raises cholesterol levels is that they don't take into account carbohydrate consumption. Saturated fat can indeed raise blood cholesterol—when it's eaten in the context of a high-carb diet.[2,3] To date, in studies looking at the Atkins protocol, saturated fat had little impact on cholesterol levels.

In these same studies, dietary fat had little or no effect on raising blood lipids. You should eat a balance of fats; fortunately, Mother Nature makes that easy for you. You may not know, for example, that in a 3½-ounce pork chop containing 22 grams of fat, only 8 grams are saturated. Another 10 grams are monounsaturated fat and the rest are polyunsaturated fat. You don't have to worry about achieving a good balance of fats if you simply eat a variety of protein foods and also consume olive oil, olives, avocados, and nuts.

Nor is there any real reason to restrict saturated fat when you're following the Atkins Blood Sugar Control Program properly. There's very little evidence to show that eating saturated fat in balance with other natural fats is harmful to your health. In fact, some studies show that even when carbs are not controlled, a moderate amount of saturated fat can raise LDL cholesterol, but it is compensated for with an increase in HDL cholesterol.[4] And recently, researchers reported to their surprise that eating a diet high in total fat or high in any particular type of fat (including saturated fat) has little or no effect on the risk of stroke.[5]

If you've been diagnosed with the metabolic syndrome, prediabetes, or diabetes, your lipid levels and insulin/blood sugar levels aren't what they should be. But avoiding foods containing cholesterol and saturated fat isn't the answer—in fact, avoiding protein-rich, fat-rich foods in favor of carbohydrates could well make your health problems worse. What will help get your blood sugar under control

RESEARCH REPORT: FATS AND DIABETES

Fat in the diet has long been blamed as a cause of diabetes. When researchers look more carefully, however, they find that the evidence actually points in the opposite direction. Dietary fat does *not* increase your risk of diabetes, and adding *certain fats* to your diet might actually help prevent diabetes. To take one example, researchers who were looking at data from the long-running Nurses' Health Study found, after following over 84,000 women for 14 years, that total fat intake wasn't associated with an increased risk of Type 2 diabetes. They also found that the level of saturated and monounsaturated fat consumption wasn't associated with a significantly higher risk of diabetes. What they did find was that higher intakes of polyunsaturated fat were associated with a *lower* risk of diabetes. In fact, all it took to reduce these women's risk of diabetes by 35 percent was getting just 5 percent more of their daily calories from polyunsaturated fats. In other words, women who got more fat from sources such as fish and vegetable oils had a lower risk of diabetes. This same study also provides another reason to avoid added trans fats. The incidence of Type 2 diabetes could be reduced by at least 40 percent if oils were consumed only in their original unhydrogenated form.[6]

and improve your blood lipids is *balancing* dietary fat in conjunction with the ABSCP.

HELP FROM THE GOOD FATS

The protective effect of dietary fat was shown in a landmark study back in 1987. Researchers compared the effects on healthy men and women of a diet high in monounsaturated fat from olive oil with those of a diet low in dietary fat and high in carbohydrates. Both diets lowered LDL cholesterol, but the low-fat/high-carb diet had the undesirable effect of both lowering HDL cholesterol and sharply increasing triglycerides.[7]

If you have the metabolic syndrome, prediabetes, or diabetes, you probably have low HDL and high triglycerides along with LDL that is normal or slightly on the high side. It's pretty clear that eating a low-fat, high-carb diet won't do much to help your blood lipids. That diet is more likely to make things worse—including your blood sugar.

PROCESSED VS. UNREFINED OILS

To prolong their shelf life and allow for heating at higher temperatures, most of the oils found in supermarkets have been heavily processed. It is best to avoid them. Instead, look for cold-pressed vegetable or nut oils, which have not been exposed to heat or treated with chemicals. Cold-pressed oils are preferable because they retain more nutrients and flavor. Expeller-pressed oils have been exposed to heat, but retain more of their flavor than refined oils do. To keep unrefined oils fresh, buy in small quantities, refrigerate after opening, and store in opaque containers. Fats become rancid when exposed to too much heat or light, are reused, or are kept too long. Eating rancid fats can increase the risk of heart disease.

GO NUTS!

Nuts are the ideal snack food when you're following the ABSCP. These delicious, crunchy morsels are crammed with unsaturated fats—in fact, up to 80 percent of the calories in nuts can come from the fat (see the chart below). They're fairly low in carbs, and because they're also high in fiber, they are low in Net Carbs. Their glycemic load is low too; on the AGR (Atkins Glycemic Ranking), most nuts are in the "eat regularly" column. (So are delicious oily seeds, such as sunflower seeds and pumpkin seeds; coconut also falls into this category.) The fiber in nuts helps slow the entry of the carbohydrates into your bloodstream, acting as a sort of time-release mechanism that delivers the carbs in a slow, steady way. Nuts also contain good amounts of trace minerals such as magnesium and selenium that may be helpful for people with, or at risk for, diabetes.

THE FAT IN NUTS

Nut	Total Fat (grams)	Saturated (grams)	MUFA (grams)	PUFA (grams)
Almond	14.5	1	10	3
Brazil	19	5	7	7
Cashew	13	2	3	8
Hazelnut	18	1	15	2
Macadamia	20	2.5	15	2.5
Peanut	14	2	7	5
Pecan	19	2	12	5
Pistachio	14	2	8	4
Walnut	18	2	5	11

Note: Amounts are for a 1-ounce serving.
Source: USDA.

EATING YOUR OMEGAS

A valuable source of dietary polyunsaturated fats is omega-3 fatty acids. You can get omega-3s from fish and from dietary supplements made from fish or algae. Many studies have shown that fish oil can dramatically help reduce the risk of heart disease.[8] The effect of these oils is so powerful that in 2002, the American Heart Association summarized research and recommended that healthy people include omega-3 fatty acids from fish and plant sources to protect their hearts.[9–11]

For those with diabetes, the value of fish also comes from the omega-3 fatty acids it contains. Omega-3s can raise HDL cholesterol slightly, have little or no effect on LDL cholesterol, and can significantly help to lower triglycerides. In fact, a meta-analysis in 1998 of 26 different studies showed that fish oil supplements, which are nothing but omega-3 fatty acids, lower triglycerides by almost 30 percent.[12] Omega-3 supplements also help in decreasing inflammatory responses which, as you know, is beneficial in the treatment of cardiovascular disease, diabetes, and the metabolic syndrome.[13]

Eating cold-water fatty fish, such as tuna, salmon, mackerel, anchovies, sardines, herring, or eel, is one way to get the benefits of omega-3 fatty acids, as is taking fish oil supplements—and we know it works because most of the studies are based on people consuming fish

SUPPLEMENTAL OILS AND BLOOD SUGAR

A few studies of omega-3 fatty acids have suggested that taking them in supplement form could raise blood sugar; a few other studies have suggested that omega-3 supplements actually improve insulin sensitivity. To find out for sure, in 1995, researchers conducted a randomized, double-blind, placebo-controlled trial using 4 grams of fish oil a day for some diabetic patients and 4 grams of corn oil for others. After 16 weeks, the fish oil had no effect on the blood sugar of the people who took it. It did, however, slightly lower their blood pressure; it also modestly lowered their triglycerides.[14]

or fish oil (not to be confused with cod liver oil). Recent tests of fish oil supplements show a lower level of mercury in the supplements than is found in the amount of fish needed to obtain an equal amount of the oil.[15] There are also plant sources of omega-3s. If you are concerned about fish as a source of environmental pollutants and/or declining supplies, you can get omega-3s from plant sources such as algae and flaxseed oil. Like fish oil, flaxseed oil and other plant sources can help control blood lipids and prevent heart attacks.[16, 17]

THE BAD FAT

Now we have to talk about manufactured trans fats—the type you should avoid whenever possible. To understand why, you'll need to know a bit more about this widely used fat.

Trans fats start out as an inexpensive polyunsaturated vegetable oils, such as corn oil. The oil is then processed to force more hydrogen atoms back into the fatty acid chains. This partial hydrogenation makes the oil thicker, less likely to go rancid, and better able to withstand high temperatures. Trans fats are also inexpensive, so they're very widely used in baked goods, in snack foods, for deep-frying, and in margarine.

The problem with overexposure to trans fats is that they can have a very dangerous effect on your blood lipids. Trans fats raise your LDL cholesterol and triglycerides, lower your HDL cholesterol, and may contribute directly to developing heart disease. A pioneering study published in 1994 showed that, overall, the people who eat the most trans fats also have the greatest risk of having a heart attack.[18, 19]

Of course, someone who eats a lot of manufactured trans fats is probably also eating a lot of low-quality carbohydrates in the form of highly processed cookies, cakes, breads, crackers, and snack foods. The latest summaries of this research indicate that the quality rather than the quantity of fat is what affects cardiovascular disease risk.[20]

By eliminating worthless high-carb foods from your diet, as you do when you follow the ABSCP, you automatically also eliminate most of the manufactured trans fats. Bear in mind, however, that these trans fats are also used in most margarines, in peanut butters, and in solid

COOKING WITH FATS

When you sauté foods or use a deep-fryer, high heat can convert a small amount of oil into trans fats. The amount is so small that it's not really a problem. To avoid accumulating trans fats in the cooking oil, however, don't reuse it, as is done in the deep-fryers found in many fast-food restaurants.

shortenings. We strongly recommend replacing these artificial fats with real butter, fresh unprocessed nut butters, and high-quality vegetable oils. (See Processed vs. Unrefined Oils, page 160.)

PUTTING FATS TO WORK

By now it should be pretty clear why good fats, meaning natural and unrefined, are such an important part of the ABSCP. The best part about adding the good fats is that it's very simple to do. Substituting extra virgin olive oil for the refined vegetable oil you might be using in salads now is not only easy, it'll make your food taste better. To get more nuts into your diet, have a handful as a snack now and then; spread a spoonful of sugar-free, nonhydrogenated peanut butter onto a piece of celery; sprinkle some slivered almonds onto green beans; or toss some walnuts in with sautéed vegetables (see Chapters 26 and 27 for more ideas). Get more omega-3s into your diet by eating canned salmon once a week at lunch, by making fish for dinner once a week, and by taking supplemental oils. Such changes are simple, but the effects on your health are profound. And as you'll learn in the next chapter, combining those good fats with protein sources is one of the best things you can do for your health.

FIND THE FAT

To test your understanding of the sources of different types of fat, answer these questions.

1. Dark green leafy vegetables contain
   polyunsaturated fat.   True ❏   False ❏
2. Which food *isn't* a good source of monounsaturated fats?
   a. olive oil
   b. salmon
   c. corn oil
   d. avocado
3. How much of the fat in a typical piece of steak is saturated?
   a. all of it
   b. almost all of it
   c. less than half
4. Cholesterol is found mostly in
   animal foods.   True ❏   False ❏
5. Essential fatty acids are found in:
   a. fish
   b. eggs
   c. nuts
   d. olive oil
   e. all of the above

Answers
1. True. 2. c. 3. c. 4. True. 5. e.

Chapter 13

THE IMPORTANCE OF PROTEIN

Protein is the main building block for every part of your body—and it's also the mainstay of the Atkins Nutritional Approach (ANA) and the Atkins Blood Sugar Control Program (ABSCP). Protein plays a vital role in stabilizing your insulin and blood sugar, making it easier to lose weight.

PROTEIN FACTS

Most of your body is made up of protein—even your bones and teeth are approximately half protein. Proteins are made up of long, very complex, intricately folded and coiled chains of some 20 different amino acids. Amino acids are small molecules made from atoms of nitrogen, oxygen, hydrogen, carbon, and sometimes sulfur. The amino acids fall into two groups: essential and nonessential.

Essential amino acids are the ones you have to get every day from your meals to maintain good health, just as you need vitamins and essential fatty acids. Nonessential amino acids can come from the food you eat, but your body also synthesizes them from essential amino acids.

You need all those amino acids from protein in order to build new cells and maintain and repair your body. Every single day, for instance, your body needs to make millions of new red blood cells to replace the ones that wear out. Without protein, it could not do so. You also need protein to make the many thousands of different enzymes, hormones, and other chemical messengers that make your body function properly. In fact, insulin is a protein—an intricate chain made of 51 assorted amino acids.

WHAT ARE AMINO ACIDS?

Just as you can make any word in the English language from some combination of 26 letters, your body can manufacture any of the many thousands of proteins it needs by combining the 20 or so different amino acids.

The essential amino acids are:

Histidine
Isoleucine
Leucine
Lysine
Methionine
Phenylalanine
Threonine
Tryptophan
Valine

The nonessential amino acids are:

Alanine
Arginine (essential for babies)
Asparagine
Aspartic acid
Cysteine (conditionally essential—in some circumstances you
may need this from your diet)
Glutamic acid
Glutamine
Glycine

Proline

Serine

Taurine (essential for babies)

Tyrosine (conditionally essential—in some circumstances you may need this from your diet)

To make your body's tissues, hormones, and other substances, your cells follow instructions from your DNA and assemble the various amino acids into different proteins. The protein chains can be as short as just two different amino acid molecules (peptides) or so complex that they contain thousands of various amino acid molecules. When exactly the right amino acids are linked together in exactly the right sequence, they coil and fold into the exact shape of that particular protein. The newly formed protein fits, just like a key into a lock, into specialized receptors in your cells—or links up with other proteins to carry out its highly specific job in your body. And when that job is done, other proteins come along and break down the "old" protein so that the amino acids can be reused. Not all the amino acids can be recycled; some are even burned for energy, which is why you need a daily supply of the essential ones.

HOW MUCH PROTEIN DO YOU NEED?

Although there's a formula to calculate the minimum amount of protein necessary for the standard low-fat, high-carb diet, the amount of protein you need to control your insulin and blood sugar and manage your weight on the ABSCP can't be calculated by a set formula. Instead, we simply—and strongly—recommend that you eat liberally of delicious high-protein foods such as poultry, fish, beef, pork, and eggs. Eat enough at each meal or snack to feel satisfied but not stuffed. Your body will tell you when you've had enough, because you'll feel satiated. You might be surprised at how quickly you feel full after eating a high-protein meal. That's because protein helps maintain blood glucose levels within the range for optimum body function. Without the dramatic highs and lows, you'll feel more energetic and less hungry.

In the end, the amount of protein you eat when you follow the

ABSCP may not be that much higher than the amount you ate before you started the program. When the dietary intake of individuals following the ANA has been studied, generally 30 to 35 percent of their calorie intake is protein. Plus, there's a very positive catch-22 here. Because you allow yourself to eat liberally of the protein foods, and protein is both very satiating and helps control the insulin/blood sugar swings that drive excess hunger, you may end up feeling too full to eat all that much of it! In fact, studies have shown that individuals who reduce their carbohydrate intake actually wind up consuming fewer calories—because they are more quickly satisfied.

PROTEIN SOURCES

The quality of the protein you eat is as important as the quantity. The ideal protein is complete—meaning it contains reasonable amounts of all nine essential amino acids. Meat, poultry, fish, eggs, dairy products, and other animal foods are complete proteins, but grains and legumes are not. Some plant foods contain all nine essential amino acids, but in most of them the quantity of at least one amino acid is very low. For this reason, most plant foods by themselves can't provide adequate amounts of all of the essential amino acids to meet our protein requirements. Grains, for instance, are generally low in lysine, and beans are low in the sulfur-containing amino acids methionine and cysteine. But people who don't eat any animal foods can still get enough of the nine essential amino acids by carefully combining different plant foods such as nuts, seeds, legumes, and whole grains. The problem for someone with an imbalanced insulin/blood sugar metabolism is that the foods full of plant proteins typically also contain lots of carbs.

Not all of your protein sources are created equal when it comes to the ABSCP, however. Meats, poultry, fish, and eggs are fair game—they're pretty much pure protein. Cheese is another good source of low-carb protein. An ounce of Swiss cheese, for instance, contains about 9 grams of protein and only 1 gram of Net Carbs. Watch out for the carbohydrates in milk and yogurt, though. A cup of whole milk or full-fat plain yogurt has 8 grams of protein, but it also contains 11 grams of Net Carbs. If you'd like to get some of your protein from milk or yogurt, try the new reduced-carb "dairy beverage" products and yogurts. The dairy beverage has extra protein and fewer carbs; 8 ounces contain 12 grams of protein and only 3 grams of Net Carbs.

EAT YOUR EGGS

Eggs are such a good source of complete protein that they're the standard against which all other proteins are compared. Because one large egg contains about 213 mg of cholesterol, however, some doctors recommend limiting or avoiding eggs, thinking they raise blood cholesterol levels. That's actually true—but the cholesterol that goes up is your good HDL cholesterol.

In a 1994 study, 24 adults who added two eggs to their daily diet for six weeks showed a 10 percent increase in their HDL levels, while their total cholesterol went up only 4 percent. The change in the ratio of total cholesterol to the HDL was not statistically significant.[1]

Two other studies published since 1999 have found that eggs aren't the issue. In both of these studies, people were fed eggs and their blood was examined. One author of the study stated that the dietary management of obesity and insulin resistance should emphasize calorie restriction rather than the restriction of fat in the diet.[2] In the second study done on healthy, postmenopausal women, Dr. G. M. Reaven stated that large amounts of cholesterol in the diet had little effect on the total or LDL cholesterol level. These results were true regardless of insulin resistance or insulin sensitivity.[3]

Unfortunately, many people have been brainwashed into thinking eggs are dangerous because they contain cholesterol. James R. came to Dr. Atkins for treatment of high blood lipids. Dr. Atkins stopped James's statin drug, put him on the Atkins controlled-carb program, and assured him he could eat eggs if he wished. James followed the program but just couldn't bring himself to believe that eggs were safe. He finally had two scrambled eggs for breakfast one morning—and spent the next ten minutes sitting white-knuckled at his kitchen table, convinced he was about to have a heart attack! He didn't, of course, and when he came in for his next checkup his blood lipids were better than they had been when he was taking the drug and avoiding eggs.

The nutritional advantages of eggs for people with diabetes are substantial. Eggs have a very low glycemic index ranking and are a good source not just of high-quality protein, but also of vitamins B, D, and E and the minerals calcium, zinc, iron, potassium, and magnesium. Egg yolks get their yellow color from the carotenoids lutein and zeaxanthin, which can help protect your eyes from the sight-robbing condition called age-related macular degeneration.

PROTEIN AND YOUR BLOOD SUGAR

We've mentioned the satiety and appetite control benefits of protein, but the advantages of swapping protein for low-quality carbs go far beyond that. Consuming protein is the signal to your body to build muscle.[4] This is obviously preferable to consuming an overabundance of refined carbs, which signals your body to store fat!

Adequate amounts of protein also help get your blood sugar under control. This was shown in a recent study that looked at the effect of a higher-protein diet on blood sugar in people with Type 2 diabetes. In this study, for five weeks 12 people with Type 2 diabetes ate a diet with 30 percent of calories from protein, 40 percent from carbs, and 30 percent from fat. They then switched for another five weeks to the standard diet recommended by the American Diabetes Association (15 percent of calories from protein, 55 percent from carbs, and 30 percent from fat). What happened? You've probably already guessed. When the patients were eating the higher-protein diet, their triglycerides were lower, their blood sugar was significantly lower, and their glycated hemoglobin (A1C) number dropped. In fact, on the higher-protein diet, the A1C went down by 0.8 percent, a significant improvement; it dropped by only 0.3 percent on the standard diabetic diet.[5]

Note that the participants ate much higher levels of carbohydrates than Dr. Atkins would have recommended for a diabetic patient. His patients typically showed a much larger drop in the A1C, a measure of blood sugar control, when they restricted carbs by following the

ABSCP. This would strongly suggest that the improvements for the patients in the study, good as they were, could have been much more dramatic had the carbohydrate amounts been lower.

Other studies have shown the benefit of protein in improving blood sugar metabolism. In one study of overweight women, 12 of the women followed a moderate-protein, reduced-carb (40 percent of calories from carbs) diet for ten weeks. Another 12 women followed the typical American diet, with less protein and 55 percent of calories coming from carbohydrates. At the end of the ten weeks, the women on the higher-protein diet had better results on both the oral glucose tolerance test and the test for fasting blood sugar. Compared with the high-carb dieters, the higher-protein dieters had much more stable blood sugar. Their blood sugar stability continued to improve over the length of the study, while the high-carb dieters experienced more blood sugar swings. And the higher-protein dieters lost more weight![6]

These women were not yet diabetic. Their improvement came from decreasing carbohydrates and increasing protein. Yet neither of these studies decreased the carbohydrates enough to show the results Dr. Atkins experienced in decades of caring for patients.[7]

IS TOO MUCH PROTEIN DANGEROUS?

For people with normal kidney function there's no evidence that the amount of protein consumed when following the guidelines of the ABSCP is harmful. In fact, there's some very important evidence to show that eating more protein, especially if it replaces carbohydrates in your diet, is good for you. To take one good example, let's look at a 1999 study that examined the diets of more than 80,000 women taking part in the Nurses' Health Study. The researchers were interested in the association between protein intake and the risk of heart attack. When they compared the women who ate the most protein with the women who ate the least protein, they found that the group with the highest protein intake had the smallest number of heart attacks. The women who ate the most protein—whether their overall diet was high-fat or low-fat—cut their risk of a heart attack by about 25 percent compared with the women who ate the least protein.[8]

In the large International Study of Salt and Blood Pressure (INTERSALT), which looked at dietary factors affecting blood pressure among 10,000 people worldwide, the researchers found something similar. The people with the highest protein intake had lower blood pressure than those with the lowest protein intake. This study confirmed what earlier studies had also shown.[9]

These studies don't mean, of course, that eating more protein will keep you from having a heart attack or getting high blood pressure, but they do suggest that getting ample amounts of protein could help prevent these problems—and that limiting your protein intake doesn't help.

HIGH PROTEIN AND YOUR KIDNEYS

Of all the myths about controlled-carb diets, the idea that you eat nothing but meat and that this will somehow destroy your kidneys is the most persistent—and has the least basis in fact. If anything, the ABSCP helps your kidneys by helping you to lose weight, lower your blood sugar, and lower your blood pressure. Contrary to the misinformation put forth about his program, Dr. Atkins recommended eating a wide variety of protein foods, including (but certainly not limited to) red meat.

As a matter of fact, a recent study showed a much greater survival rate in patients with severe diabetic kidney disease who decreased their carbohydrate intake. In this study, one group of nearly 100 patients got 25 to 30 percent of their calories from protein and 35 percent of their calories from carbs. They were allowed to eat protein in the form of chicken, fish, eggs, soy, and dairy sources without restriction; beef and pork were not permitted to decrease iron intake. Another group of nearly 100 patients followed the standard restricted-protein diet for kidney patients, getting only 10 percent of their calories from protein and 65 percent from carbohydrates. Over roughly a five-year period, the high-protein, low-carb patients did much better. In these patients with severe kidney disease, iron intake was also restricted. The researchers concluded that this approach was 40 to 50 percent more effective than standard protein restriction in prolonging kidney function, delaying end-stage kidney disease, and reducing the rate of death from all causes.[10]

I have seen cases among my patients with diabetes and the metabolic syndrome, whose urinary protein level decreased on a low-carbohydrate plan. Two of my patients are highlighted in this book—Joe McCoy and Pia S. in Chapters 9 and 10 respectively. I monitor urine protein excretion on all of my patients with the metabolic syndrome and diabetes. I have yet to see a case in which urinary protein excretion increased on Atkins. As a matter of fact, I have several patients who have kidney damage from a variety of causes whose protein excretion improved when carbs were controlled. I continue to perform the 24-hour urine test for protein every three months until I have two tests that are stable. Less frequent monitoring occurs as circumstances dictate. If I reach a point where no further improvement in kidney function occurs, kidney-protective medication may be needed.   —MARY VERNON

What if you already have Type 2 diabetes? Will eating protein increase your risk of developing kidney disease? It's very unlikely. There's little if any evidence to show that normal or even high-protein intake will increase your risk of developing protein in the urine, an indication of kidney disease.[11] A recent article points out that severe protein restriction in those with diabetic nephropathy (kidney disease caused by diabetes) does not seem to slow the progression of kidney disease but rather can cause malnutrition.[12]

Kidney disease is a serious complication of diabetes, but only some people with diabetes go on to have severe kidney disease. Study after study has shown that those who do develop nephropathy eat no more protein than those who don't. Study after study has also shown that the major cause of kidney disease among people with diabetes isn't protein in the diet. It's the combination of high blood pressure, high blood sugar, and high insulin that is deadly—this trio can do a lot of damage to the tiny blood vessels in your kidneys that filter waste products from your blood. Kidney disease in Type 2 diabetics is the perfect example of the vascular consequences of the metabolic syndrome. If you want to prevent damage to the kidneys, controlling your carbs is your strongest defense in the battle to maintain healthy blood vessels throughout your body, as well as in your kidneys. People diagnosed with kidney disease must follow the ABSCP only under medical supervision.

PROTEIN AND YOUR BONES

The next most common myth about the controlled-carbohydrate program is that eating large amounts of protein weakens your bones by leaching calcium from them. Just the opposite is true: A diet high in protein strengthens your bones and can slow down the process that leads to osteoporosis, a condition leading to thin, brittle bones that break easily.

Let's look at how this myth got started. Several studies in the 1970s and 1980s showed that a high-protein diet might change the amount of calcium excreted from the body, but the results were inconclusive. One study of young men in 1981, for instance, showed that a high-protein diet increased urinary excretion of calcium.[13] Another study, however, showed that a high-protein meat intake did not cause excess calcium excretion.[14]

Some nutritionists use these inconclusive studies to "prove" that a high-protein diet is bad for your bone health. What these people neglect to mention is that the value of dietary protein for building and maintaining strong bones as you get older has been powerfully shown by several recent studies.

In 1998, a carefully conducted study of seven young women compared the effects on calcium absorption of a low-protein and a high-protein diet. The result? Calcium absorption from food was much *lower* on the low-protein diet.[15]

Results from the long-running Framingham Osteoporosis Study, published in 2000, showed that eating a diet high in protein has a *protective* effect on your bones as you get older. Among the 615 elderly people in the study, the ones who ate the most protein had the strongest bones—and the ones who ate the least protein had the weakest bones. And over the four-year study period, the people who ate the least protein lost significantly more bone mass than the people who ate the most protein. The connection held up regardless of age, weight, smoking habits, calcium intake, and even estrogen use.[16]

Further evidence that protein helps preserve your bones came in 2002, when an important study showed that the combination of a high-protein intake and calcium and vitamin D supplements significantly *slows* bone loss in older adults. The study followed nearly 350 men and women, aged 65 or older, over a three-year period. The participants all ate their usual diet, but half were also randomly assigned to take two supplements containing 700 IUs of vitamin D and 500 mg of calcium. Others ate their usual diet and took two dummy pills, as the study was double-blind: Neither the participants nor the researchers knew which group they were in. At the end of three years, the researchers found that among the people taking the calcium and the vitamin D supplements the ones who also ate the most protein had the strongest bones. Among the people taking the dummy pills, there was no connection between the amount of protein in the diet and the amount of bone loss.[17]

What this study shows very clearly is that when a high-protein diet is *combined* with high-calcium intake, calcium absorption is increased and bones stay stronger. The amount of calcium needed isn't very large. In fact, the study participants with the strongest bones took in an average of 1,300 mg of calcium each day—only 100 mg a day more than the recommended daily amount for adults over age 50.

A study published in 2004 was designed to answer questions about calcium balance and dietary protein. After studying 32 people for 63 days on either a lower-protein diet or a higher-protein diet, the researchers concluded that exchanging protein for carbs in the diet, calorie for calorie, may have a favorable impact on the skeletons of healthy men and women.[18] This study supports the idea that replacing carbs with protein may be important to maintaining healthy bones.

When you follow the ABSCP, you get plenty of protein *and* plenty of calcium. The calcium comes from cheese (just one ounce of Cheddar cheese contains 204 mg of calcium) and from all those green leafy vegetables, nuts, and legumes you're eating now. Along with the calcium you're getting other nutrients important for bone health, including magnesium, phosphorus, and folic acid. You also get plenty of vitamin D from your food—it's abundant in eggs, butter, cheese, and fish. To account for individual differences in intake and absorption,

THE STORY ON SOY

In 1999, the FDA approved a heart health claim for soy protein. The agency began allowing food companies to put a statement on foods that provide at least 6.25 grams of soy protein per serving, saying that eating the food could help reduce your risk of heart disease. Does this mean you should eat a lot of soy foods? It's hard to say. There's a possible downside to large amounts of soy—among other things, it may increase the risk of breast cancer in women at high risk, such as postmenopausal women and those who have a personal or family history of breast cancer. That's because soy contains a family of substances called isoflavones, which have an estrogenic effect; in other words, they weakly mimic the effects of the hormone estrogen in the body, which may trigger breast cancer in susceptible women. Until further research is done, we recommend no more than two servings of soy products of any sort per day for those who may be at risk from excessive estrogen.[19]

we recommend that you take a balanced supplement containing calcium and phosphorus (we'll discuss supplements in more detail in Chapter 20).

When it comes to protein, we suggest that you get it from a variety of sources, including soy foods now and then (see The Story on Soy above). As mentioned in Chapter 12, eating fish up to twice a week is valuable both for its high-quality protein and the omega-3 fatty acids. Eating a wide selection of protein foods gives you a variety of nutrients, flavors, and cooking possibilities, too—it helps keep your menus interesting.

We recommend that, when choosing your proteins, you select organic meats and eggs. These foods are more expensive, but they make up for it by being more flavorful—and, more important, they do not contain hormones and antibiotics. (And when you buy these products you're helping to support sustainable agriculture.) Go easy on processed meats such as salami. Even when you choose high-quality brands that don't contain added carbohydrates as filler, they often contain nitrates and other additives and preservatives, all of which are best consumed rarely.

To avoid the mercury and other toxins that may be in fish, limit your consumption to just two portions a week. A recent FDA/EPA advisory emphasized the benefits of eating fish; however, for young children or those who are planning to get pregnant, are pregnant, or are nursing, certain precautions should be taken to minimize exposure to mercury. The advisory states that these individuals should avoid shark, swordfish, king mackerel, and tilefish because these varieties contain high levels of mercury. When consuming fish, this group should eat a variety of fish and seafood that are lower in mercury and limit their intake to two meals per week. Five of the most common fish that are lower in mercury are shrimp, canned light tuna (albacore white tuna should be limited to once a week), salmon, pollack, and catfish. Check local EPA advisories concerning the safety of fish caught in local lakes, rivers, and coastal areas. As we have discussed, supplemental oils may have the nutritional benefits with fewer potential risks (see page 162).

We hope that after reading this chapter and the last, you now real-

ATKINS WITHOUT MEAT

Pictures of juicy grilled steaks appear so often in articles about Dr. Atkins that many people believe only confirmed carnivores can follow the program. Not so! Many vegetarians have improved their health by doing Atkins. Vegetarians who will eat dairy products and eggs (lacto-ovo vegetarians) have no trouble at all getting enough high-quality protein to replace the carbs in their diets. Stricter vegetarians and even vegans, who eat no animal products at all, have to be a little more creative to get their protein, but it can still be done by eating soy foods and carefully combining whole grains, nuts, and legumes. If you don't eat animal foods, you also need to be very vigilant about getting enough dietary fat and vitamins, such as vitamin B_{12}.

ize the essential roles of both dietary fat and protein in the Atkins Blood Sugar Control Program. However, the ABSCP isn't just about fat and protein—other foods, including plenty of vegetables and some grains and fruits, are a big part of the program! The next six chapters will tell you all about the wonderful variety of delicious, high-nutrient, low-carb foods you can eat.

PICK THE PROTEIN

1. Which food *isn't* a complete protein?
   a. chickpeas
   b. hard-boiled egg
   c. shrimp
   d. baked chicken leg
2. How many essential amino acids do humans need?
   a. 6
   b. 9
   c. 22
3. When you follow the Atkins Blood Sugar Control Program, you:
   a. limit protein to 1 gram per pound of body weight
   b. eat enough protein foods to assuage hunger
   c. eat equal amounts of protein and carbohydrates
4. Protein is valuable for:
   a. stabilizing blood sugar
   b. satisfying hunger
   c. building muscle
   d. all of the above

Answers
1.a, 2.b, 3.b, 4.d.

Chapter 14

THE ATKINS GLYCEMIC RANKING

In previous chapters, we've made reference to the Atkins Glycemic Ranking (AGR). This simple but powerful tool will help you choose the carbohydrate foods that minimize the impact on your blood sugar. All carbohydrates in your diet trigger a rise in blood sugar, but how large that rise is depends a lot on the type of carbohydrate. The way to keep that rise to a minimum is to choose carbs with a low AGR. The AGR is based on important recent research into the effects of carbohydrates on your blood sugar. It's a cutting-edge concept that takes a little explaining to be understood.

SIMPLE VS. COMPLEX CARBS

We talk a lot about carbohydrates in this book, but what are they? When you remove the protein, fat, water, and ash (minerals) in a food, anything that is left is considered carbohydrate—the sugary or starchy part of the food plus any dietary fiber. For decades, a basic concept in nutrition was that sugary foods are simple carbohydrates and starchy foods are complex carbohydrates. Simple carbohydrates were assumed to be digested quickly, complex carbohydrates more slowly.

That would mean that simple carbohydrates affect your blood sugar more quickly than complex carbs. But do they?

Researchers began questioning that basic premise in the early 1980s, and ever since then a growing mountain of scientific studies tells us that the traditional simple/complex carbohydrates division just doesn't hold up. For instance, under the old theory, eating a starchy complex carbohydrate such as a baked potato should raise your blood sugar slowly. It doesn't. In fact, eating a baked potato raises your blood sugar even more speedily than eating a few spoonfuls of table sugar!

Unfortunately, current standard nutritional guidelines, which tell you to eat less fat and more carbohydrates, imply that all carbs are pretty much the same. They don't even consider how different carbohydrate foods impact blood sugar.

THE GLYCEMIC INDEX

There's a much better way to think about the way carbs act on your body: It's using what's called the *glycemic index*.[1] The thinking behind the glycemic index (GI) is pretty simple. The GI is a measure of how quickly a carbohydrate food affects your blood sugar. Because pure glucose raises your blood sugar very quickly, 50 grams of glucose (about 3 tablespoons) is the standard reference food for the glycemic index—it's ranked 100. (The more recent versions of the glycemic index use a slice of white bread as the standard reference.) The effect on your blood sugar of other carbohydrate-containing foods can then be compared with the effect of glucose or white bread to ascertain a particular food's glycemic ranking. An apple that contains 50 grams of carbohydrates, for example, raises your blood sugar to 55 percent of the level caused by eating 50 grams of glucose, so an apple has a glycemic ranking of 55. (To determine a food's GI, a volunteer eats a portion of the food large enough to contain 50 grams of carbs; then his blood glucose is measured frequently over the next few hours.)

Instead of thinking of carbohydrates as simple or complex, sugary or starchy, you could think of them as fast-acting and slow-acting. Obviously, if you need to keep your blood sugar normal, slow-acting carbohydrates—those with a lower GI ranking—are the ones to choose. They're the ones that are digested slowly and cause a gradual rise in blood sugar, followed by a gradual fall.

There's been a lot of research into the glycemic index over the past few decades, so we now have a pretty good idea of the rankings for hundreds of common carb-containing foods. As a rule of thumb, foods ranked from 0 to 55 are considered low GI; foods ranked from 56 to 69 are medium GI; and those at 70 and above are high GI. Amazingly, there are some foods that have a GI ranking above 100, meaning they elevate your blood sugar even faster than when you eat pure glucose. Remember that baked potato we mentioned earlier? A baked potato served without fat (no butter or sour cream) has a GI ranking of 102!

A major criticism of the GI concept is that it doesn't take mixed meals into account. After all, you're not very likely to eat a baked potato all by itself—it would generally be part of a larger meal that would include protein, fat, and perhaps fiber from other foods, all of which slow digestion and your absorption of glucose. That's true, but it doesn't diminish the usefulness of the glycemic index. When researchers do studies that involve mixed meals, they use a formula for calculating the amount and type of carbohydrate in the meal so they can factor in the effects of the other foods.

THE GLYCEMIC LOAD

The glycemic index is certainly a useful tool, but it does have some limitations. One big problem is that it's based on food portions that contain 50 grams of carbohydrate. That means that if a food is low in carbs to begin with, the portion itself has to be large. Also, even within a single food, the GI also doesn't fully account for the fiber and fat content, which slow the entry of glucose into your bloodstream. For some foods, such as carrots, the extra-large portion size required to comprise 50 grams of carbohydrate makes the GI number misleading.

To solve the problem of misleading GI numbers, researchers have come up with a number that's even more valuable: the glycemic load (GL).[2,3] The GL numbers are more realistic because they take into account the fiber content and portion size of a food. To calculate the GL of a food, take the GI ranking and multiply it by the number of grams of carbohydrate per serving, and then divide that number by 100. Using this calculation, the GL of that baked potato would be about 38.

The GL is a measure of the quantity of carbs in a typical portion, which makes it a very useful tool for deciding which carbs to eat. However, the portion sizes used to determine the GL are small, so it's easy to eat more and have your carbs add up faster than you realize. Even when you're eating high-quality carbs, you still need to keep an eye on your total carb intake.

USING THE ATKINS GLYCEMIC RANKING

How can you choose the right carbs for you, in the right amounts, without juggling a calculator, a measuring cup, and a carb counter? By using the Atkins Glycemic Ranking. This is a three-tier system that Dr. Atkins and nutritionists working with him developed for ranking foods, based on a combination of their glycemic index, glycemic load, and Net Carbs. This easy-to-follow guide is very helpful when counseling patients about their carbohydrate choices, and we believe you, too, will find it helpful (see Appendix 4, page 467).

The Atkins Glycemic Ranking sorts carbohydrate-containing foods into three categories:

1. Low AGR: eat regularly
2. Medium AGR: eat in moderation
3. High AGR: eat sparingly

Remember that the AGR ranking is based on a food's impact on your blood sugar, not on how many carbs it has, so it's still crucial to keep an eye on portion size and count your daily carbs. A food such as lentils can have a low AGR per serving, but each half-cup serving still packs about 12 grams of Net Carbs. On the other hand, a low-AGR food, such as broccoli, is very low in carbs and, because it's relatively high in fiber, it's ranked zero on the GI and GL scales.

When you combine the AGR charts that start on page 467 with your carb gram counter, you have the necessary tools for choosing the foods and portion sizes that will help control your blood sugar. As you'll see from the charts, you're not in danger of going hungry or getting bored by your food even if you stick to nothing but the low-AGR foods. And remember, to slow the entry of glucose from any carbohydrate food, even the low-AGR ones, eat them as part of meals and snacks that also contain fat and protein.

By using the AGR categories to choose your carbs, you'll be well on your way to weight loss. More important, you'll be traveling down the road to stable blood sugar, better blood lipids, and a reduced risk of heart disease.

"I'M STILL HUNGRY": THE HIGH-GI DIET

Almost by definition, a high-GI diet will cause obesity because of its major effect on appetite. Here's why: When you eat foods that have a high-GI ranking, your blood sugar shoots up. That makes your pancreas pour out insulin to clear away the extra blood sugar; at the same time, your body suppresses the hormone glucagon, whose role it is to counteract a drop in blood sugar. For several hours after the high-GI meal, then, you end up with high levels of insulin and low levels of glucagon. That makes your blood sugar drop too low, which means you get hungry, crave more high-GI carbs, end up eating too much—and start the whole cycle all over again.

RESEARCH REPORT: HEART DISEASE, GI, AND GL

Researchers have known for years that a diet high in refined carbohydrates can raise your triglycerides—a risk for heart disease. More recently, they've come to realize that a diet high in refined carbohydrates is also a diet that has a high overall glycemic index. Several studies have looked at how a high-GI diet relates to heart disease. Not surprisingly, there's a strong connection. In a 2000 report that looked at results from the Nurses' Health Study, the women whose diets were made up of foods with the highest glycemic load had the highest risk of heart disease. These women had almost double the risk of heart disease as the women whose diets had the lowest glycemic load. The heaviest women in the study had the highest risk, but they didn't have to be overweight for their risk to go up. The increased odds of heart disease from a high-glycemic load diet started at BMIs of just 23.[4]

Another study in 2001, based on data from the Third National Health and Nutrition Examination Survey, looked at the relationship between the glycemic index and levels of HDL cholesterol in the blood. Nearly 14,000 people participated in that study, and sure enough, the ones whose diets were highest in high-GI foods also had the lowest HDL levels.[5] (A reminder: HDL cholesterol is known as the "good" cholesterol, so lower levels are more dangerous to your heart health.)

As you already know, the combination of low HDL cholesterol and high triglycerides signals the metabolic syndrome. In a 2001 study of nearly 300 women, researchers found that the women whose diets were made up of foods with the highest glycemic load also had the lowest HDL and the highest triglycerides compared with the women whose diets were made up of foods with the lowest glycemic loads. The triglyceride difference was particularly notable among the heavier women who ate high-GL diets—their mean triglyceride level was 198, above the recommended level of 150. The researchers concluded that a high-GL diet is a potential risk factor for heart disease, particularly in women who are prone to insulin resistance.[6]

Once again, it is gratifying to see research catch up to Dr. Atkins' clinical observations. Perhaps this means that we will soon see the national nutritional guidelines recognize the importance of controlling the quality and quantity of carbohydrate intake. But there is no need for you to wait for them: You can take action right now.

WHY ARE AMERICANS OBESE?

If you follow the standard advice to control your fat intake rather than your carbs, you're likely to end up as a statistic in the worldwide obesity epidemic—if you're not there already. By replacing the fat in your diet with carbohydrates high on the glycemic index, you've unwittingly fallen into the obesity trap. The very same low-fat carbohydrate foods your doctor suggests you eat—potatoes, pasta, bread, rice—are exactly the foods that are high on the glycemic index. That makes them the foods that are most likely to make you hungry and cause you

TWENTY MOST COMMON CARBOHYDRATE-CONTAINING FOODS

Food	GI	GL
1. Cooked potatoes (mashed or baked)	102	38
2. White bread	100	13
3. Cold breakfast cereal	varies	varies
4. Dark bread	102	12
5. Orange juice	75	15
6. Banana	88	24
7. White rice	102	46
8. Pizza	86	68
9. Pasta	71	28
10. English muffin	84	22
11. Fruit punch	95	42
12. Cola	90	35
13. Apple	55	12
14. Skim milk	46	5
15. Pancake	119	67
16. Table sugar	84	3
17. Jam	91	12
18. Cranberry juice	105	20
19. French fries	95	33
20. Candy	99	28

Note: Standard reference (GI = 100) is white bread.

to overeat! Take at look at the following table from the Nurses' Health Study from 1984. It lists the 20 most commonly eaten carbohydrates in the United States, along with their glycemic ranking and glycemic load. Could there be a better illustration of why waistlines today are so large? Almost all these foods are high in carbohydrates, high on the GI and GL rankings, and low in overall nutrition.

Study after study since the late 1970s has shown that eating a low-GI diet increases satiety, decreases hunger, and lowers the amount of food eaten. Here's one good example: A study of obese teenage boys published in 1999 looked at the effect of eating meals containing different GI levels but the same number of calories. The teens ate the meals for breakfast and lunch; then they were followed for five hours to see how soon they got hungry again and asked for snacks. When the boys ate the high-GI meals, they were hungry again in well under three hours—and ate snacks that provided a lot of calories. After the low-GI meals, they weren't hungry again until nearly four hours later—and they ate 81 percent fewer calories from snacks.[7]

This response to a low-GI diet might seem familiar. It's exactly what happens when you start following the ABSCP, which by definition is a low-GI way of eating. It's pretty clear that controlling your carbs increases satiety, reduces hunger, and improves your overall nutrition. When you choose low-GI, low-AGR foods, you're eating fewer carbs overall. The carbs you do eat are high-quality, low-GI carbohydrates from fresh vegetables, fruits, and relatively unprocessed foods—and they're part of a meal that contains protein and healthy fats. You fill up fast and stay full longer—and you get lots of vitamins, minerals, and other valuable nutrients in these foods.

DIABETES AND THE HIGH-GI DIET

It seems pretty obvious that if foods high on the glycemic index are a big part of your diet, your risk of getting diabetes goes up. Cut back on the high-GI foods and you'll probably lose weight, improve your insulin re-sistance and blood lipids, and lower some other markers for heart disease and diabetes. That could go a long way to preventing diabetes.

What if you already have diabetes? In that case, getting away from a high-GI diet is no longer an option—it's a necessity. A very important 1999 study makes the point clearly. The study looked at how two identical diets with different GIs affected people with Type 2 diabetes. The 20 patients in the study were randomly assigned to eat preweighed diets with different GIs—one high, one low—for 24 days. After the 24-day period, they then switched to the other diet. Each diet was exactly the same in terms of protein, fat, carbohydrates, and dietary fiber. The study was designed simply to change the types of foods eaten, not to cause any change in the participants' weight. The different GI levels came from the way the starchy foods were prepared.

When the patients ate the low-GI diet, their blood sugar numbers averaged 30 percent less. On both diets, LDL cholesterol dropped significantly, but it dropped a lot more on the low-GI diet. Perhaps even more important than the drop in blood sugar and LDL cholesterol was the change in plasminogen activator inhibitor-1 (PAI-1) activity. High PAI-1 levels mean that your blood is more likely to clot and cause a heart attack—and people with diabetes tend to have dangerously high PAI-1 levels. On the low-GI diet, PAI-1 was normalized; on the high-GI diet, it stayed the same.[8]

We could go on a lot longer about all the studies that show how effective a low-GI diet is in controlling diabetes, but we think you get the idea. So do health authorities around the world. The GI concept is now widely used internationally as the basis for healthy eating recommendations for people both with and without diabetes.

There's one major exception: the United States. The American Diabetes Association (ADA) and other organizations still don't think there's enough scientific evidence in favor of the glycemic index concept. Instead, they focus on the total amount of carbohydrate (and calories) in the diet, not the type of carbs or where they come from, and they recommend that you get 55 percent of your calories from carbohydrates. They also appear to think the GI approach is too complicated for the average person to understand. That's why the exchange system recommended by the ADA (which itself is complicated) includes all sorts of high-GI foods made from refined carbohydrates—and that's why it doesn't help most of the people who follow it. But we think you're intelligent enough to grasp this concept. Using the Atkins Glycemic Ranking to choose your carbs is simple and effective. We hope you'll stick to it as you follow the dietary recommendations in the next five chapters.

TEST YOUR GLYCEMIC KNOW-HOW

How well do you understand the AGR rankings? Can you pick the food with a lower AGR?

1. Choose your vegetables:
    a. cabbage or baked beans?
    b. broccoli or baked potato?
    c. sweet potato or mustard greens?
    d. corn or cauliflower?
2. Choose your fruit:
    a. orange juice or grapefruit?
    b. strawberries or prunes?
    c. pear or raisins?
    d. plum or banana?
3. Choose your grains:
    a. barley or cornflakes?
    b. soy pasta or semolina pasta?
    c. old-fashioned oatmeal or English muffin?
    d. brown rice or white rice?
4. Other choices:
    a. lentils or baked beans?
    b. Swiss cheese or skim milk?
    c. macadamia nuts or cashews?

Answers

1. a, cabbage; b, broccoli; c, mustard greens; d, cauliflower. 2. a, grapefruit; b, strawberries; c, pear; d, plum. 3. a, barley; b, soy pasta; c, old-fashioned oatmeal; d, brown rice. 4. a, lentils; b, Swiss cheese; c, macadamia nuts.

FIGHTING HIS OWN WAY

Mark Anthony Montaquila says a low-fat diet had him nodding off after meals, with less than optimal cholesterol and triglycerides, and unable to build muscle despite a vigorous exercise program that includes martial arts. Atkins pointed him in a new direction and helped him battle back to health and fitness, decreasing his body fat to 12 percent.

NAME: Mark Anthony Montaquila
AGE: 38
OCCUPATION: Corrections officer
HEIGHT: 5 feet 8 inches
WEIGHT BEFORE: 189 pounds
WEIGHT NOW: 175 pounds

I'm a longtime practitioner and teacher of aikido, a martial arts discipline whose founder proclaimed, "True victory is victory over the self." Maybe that mind-set is what kept me faithfully adherent to a fat-free diet for years, even though it didn't seem to be doing me any good.

I ate pasta and potatoes, avoided fat, and avoided meat because I believed the low-fat junk. But I didn't like the way I looked. I'd always been an exercise person and that's why it drove me nuts. Even when I was training for boxing, doing round after round and running three miles,

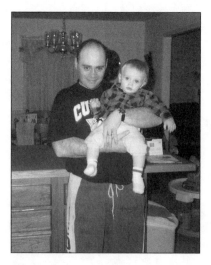

BEFORE

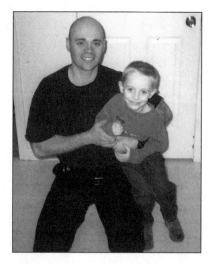

AFTER

nothing would happen. I couldn't get ripped and the reason why was that I was eating carbs.

But worse than the way I looked was the way I felt. I didn't know why I'd fall asleep for two hours after breakfast and feel sleepy after every meal. Now I look back and realize it was because my blood sugar was all out of whack. I was having two or three cups of sugary, black coffee that left a sludgy residue on the bottom of the cup, along with some pancakes and syrup. I figured that since it didn't have any fat, it must be okay.

I didn't have any serious health problems. My blood pressure was normal and, thanks to an intense cardio routine, my heart rate was in the 40s. Still, given my intense exercise regimen, my borderline-high cholesterol and elevated triglycerides didn't make sense. I was worried that I was headed for diabetes by the time I reached my forties. Some of my relatives were diabetic at that age, and I sensed that my starch-filled diet might be sabotaging my healthy lifestyle. When you exercise, that's two steps forward. When you eat junk, that's three steps back.

I shared my concerns with my brother, who suggested that I look at Dr. Atkins' New Diet Revolution. When I read the chapter that asked, "Is this you?" I was hooked. I read a third of the book that night and decided to start doing Atkins right away. I went on Induction and had absolutely no problem sticking to it. I was so upset by what I read that it was easy to give up my pasta and rice. Because I knew what they were doing to me, I never missed them and I never looked back. I was on a mission.

Within three months, I went from 189 pounds to 159. I subsequently gained some 15 pounds of lean body mass through weight lifting. My sludgy coffee and pancake breakfasts were history. I ate eggs and cheese every morning for three months and it was great! I stayed on Induction for two weeks and then gradually added back modest amounts of carbs to my diet, eventually reaching my current maintenance level of approximately 30 grams per day. I also started taking some of the nutrients Dr. Atkins recommends: selenium, zinc, chromium, and green tea. Pretty soon, my cholesterol and triglycerides were down and my energy was up.

The weight loss set off a wonderful chain of events. First, I got certified as a personal trainer and golf-conditioning specialist. Then, I made some golf instructional videos and hosted my own local TV show on golf. Losing weight gave me a lot of confidence, and I was also very inspired by Dr. Atkins. He always stood up for what he believed, even when the medical *establishment ridiculed him. I had unconventional beliefs about how one should train for golf and he inspired me to make those videos.*

All of my video work and TV experience made me a better presenter. I believe that's what catapulted me to my current job. About a year ago, I was hired to teach fitness, nutrition, and wellness classes at a corrections facility. It was my dream job ever since I joined the academy. I have to give Dr. Atkins a lot of credit for my success. My life has really changed and it's all because I bought that book.

Note: Your individual results may vary from those reported here. As stated previously, Atkins recommends initial laboratory evaluation and subsequent follow-up in conjunction with your health care provider.

Chapter 15

FIBER FACTS

When your diet is rich in fiber, your blood sugar stays steadier, and your food is more filling. And because fiber-rich foods are also usually rich in vitamins, minerals, and other valuable nutrients, you get an extra nutritional boost from eating them.

WHAT IS FIBER?

Dietary fiber comes from plant foods and falls into two main categories: digestible and nondigestible.

Nondigestible fiber (sometimes called insoluble fiber) comes in the form of cellulose, which makes up the cell walls of plant foods. Cellulose absorbs water, but it doesn't dissolve in it. Nondigestible fiber is found in wheat bran, nuts, the skins of vegetables and fruits, crunchy vegetables such as celery and bell peppers, and leafy green vegetables such as collards and lettuce.

Digestible fiber (sometimes called soluble fiber) comes from the various gums, pectins, lignans, and other natural substances found in plant foods. Although it's never actually digested—like nondigestible fiber, it cannot be broken down by your digestive system and simply passes through you—digestible fiber dissolves in water to form a soft gel in your intestines. Good sources of digestible fiber include beans, oatmeal, oat bran, apples, and pears.

Most plant foods contain at least some of both forms of fiber. The more fiber a food contains, the more likely it is to fill you up quickly—and keep you feeling full longer. High-carb, low-fiber foods—brownies, for example—don't really satisfy your hunger for long. The sugar from these foods enters your bloodstream almost instantly, giving you a temporary feeling of satiety that quickly disappears as your blood sugar drops. You could eat five brownies in a row and still end up ravenously hungry—to say nothing of irritable, shaky, and mentally foggy—several hours later.

But what if you ate a protein-and-fat snack along with some fiber—a stick of celery stuffed with cream cheese, for instance? You'd be getting about 2 grams of protein and about 10 grams of dietary fat from the cream cheese, along with about 1 gram of fiber. This crunchy, easy-to-make snack will fill you up without sending your blood sugar up and down—in fact, it will help stabilize your blood sugar so you won't be hungry or cranky later.

As you just learned in Chapter 14, fiber slows the rate at which glucose from your food enters your bloodstream. Generally speaking, foods that are low on the glycemic index and have a low glycemic load also have a lot of fiber. Review the AGR charts beginning on page 467 and you'll see an extensive list of high-fiber vegetables—such as broccoli, cabbage, and zucchini—in the "eat regularly" column.

NET CARBS: THE ATKINS ADVANTAGE

Net Carbs have been explained briefly in earlier chapters, but we'd like to elaborate on this important concept. When you follow the Atkins Nutritional Approach (ANA) or the Atkins Blood Sugar Control Program (ABSCP), you need not count the dietary fiber in a food when calculating the amount of carbohydrates in a portion. In other words, the Net Carbs are the total grams of carbohydrate content per serving *minus* the fiber content (also minus the sugar alcohols and glycerine found in some reduced-carb foods). Why don't you count the fiber?

Because although fiber is technically classified as a carbohydrate, your body can't break it down and convert it to blood sugar.

In most cases, the number of grams of Net Carbs per serving will be lower than the number of grams of total carbs. The only exceptions are foods that have virtually no fiber content, such as eggs and cheese. For these foods, the grams of total carbs and Net Carbs are the same.

How can you find the carb and fiber content of a food to calculate the grams of Net Carbs? On packaged foods, check the food facts panel, being careful to note the (often underestimated) definition of a serving that tops the list. Then look a little further down on the panel for the total carbohydrates listing—this gives you the grams of carbs per serving. Indented just below the total carbohydrates listing are the grams of dietary fiber per serving. To find the Net Carbs per serving, subtract the fiber per serving from the total carbs for that serving. To take a good example, consider the carbs in a 1-ounce serving of macadamia nuts. There are 3.2 grams of carbs in the serving and 1.9 grams of fiber. To find the Net Carbs, subtract 1.9 from 3.2 to get 1.3 Net Carbs per serving ($3.2 - 1.9 = 1.3$). The Net Carbs are less than half of the total carbs.

Reading the food facts panel only works with packaged foods, of course. For foods such as fresh vegetables, or when you're eating out, you'll need a little extra help. We suggest carrying *Dr. Atkins' New Carbohydrate Gram Counter* with you or checking the free online carb counter at www.atkins.com.[1]

It's tempting to think that a high-carb, high-fiber food is more acceptable when you look at it on a Net Carb basis. That's almost always not the case, however. Foods that tout their healthful high-fiber content often still turn out to be very high in Net Carbs. Half a cup of bran cereal (not to be confused with unprocessed bran), for instance, has about 15 carb grams, but only about 3 fiber grams, so the grams of Net Carbs per serving still are about 12. If your carb threshold is 60 grams of Net Carbs or less a day, those 12 grams of carbs are a big part of your daily allowance.

If you have diabetes and are watching your blood sugar response with a glucose meter, observe closely for signs of elevation any time you eat a carbohydrate-dense food, regardless of the fiber content. If you have questions about the effect of a new food, check your blood sugar 90 minutes after eating the food. Your aim is to keep your blood sugar below 140 mg/dL after this interval. If your sugar spikes higher than that, you should probably avoid the food. But why even risk a blood sugar spike and the unpleasant blood sugar dip that will almost certainly follow? Instead, turn to the AGR list to help you choose carbohydrate foods wisely.

HOW MUCH FIBER IS ENOUGH?

New dietary guidelines from the Institute of Medicine recommend that women should get 21 to 25 grams of fiber daily and men 30 to 38 grams daily.[2] Not surprisingly, given our high refined-carbohydrate diet, the average American typically gets only 16 grams of fiber a day.[3] Although it's obvious that the average American is not getting enough fiber to fulfill the standard recommendations, it's difficult to put a number on exactly how much fiber you really need. Keep in mind that these recommendations were developed based on studies of people whose diets did not restrict carbohydrate intake.

If you eat at least five standard servings of fresh vegetables and salad greens every day, you still might not take in the recommended amount of dietary fiber, but you would, so long as you're doing it properly, be getting excellent nutrition and probably more high-quality fiber than most Americans. Even if you need to restrict your carbs to the Induction level of 20 grams, you'll still be getting five servings per day.

At the very least, the amount of fiber in your diet should be the amount necessary to maintain comfortable bowel movements. That amount can vary considerably from person to person. When you follow the ABSCP, you may well end up eating more fiber than you did on your high-carb diet. Once you remove the refined carbs and start eating a lot of leafy greens, low-glycemic-index vegetables, nuts and seeds (see the AGR charts beginning on page 467), you've already made a beneficial change.

You may certainly add a fiber supplement to increase your fiber intake. Remember that any dietary change may change your bowel pattern temporarily. Attempt to maintain a bowel pattern that is normal for you—most people will have a comfortable bowel movement at least every other day. If you had frequent diarrhea prior to starting the ABSCP, you may experience fewer loose stools.

Sheila W. is a patient of mine who had part of her colon removed. For several years she avoided lettuce and other raw veggies because of rapid onset of diarrhea after consuming these foods. She began the ABSCP to support a family member who was using it to address metabolic problems. To her amazement, Sheila's bouts of diarrhea disappeared with a controlled-carb plan. She was able to reintroduce salads and other raw veggies without needing to stay near a restroom. —MARY VERNON

For proper bowel function, be sure to drink eight 8-ounce glasses of water each day and engage in regular exercise. As you know, these are integral components of both the ANA and the ABSCP. Experiment a bit with your vegetables to find higher-fiber choices you enjoy. You might try substituting chicory for some of the other salad greens, for example. One cup of chicory has 7 grams of fiber and only 1 gram of Net Carbs. Compare that with 1 cup of shredded romaine lettuce, which has only 1 gram of fiber and about ½ gram of Net Carbs. With such small adjustments, you come out way ahead on fiber without adding very much at all to your Net Carb count for the day.

To increase dietary fiber, try a dose of crushed flaxseeds or unprocessed bran. Both these excellent natural remedies for constipation are available at any health food store. Stir 2 teaspoons of flaxseeds into a glass of water and drink it down in the evening, or sprinkle them on your salad at dinner—you'll probably get results the next morning. The advantage of flaxseeds is that in addition to your dose of fiber you get some additional omega-3 fatty acids, plus some extra magnesium and zinc. If you don't like flaxseeds or find them inconvenient, an alternative is a bulk-forming fiber supplement made from psyllium (Fiberall, Metamucil). To avoid adding sugar, select only the unflavored, sugar-free form of these products and follow package directions. Because the digestible fiber from flaxseeds and psyllium passes through you instead of being absorbed, the Net Carbs per dose are basically zero. (Have your flaxseed or psyllium dose a few hours apart from any medications and supplements. If you take them together, the fiber may block your absorption of drugs or supplements.)

Increasing your fiber intake too rapidly, whether from high-fiber foods or from a supplement, can cause digestive upset, including gas, bloating, cramps, and diarrhea. To minimize these problems, increase your intake gradually by adding a little more fiber every few days and giving your digestive system a chance to adjust.

When you eat fresh, low-carb vegetables, nuts, seeds, and low-glycemic fruits, you get not only fiber the natural way, but also lots of other important nutrients. Read on to the next chapter to learn more and realize how varied and delicious your diet will be as you follow the Atkins Blood Sugar Control Program.

WHAT'S YOUR FIBER IQ?

1. The two kinds of dietary fiber are:
   a. digestible and nondigestible
   b. edible and inedible
   c. fructose and sucrose
2. How do you find the Net Carbs per food serving?
   a. subtract the carbs from the fiber
   b. subtract the fiber from the carbs
   c. add the fiber and the carbs
   d. divide the carbs by the fiber
3. Which foods are good sources of digestible fiber?
   a. chicory
   b. peas
   c. apples
   d. beans
4. Which foods are good sources of nondigestible fiber?
   a. celery
   b. nuts
   c. collards
   d. oranges

Answers
1. a. 2. b. 3. all of them. 4. a, b, c.

Chapter 16

THE BOUNTIFUL HARVEST

Vegetables offer an amazing variety of flavors, colors, and textures. But there's more to vegetables than just their great looks and tastes. A basic principle of the Atkins Blood Sugar Control Program (ABSCP) is that you trade in low-quality, low-nutrient foods (such as refined carbohydrates) for high-quality, high-nutrient foods—and the majority of vegetables fall into the latter category.

Simply replacing poor-quality carbs with high-quality veggies may be enough to make an improvement in your blood sugar. It's a win-win situation: When you begin eating a greater variety and quantity of vegetables, you realize that they taste so good you won't really miss refined carbs. Plus, vegetables are packed with the nutrients that are missing in most refined carbohydrates. And they're a rich source of fiber, which can help to stabilize your blood sugar levels. If your daily carb allowance will let you, you can also enjoy many of the same benefits from low-glycemic fruits.

LAYING THE FOUNDATION

Fresh vegetables and low-glycemic fruits are important in the ABSCP because eating these foods can help stabilize your blood sugar—if you

RESEARCH REPORT: VEGETABLES AND HEART HEALTH

In addition to helping to prevent and treat diabetes, all those servings of asparagus, broccoli, cauliflower, and their kin are essential for helping prevent cardiovascular disease. If you have the metabolic syndrome, prediabetes, or diabetes, you know your risk of heart disease and stroke is sharply elevated—and you can use all the help you can get in this area. Let's look at the results from a recent study that examined the connection between vegetable and fruit intake and the risk of cardiovascular disease. The study, published in 2002 in the *American Journal of Clinical Nutrition*, looked at almost 10,000 adults who had been followed for nearly 20 years as part of the first National Health and Nutrition Examination Survey.[1]

Among the study participants, those who ate vegetables and fruits three or more times per day had a 42 percent lower risk of dying from a stroke compared with those who ate produce once a day or not at all. The produce eaters also had a 27 percent lower risk of dying from cardiovascular disease, a 24 percent lower incidence of death from clogged arteries causing heart disease, and a 15 percent lower risk of dying from any cause.[2]

eat them instead of refined carbohydrates. People who choose to eat this way early on may actually protect themselves from developing blood sugar problems.

A study published in 1999 helped to provide more support for the importance of eating vegetables. Eleven hundred subjects completed a food frequency questionnaire and underwent a glucose tolerance test. Those who ate salad and raw vegetables had significantly less incidence of Type 2 diabetes and impaired glucose tolerance than those who ate salad and raw vegetables infrequently. Notably, there was not a statistically significant difference recorded in glucose measurements for those who ate fruit.[3] This confirms the benefits Dr. Atkins observed in his patients when they consumed the minimum recommended amount of vegetables. When you're doing Atkins properly, of course, you should be eating a minimum of five servings of vegetables a day.

VEGETABLES AND BLOOD SUGAR

What is it about vegetables that makes them so good for you? Well, they are generally pretty low in carbs, and almost all nonstarchy vegetables are both low on the glycemic index (GI) and low in glycemic load (GL). Just by replacing high-carb, high-GL foods with low-carb, low-GL foods—substituting broccoli for a baked potato, for instance—you will improve your blood sugar levels. But there's more to it than that. What may be just as important is that these foods are packed with fiber, antioxidants, vitamins, minerals, and phytonutrients. We know that these nutrients are particularly important if you have the metabolic syndrome, blood sugar abnormalities, or diabetes.

FANCY FRUIT—IN MODERATION

Now let's take a detour to talk about fruit, before we return to vegetables. Overall, fruits are higher in carbs than an equivalent serving of vegetables. That's why when you do eat fruits, you should have them as a snack with a food containing protein and fat, or eat them as dessert after a meal that contains protein and fat. Doing so helps keep the sugar in the fruit from entering your bloodstream too quickly. To avoid getting too many carbs from fruits, be aware of portion size. A typical fruit portion on the ABSCP is one small apple, half an orange, or a ½ cup of red grapes or blueberries.

When you get to the point in the program where you can add fruits, begin with those on the "eat regularly" list of the AGR (check the AGR charts beginning on page 467). If you need to limit your carbs, these foods must now be only occasional treats that are always eaten with protein and fat. The few fruits, such as bananas and raisins, that fall into the "eat sparingly" category are basically off-limits if your carb threshold is 60 grams of Net Carbs a day or less.

When you begin to add fruit to your diet, start with only a few servings a week, carefully observing your symptoms and blood sugar response. If you notice that your blood sugar goes above 140 mg/dL 90 minutes after a meal, or if you experience sensations that you associate with blood sugar ups and downs, then hold off on fruit. Perhaps your metabolism has not yet improved enough to allow the level of natural sugar in fruits. In that case, if you're at the stage where you want to add more carbs to your daily allowance, opt for more low-glycemic vegetables instead and then try adding small amounts of fruit again at some point in the future.

If your insulin/blood sugar metabolism is severely compromised, you may at best tolerate only one serving of fruit a day. As time goes by and your insulin/blood sugar improves, you may be able to increase the amount of fruit you eat, but you'll probably always have to be aware of portion size.

WHAT'S A SERVING?

We strongly recommend that you eat, at the very least, five servings a day of fresh low-glycemic, low-carb vegetables—more if your daily carb budget allows. We also recommend that if you are consuming between 20 and 40 grams of Net Carbs a day, you eat no more than two daily servings of fruit (other than olives, avocados, or tomatoes, which are regarded as vegetables even though they are actually fruits). What's a serving? In the ABSCP, a vegetable serving is 1 cup of raw leafy greens or ½ cup of cooked nonstarchy vegetables, such as broccoli or Brussels sprouts. In the case of vegetables like tomatoes or spinach, which cook down significantly, be sure to measure them raw to avoid overconsumption of carbs. A fruit serving is one small fruit, such as an apple, or ½ cup of berries. Be aware of portion size and check your carb gram counter when in doubt.

HOW ARE WE DOING?

After more than a decade of advertising and public education about the nutritional value of vegetables and fruits, how is the average American doing? Not that well. Between the years 1990 and 1996, according to a 2000 study, only about 45 percent of Americans actually ate five or more servings a day. This is up from 32 percent between 1989 to 1991.[4] That is an improvement, yet more than half of American adults are still below the minimum recommended amount.

But here's the bad news: The nutritional quality of those fruits and vegetables is still low. Only five fruits and vegetables accounted for 30 percent of consumption: iceberg lettuce, tomatoes, French-fried potatoes, bananas, and orange juice. In other words, a significant portion of the fruits and vegetables the average American eats is either very low in nutrients (iceberg lettuce) or high in carbohydrates (bananas and orange juice), or both (French fries). While tomatoes are fairly low in carbs and are a good source of vitamin C, lycopene, and fiber, the average daily amount eaten was only half a standard serving, or about the amount that comes on top of a fast-food burger.

In the same study, the researchers found that for the average person, white potatoes represented 30 percent of total vegetable intake. Of that 30 percent, one-third was French fries. By comparison, broccoli made up only 0.4 percent of vegetable intake. Only 3 percent of the population eats any broccoli on any given day! Although nutritionists classify the potato as a vegetable, it really belongs in the same category as other high-GI carbohydrates such as pasta. In terms of glycemic response, eating potatoes is almost exactly the same as eating an equivalent amount of pure sugar. In fact, it's worse—a baked potato or a serving of French fries will spike your blood sugar and insulin levels even faster and higher than eating a candy bar.[5]

How does your intake of vegetables and fruits compare with that of the average American? If you're following the Atkins Blood Sugar Control Program properly, you rank far above average. Your intake of high-quality vegetables is not only significantly higher, it's significantly more varied. And that means you're getting above-average amounts of a variety of vitamins, minerals, antioxidants, and phytonutrients that are known to help your body fight off virtually all the most common life-threatening diseases.

VARY YOUR VEGGIES

Okay, it is understandable that broccoli and spinach may not be your favorite foods. And even favorite foods can get a little dull if you eat them all the time. To keep your taste buds happy, go for variety. Today there's a whole world of interesting vegetables in the produce section of just about every supermarket. Bored with Brussels sprouts? Try chayote (a sort of squash from Central America), snow pea pods, or turnip greens. Or try a mix of different vegetables, in a stir-fry, for example. You'll be happy to know that fiber isn't really affected much by cooking. In fact, many high-fiber vegetables are more digestible when they're cooked, so try adding them to soups, stews, and casseroles—there are some great vegetable recipes in Chapter 27, as well as at www.atkins.com.

We prefer that you not drink most veggies or fruit—you lose a lot of the valuable fiber that way. Fruits are much higher in carbs, mostly in the form of fructose, and dumping all that sugar into your bloodstream can really make your blood sugar jump. Be wary of fruit juice "drinks," which often contain a tiny amount of real fruit juice and lots of water and sugar, in the form of high-fructose corn syrup.[6–8]

ANTIOXIDANTS AND FREE RADICALS

Every second of every day, the trillions of cells in your body are hard at work. One of their jobs is to create energy by burning glucose or fat for fuel. A perfectly normal by-product of this process is the free radical—an unstable atom missing an electron. When an atom is missing an electron, it blunders around, looking for another electron it can grab—and often it steals that electron from another molecule and damages it in the process. To quench free radicals before they can seize electrons from places where they might do damage, your body employs antioxidants. These chemicals capture the free radicals and, in a

SALAD DAYS

When you do the ABSCP, you can and will—and should—eat a lot of salad. Salads are a great way to get more of those fiber-rich leafy greens we keep talking about without racking up a lot of carbohydrates. In general, 1 cup of any salad green has less than 1 gram of Net Carbs. You also get to dress those salads with your favorite low-carb dressings. That gives you a good way to get in the good fats, like olive oil. (See Chapter 12 for more on the value of dietary fats.)

Unfortunately, the most commonly eaten salad green is iceberg lettuce—the variety that's probably the lowest of all in terms of fiber and nutrients. It's hard to escape this bland lettuce when you eat out, but you can easily make your salads at home a lot more interesting and nutritious by trying the many other lettuce varieties now available in the produce section. You can also add extra fiber, nutrients, and taste to your salads by tossing in some nuts and seeds—slivered almonds and sunflower seeds, for example—but only if you stay within your daily carb gram allowance.

complex series of steps, quickly neutralize them. To ensure that this defense team can do its job properly, your body needs plenty of vitamins—particularly beta-carotene (the natural precursor to vitamin A), vitamin C, and vitamin E—and trace minerals, especially selenium and zinc.

Everyone produces free radicals all the time; they're a normal part of your metabolism, and for the most part your body is able to cope with them. The process of metabolizing big doses of carbohydrates, however, generates oxidative stress by producing an abundance of free radicals. Excess body fat also adds to your free-radical production and puts a strain on your body's antioxidant system. In addition, if you're overweight and you've become insulin resistant (even if you don't know it yet), you may have excess glucose circulating in your bloodstream, and that causes a *lot* more free radicals and oxidative stress. Many researchers believe, in fact, that oxidative stress from free radicals plays a big part in many of the complications of diabetes and also in heart disease. Oxidative stress may also speed the destruction of the insulin-producing beta cells in your pancreas.[9]

Free radicals also are involved in the formation of what are known as advanced glycosylation end products, or AGEs. Over time, glucose attaches to proteins in your body and gums them up. The results, the AGEs, are believed to damage tiny blood vessels in your eyes, kidneys, and elsewhere. Many researchers believe that free radicals participate in this process, too.[10]

Of course, losing weight and getting your insulin and blood sugar under control are the clearest ways to reduce free-radical production. Eating antioxidant-rich fresh vegetables and fruits within your individualized carbohydrate limit can help, too. If you implement the ABSCP, your production of free radicals should drop automatically, because your oxidation of carbohydrates drops.[11] (Supplements can help too—we'll discuss them in more detail in Chapter 20.)

RESEARCH REPORT: ANTIOXIDANTS AND THE METABOLIC SYNDROME

A recent study comparing adults with and without the metabolic syndrome showed that those with the syndrome had low levels of important antioxidants, especially vitamin C and vitamin E. The researchers agreed that in addition to nutrient-dense foods, supplements could be beneficial in raising antioxidant levels in adults with high oxidative stress caused by the metabolic syndrome.[12] As you know, controlling carbohydrates goes a long way toward controlling the metabolic syndrome. Carbohydrate-laden diets (filled with foods such as French fries) fuel the fire of oxidative stress, using up antioxidants at a high rate. On top of that, you're not getting enough antioxidant nutrients to begin with, because all those refined carbohydrates have had most of their nutrients processed out of them. This dangerous combination—higher levels of oxidative stress, lower antioxidant intake—causes further blood vessel injury.

THE ATKINS RATIO

All vegetables and fruits contain good amounts of antioxidants, but some contain more than others. If you're watching your carbs, you want to choose the vegetables and fruits that are highest in antioxidants and lowest in carbohydrates. Figuring that out on your own would be a complicated exercise in chemistry, so we've done it for you by listing the Atkins Ratio for the top ten vegetables and fruits (see page 208). This ranking tells you how much antioxidant bang you get for your carbohydrate buck. (The higher the Atkins Ratio, the greater the antioxidant content relative to the carb count.) Whenever you can, choose at least two of your daily vegetable servings and at least one of your fruit servings from these foods, provided that you do not notice a change in your blood sugar level or associated symptoms. (For drinks that are high in antioxidants, see Chapter 19.)

OTHER GOOD STUFF

Magnesium

Fiber and antioxidants are reason enough for veggies and fruit to be valuable foods on the Atkins Blood Sugar Control Program, but there are even more reasons. Here's one good one: Overall, vegetables and fruits are good sources of the mineral magnesium. For reasons that aren't fully understood, many people with diabetes and blood sugar abnormalities are low in magnesium, which is needed for a wide variety of normal body processes (we'll talk more about the role of magnesium in Chapters 20 and 21).[13] Adding magnesium to the diet may help you control your blood sugar better. Good choices include broccoli, okra, spinach, and Swiss chard. Nuts and beans are also good sources of magnesium, as are fruits, but they're not as rich a source as vegetables—and beans are relatively high in carbs.

Phytonutrients

Every plant food also contains a large number of other natural chemicals that go under the general heading of phytonutrients or, some-

VEGETABLES

Food	Atkins Ratio	Total Carbs (grams)	Net Carbs (grams)
Garlic (1 clove)	23.2	1.0	0.9
Leaf lettuce (1 leaf)	8.2	1.0	0.5
Kale	6.5	3.4	2.1
Onion (1 tablespoon)	6.2	1.1	1.0
Spinach	5.0	5.1	2.2
Broccoli	3.2	4.9	2.2
Red bell pepper (raw)	2.5	4.8	3.3
Brussels sprouts	2.3	6.8	4.7
Beets	2.1	6.1	4.7
Cauliflower	1.8	2.6	0.9

All servings are ½ cup cooked unless otherwise noted.

FRUITS

Blueberries	2.3	10.2	8.3
Strawberries	2.3	5.1	3.4
Blackberries	2.2	9.2	5.4
Plum	1.0	3.7	3.3
Orange	0.8	10.6	8.4
Kiwifruit	0.5	11.3	8.7
Pink grapefruit	0.5	9.5	7.8
Red grapes	0.5	14.2	13.4
Tomato	0.5	4.2	3.2
Green grapes	0.4	14.2	13.4

All servings are ½ cup raw.

times, flavonoids. These substances are often what give a food its characteristic taste and color—and they also have numerous health benefits. The phytonutrient list is long and getting longer all the time as research continues in this exciting area. Here are just a few beneficial phytonutrients:

- *Lycopene.* Found abundantly in tomatoes, lycopene may help prevent prostate cancer.
- *Resveratrol.* Red wine and red grapes are the best source for this phytonutrient; high levels in your blood are associated with a reduced risk of heart disease.
- *Quercetin.* This powerful antioxidant is found in onions and garlic; it can also be helpful for allergy relief and to enhance the immune system.
- *Lutein and zeaxanthin.* These phytonutrients, found in dark green leafy vegetables such as kale and collard greens, can help protect your eyes against age-related macular degeneration, a leading cause of blindness in older adults.[14]

All this and more are the bonus you get from eliminating low-quality carbohydrates and replacing them with high-fiber, nutrient-rich plant foods.

Need we say more? We don't think so—the evidence is pretty convincing. And now that you've got a good grasp of why you need to eat those fresh leafy greens, in the next chapter we'll move on and explain how to choose other good carbs.

WHAT'S YOUR VEGGIE IQ?

1. A standard serving of a cooked vegetable is:
   a. 1 pint
   b. 9 pieces
   c. ½ cup
   d. 100 grams
2. Vegetables are a good source of:
   a. dietary fiber
   b. vitamin C
   c. magnesium
   d. phytonutrients
   e. all of the above
3. Which vegetable is *not* on the low-carb, low GI/GL list:
   a. Brussels sprouts

    b. broccoli

    c. potato

    d. salad greens

    e. cabbage

4. The top five vegetables for antioxidant power are:

    a. zucchini

    b. cabbage

    c. garlic

    d. leaf lettuce

    e. onions

    f. string beans

    g. kale

    h. cauliflower

    i. spinach

    j. carrots

Answers

1. Trick question—c (American units) and d (metric units) are both correct. 2. e. 3. c. 4. c, d, e, g, i.

MAN ON A MISSION

Since childhood, Steve Horstman battled futilely to lose weight. Once he realized he was a carb addict and well on his way to diabetes, he took the steps necessary to win back his life.

NAME: Steve Horstman
Age: 37
Height: 6 feet 1 inch
Weight Before: 571 pounds
Weight Now: 250 pounds

Total Cholesterol Before (6 months in): 230
Total Cholesterol Now: 151
LDL Now: 85
HDL Now: 66
Triglycerides Now: 132
Blood Pressure (6 months in): 140/90; resting heart rate: 88
Blood Pressure Now: 115/65; resting heart rate: 56

I started doing Atkins on April 28, 1999. I'll never forget that date—for me, it has the same importance as the days your kids are born. I'd carried extra weight even as a child and had tried every diet in the world. But I'd always lose/regain, lose/regain. In the late eighties, I actually had the most success. I got myself down to 200 pounds by starving myself. Looking back, I was also eliminating carbs without knowing it. But I was so hungry all the time I just couldn't stick to it. I became a cynic about all diets.

One day I noticed that my wife, Melissa, had bought Dr. Atkins' New Diet Revolution *and put it on top of my dresser without saying anything. Well, it just sat there for two days. I happened to be home on a day off having lunch, which I remember was six hot dogs with buns and two cans of Coke. I like to read while I'm eating, so I decided to take a look at the book. When I finished the chapter "Is This You?" I said, "Wow! That is me." By 6:30 that evening I had read the entire book twice and started it a third time when I called my wife at work. "We are going to try this diet." She splurged and brought home steaks and lobster tails for our first Atkins dinner.*

The next day I weighed myself at a local store in our town of Burlington, Kentucky, a suburb of Cincinnati, which had an old-fashioned grain scale. I already knew that conventional scales don't exceed 300 pounds, so this was my only option. I thought I'd weigh in a little over 400 pounds. The scale read 571 pounds. I also had a 70-inch waist and had begun to develop all the signs of Type 2 diabetes.

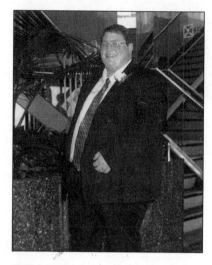

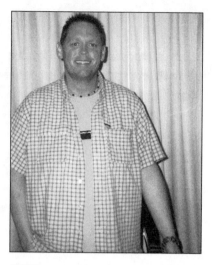

BEFORE   **AFTER**

Even though I was still very skeptical about the program, I decided to give it a try, staying at or under 20 grams of Net Carbs per day as required in the Induction phase. Weighing in on the same scale nine days later, I realized I had lost 30 pounds. "Okay, that's it; I'm hooked," I said.

Then I found an electronic scale that could handle my weight at a GNC store. I went there every day to track my progress. Within the first two months, I had lost 100 pounds. That's when I started exercising by walking to the end of my block and back, stopping to rest halfway each way. The first year, I stayed on Induction for the entire time and lost 273 pounds. I've been watching carbs at the Ongoing Weight Loss level since then and have lost an additional 48 pounds. I still have 25 pounds to go to reach my goal weight of 225.

It amazes me now to think about what I used to eat. I skipped break-fast, but for lunch I'd go to a fast-food restaurant and consume four sand-wiches, two large fries, and a large Coke. Then I'd go to another fast-food restaurant, eat three or four more sandwiches, maybe a bag of onion rings, and another large Coke. I made two stops because I was embarrassed by the amount I was eating and I was looking for taste variety, too. I would down four or five peanut-butter-and jelly sandwiches or a bag of Doritos while waiting for the lasagna and garlic bread I would have for dinner to be ready. I probably drank the equivalent of 12 large Cokes per day.

Now I've really developed a taste for veggies. Broccoli, cauliflower, as-

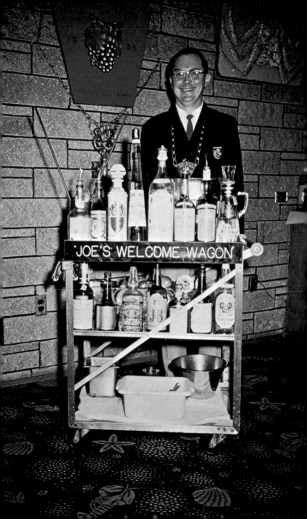

Joseph G. Pittenhedd

Joe holds a degree of International Wine Sommelier (Counsellor) and is privileged to wear the Gold Medallion for having passed advanced study and tests given him on wine knowledge, preparation of food and mixology technique. He received 2nd honors in 1953 for the National Wine-Week promotions, in which over 28,000 restaurants participated.
Joe is also a member of the Society of Bacchus in America (a research group starting a Wine Museum in the U.S.A.), and the Guild of Sommeliers of London, England, and Sidney, Australia.

QP-304

1402 Grant, San Francisco, CA 94133   Tel (415) 986-8866

QUANTITY POSTCARDS

Mfr. Pub./Wholesale/Retail/Mail Order

Catalogue
available

paragus, spinach, mixed greens—these are all new foods for me. Even though I hate the cold days in winter, I continue to walk with my wife, Melissa, who has lost about 100 pounds herself on Atkins, with 35 more pounds to go. We shoot for three to four miles, five to six days per week. I know I need to add some more aerobic activity to get my heart rate up, and I plan to do so.

It is absolutely fun to go shopping for clothes now. I used to have to get everything by mail order. It was a pretty big day for me when I finally shopped at a regular department store and bought a real pair of blue jeans without an elastic waistband. My waist is now 38 inches. I've gone from a 6X to an extra-large shirt. My shoe size has dropped from a 14 to an 11½. And my ring size has gone from a 14 to an 11½. I had been wearing my wedding ring on my thumb!

I've been working in restaurant management for most of my career. Recently, a young lady came in to apply for a job at my location. "Do you know who I am?" I asked. "You worked for me for four years," I said. I showed her my ID and she was so happy about how I looked she started crying and gave me a big hug.

I've actually become a bit of a celebrity, appearing on the Today show and the area news. About a week after I appeared locally, I was shopping for groceries and bought a lot of Atkins products. I started talking to the manager, who happened to be at the register, and I asked her if low-carb products were selling. "Can't keep it on the shelves since that guy from around here was on TV." "I'm that guy," I said, and she asked me for my autograph!

I have helped counsel about 100 people through the approach. Everybody who does Atkins—and does it right—loses weight. I've turned into a walking carb-counter. I help other people find the hidden carbs in what they have been eating. "You can lie to everybody, but you can't lie to yourself," I tell them. My three kids are really proud of me. When my youngest, a nine-year-old, sees an old picture of me, she can't remember that I looked so fat. Diabetes, heart attack, stroke—I might not be here for my kids today if it wasn't for Atkins.

Note: Your individual results may vary from those reported here. As stated previously, Atkins recommends initial laboratory evaluation and subsequent follow-up in conjunction with your health care provider.

Chapter 17

CONTROLLING YOUR CARBS—
AND LIKING IT

All carbohydrates are most definitely not created equal. The right carbohydrates in moderate amounts can help you stabilize your blood sugar and may even help prevent diabetes; the wrong carbs (particularly when consumed in excess) can send your insulin and blood sugar levels soaring out of control.

We can look at carbs in a number of different ways. The traditional nutritional division is simple and complex carbohydrates. But as we've said, these terms are misleading. For example, berries are classified as simple carbohydrates, because fructose, the sugar in fruit, breaks down easily. Meanwhile, a high-carbohydrate granola bar full of added sugar is regarded as a complex carbohydrate because it contains whole grains, which don't break down as quickly. In this case, the nutritional recommendation to eat more complex carbohydrates would mean eating more of some pretty unhealthy foods and less of some very healthy ones.

GOOD CARBS, BAD CARBS

As you learned about the Atkins Glycemic Ranking (AGR) in Chapter 14, the glycemic load (GL) and glycemic index (GI) are a much more helpful way to look at the carbohydrates in your diet. Now let's take a closer look at carbohydrates to better understand why we suggest eating some carbs on a regular basis, others in moderation, and certain carbs rarely or never. Whichever carbs you eat on any given day, you must keep your Net Carb count within your personal threshold.

We have talked a lot in this book about how carbs can raise your blood sugar; but that does not mean that all carbs are bad. The ones that raise your blood sugar too quickly and too high are high-GI foods that also have a high GL. These are mainly foods that are highly refined, highly processed, and low in fiber: white rice, bread made with bleached white flour, pasta, French fries, grits, and so on. But we also have to be aware of unrefined carbs that have a high GI, such as wild rice and millet. While those are inherently good foods, it's important for people with blood sugar problems to choose unrefined, high-fiber, low-GI/low-GL carbs—the ones that end up having a low AGR. Lots of unrefined, delicious carbs can be found on the AGR "Eat regularly" and "Eat in moderation" lists (see Appendix 4, page 467)—acorn squash, lentils, peanuts, and nectarines, for instance.

ADD CARBS WITH CAUTION

All carbs always count, however, and even large portions of low-AGR foods could cause an undesirable jump in your blood sugar. To moderate the impact, add small portions of low- and moderate-AGR foods back into your diet as part of a meal that also contains protein, fat, and dietary fiber. As you do so, keep an eye on your weight, blood sugar, triglycerides, symptoms, and appetite control. If weight loss stops suddenly or you regain weight, if you get jittery and hungry, or if your blood sugar or triglyceride levels go up, cut back on your servings of these carb foods. On the other hand, if these indicators remain stable, go ahead and have an occasional serving. Be extremely aware of portion size, however. The standard portion of, say, cooked acorn squash is only ½ cup. If you're very carb-sensitive, you may have to limit even that amount to just a few times a week. For ideas on how to use small amounts of higher-carb veggies, legumes (beans), and even grains, check out the meal plans and recipes in Chapters 26 and 27.

CARB CRAVINGS: HOW TO FIGHT BACK

For some people, eating even a small portion of a high-quality carbohydrate such as brown rice is very difficult—it triggers their carbohydrate cravings. This can lead to a serious detour off the ABSCP and back onto the blood sugar roller coaster. What happens then? Rapid changes in insulin and blood sugar levels, mood swings, weight gain, gas and bloating, preoccupation with food—in short, eating those carbs could trigger your addiction (let's call a spade a spade) and cancel out all the health gains you have made.

When carbohydrates beckon, fight back with some simple strategies:

- Admit that you're tempted and then consciously remind yourself of how much better you feel when you limit the carbs in your diet. Say it out loud if that helps.
- Eat a snack containing protein and fat. Your cravings could be coming from low blood sugar; the snack will stabilize it.
- Consider eating frequent, smaller meals including protein, fat, and fiber on a regular schedule. Don't ever let yourself get too hungry.
- Substitute a low-carb food for the food you crave. If you must have chocolate, try a low-carb bar or a chocolate shake.

Once the craving is past, understanding what set it off can help you avoid it next time. Did you go too long without eating, triggering a drop in blood sugar? Try not to go more than four waking hours without a meal or a protein snack—a slice of turkey, a chicken drumstick, or a small piece of cheese, for instance. Did you eat because of stress or anxiety, not hunger? Simply being aware of why you're eating can help here. And if you find yourself eating because you're stressed, again, choose a high-protein food to snack on—this helps stop stress-related cravings. Did you let someone pressure you into eating? You've probably heard this all too often: "Go ahead, a little bit won't hurt you." You know a little bit *can* hurt you, so simply say, "I'm being more careful about what I eat these days."

CHOOSING GRAINS WISELY

Even unprocessed whole grains are relatively high in grams of Net Carbs per serving. Some are relatively low in GI and GL, however, which is why certain whole grain foods, such as kasha (buckwheat groats) and whole wheat couscous, fall into the "eat in moderation" category on the AGR. For people who need to keep their carbs in the 20- to 40-grams-a-day range, however, eating even these foods may not be possible. If you're still in the Ongoing Weight Loss phase of the Atkins Blood Sugar Control Program or you don't have your blood sugar under control, you'll have to be very cautious about adding grains back into your diet.

Old-fashioned oatmeal and barley, whole grains that are on the "eat regularly" AGR list, are both high in beta glucan, a type of digestible fiber. Beta glucan helps keep the carbohydrates in oatmeal and barley from having a big effect on your blood sugar, and it also helps slow down your absorption of carbs from other foods as well.[1] Once you can handle whole grains, a bit of barley is a great addition to soups and casseroles, and oatmeal—the original comfort food—makes a warm and filling breakfast food or snack. The value of oatmeal comes only from whole oats, however. Look for "steel-cut," "old-fashioned," or "rolled" oats and enjoy their chewy texture and nutty flavor. The processes involved in making quick-oatmeal and instant-oatmeal products remove a lot of the fiber and beta glucan, which means the carbs enter your bloodstream too quickly. Instant oatmeals also usually have sweeteners and other high-carb additions.

GRAINS FOR BREAKFAST

Many ready-to-eat breakfast cereals claim to be healthful, but a quick check of the ingredients label reveals that they are made mostly from refined grains and added sugars; many also contain trans fats. Cornflakes have a higher GI than a slice of white bread![2] If your daily carb allowance is above 60 grams of Net Carbs, you might be able to have a good whole grain choice for breakfast now and then. But check the ingredients label, and remember to combine protein and fat with the

FOOD INTOLERANCES

It's surprisingly common for people to have an intolerance for grains and yeast, which is used in bread and other grain products as well as in fermented foods such as yogurt. Symptoms may include diarrhea, heartburn, gas and bloating, headaches, chronic tiredness—and unstable insulin/blood sugar. Paradoxically, food intolerances can provoke cravings for the very food that causes the symptoms. In the case of wheat sensitivity (one of the most common), it means frequent cravings for high-carb foods like bread, bagels, and pasta, which aggravate unstable blood sugar. Food intolerances, also known as food sensitivities, can be isolated by keeping a food diary, which will allow you to associate symptoms with eating a particular food. A trial period in which you eliminate the offending food from your diet can help you confirm an intolerance or sensitivity.

If you notice that certain symptoms improve when you're on Induction—during which you consume almost none of the common offenders—and recur at higher levels of carbohydrate intake, consider eliminating any recently introduced food, which may well be the culprit. After a symptom-free period, it might be possible occasionally to add small amounts of offending foods without symptoms returning.

grains, and watch your blood sugar and symptoms afterward. Good options include Fiber 1, old-fashioned oatmeal, and unsweetened müesli (a mixture of oatmeal, wheat germ, other grains, and nuts). As an alternative you could try one of the low-carb breakfast cereals that use soy instead of grains. What to pour on that cereal? There are several options other than milk, which contains the sugar lactose, making it high in carbs (and many people have trouble digesting it). You can add cream by itself or diluted with water, or use low-carb soymilk or a reduced-carb dairy beverage.

BEANS AND BLOOD SUGAR

Beans, peas, and lentils—also known as legumes—in all their many colors and flavors, are another delicious source of low-GI/low-GL carbohydrates. (Technically speaking, peanuts are legumes, too, but for all practical purposes they're treated as nuts.) Like whole grains, beans are rich in digestible and nondigestible fiber, vitamins, minerals, and other nutrients.

On the plus side, beans are very low on the GI ranking, and their high fiber content means they also have a very low GL. In the AGR, some beans, including bean products such as tofu (bean curd) and unsweetened soymilk, fall into the "eat regularly" category. A few that are slightly higher on the GI/GL rankings, including roasted soybeans, chickpeas, and kidney beans, fall into the "eat in moderation" category. The beans to avoid are baked beans and similar dishes—but not because of the beans. Baked beans, barbecued beans, and similar dishes contain molasses and other added sugars that add a lot of empty carbs, which can put you back on the insulin/blood sugar roller coaster.

On the negative side, beans are relatively high in Net Carbs, meaning you need to keep your portions to a ½ cup or so—and only if your daily carb threshold allows it. Your best bet is to find ways to use beans in small portions. For instance, add some chickpeas to a tossed salad, lentils to a beef-vegetable soup, or cooked black beans to a pork and veggie stir-fry.

THE GRAINS—AND MORE—TO AVOID

Review the AGR list for grains on pages 471–472. A lot of these grains, including brown rice and brown-rice cakes, are in the "eat sparingly" category. On the AGR list for vegetables on pages 468–469, you'll also see that sweet corn and white potatoes in any form (French fried, baked, mashed) are in the "eat sparingly" column. All these foods are very high in carbohydrates and relatively low in nutrients; their GI rankings are very high, and so are their GL rankings. Even once you have reached your weight goal and normalized your blood sugar, we advise that you still treat these foods as very rare treats—in the same

STARCH-BLOCKING BEANS

An extract made from white kidney beans is now widely sold as an over-the-counter "starch blocker." These heavily advertised products claim to "neutralize" the starch in high-carb foods. All you have to do, the ads claim, is take a couple of these pills at the start of a meal, and they'll block your absorption of about 75 percent of the calories you eat from carbo-hydrates. Starch-blocking products do contain a substance found natu-rally in white kidney beans (as well as some other beans and also wheat) that inhibits or blocks amylase, the enzyme your body uses to break down carbohydrates in your intestinal tract. In fact, the starch-blocker supplements work in a similar way to the prescription drug acarbose (Precose or Glyset).

Both the supplements and the prescription drugs have serious draw-backs. They're not meant to aid weight loss—they're designed to help control blood sugar—but that doesn't stop unscrupulous manufactur-ers from pushing the supplements as a way to lose weight while eating all you want of anything you want. No studies of acarbose have shown that the drug causes weight loss, although a few studies have shown that some people with impaired glucose tolerance are less likely to become diabetic if they take the drug.[3, 4] The side effects of blocking carbohy-drate digestion can be very unpleasant. Severe cramps, diarrhea, and gas are likely. Many people using acarbose experience flatulence. Dr. Atkins never prescribed acarbose. Why take a costly drug with nasty side effects when you can benefit your health considerably more by controlling the carbs in your diet to begin with?

category as birthday cake. They can never again become a regular part of your diet without your suffering immediate consequences. Nearly eliminating these foods from your diet may take some getting used to, but as you continue to feel the improvements in your health the ABSCP brings, you'll find there's little room on your plate for low-quality carbs.

WHAT'S YOUR CARB IQ?

1. Which beans are preferable?
   a. lentils or black-eyed peas
   b. chickpeas or pinto beans
   c. baked beans or kidney beans
2. Which grains should you choose?
   a. white rice or barley
   b. old-fashioned oatmeal or instant oatmeal
   c. brown rice or buckwheat groats (kasha)
3. Which fruits should you choose?
   a. mango or apple
   b. raspberries or banana
   c. strawberries or grapes
   d. kiwifruit or blueberries

Answers

1. a, lentils; b. chickpeas; c. kidney beans. 2. a, barley; b. old-fashioned oatmeal; c, buckwheat groats. 3. a, apple; b, raspberries; c, strawberries; d, blueberries.

Chapter 18

SUGAR NATION

The amount of sugar we consume in this country is incredible. In one year, the average person eats about 150 pounds of added sugar![1] Sugar comes in all different forms: table sugar (sucrose), high-fructose corn syrup, honey, and maple syrup, to name just a few. Unfortunately, almost all of that sugar, no matter what its form, is consumed in low-quality, high-carb foods or soft drinks. All those sweet, nutritionally empty foods go a long way to explaining our frighteningly high rates of obesity and diabetes. It also helps explain why today's kids and teenagers are at such high risk of becoming overweight—an outrageous situation that grows more dire with every passing year.

Sugars of all sorts, with a few exceptions, raise your insulin and blood sugar levels almost instantly. That's not a good idea for anyone, but it's especially risky for people with the metabolic syndrome, prediabetes, and diabetes. Fortunately, today's sugar substitutes include some good-tasting, safe alternatives. On the Atkins Blood Sugar Control Program (ABSCP), you can easily eliminate added sugar (as opposed to naturally occurring sugars in vegetables, fruits, and other carbohydrates) from your menus and still enjoy a healthy, varied diet.

BREAKING THE SUGAR ADDICTION

For some people, however, sugar is more than a sweet taste—it's an "addiction." Here's what happens: When your blood sugar drops, you instinctively seek something rich in carbohydrates—usually a sugary snack—to bring it back up. That's the insidious beginning of the sugar addiction that plagues so many of us today. If you have the metabolic syndrome, prediabetes, or diabetes, you're a lot more likely to have unstable blood sugar. When your blood sugar drops, you may feel tired, irritable, or shaky, or experience mood swings—feelings you know you can soothe by eating high-carb foods. But when you bring your blood sugar back up by eating those foods, you're likely to overshoot and have your blood sugar spike higher than normal (hyperglycemia). What happens then? You might feel better for a couple of hours, until the extra insulin your body pumps out causes your blood sugar level once again to drop too low (hypoglycemia)—and the roller-coaster cycle starts all over again. You end up craving and eating sugary foods as a way to treat your blood sugar swings and the many symptoms that come with them.

By controlling your carbs and sharply reducing the amount of sugary foods you eat, as you do on the ABSCP, you break the sugar cycle. You don't get the ups and downs that make you crave high-carb foods, your energy stays steady, and mood swings end. Your blood sugar is under control—and that helps you get other aspects of your health under control as well.

COPING WITH CRAVINGS

When you switch to the ABSCP, you're giving up added sugar, including natural sweeteners such as honey or molasses. You can still enjoy plenty of delicious treats, but the sweet taste will come from substitute sweeteners and from the naturally occurring sugars found in low-GI fruits such as berries. When you start the program, however, you'll be cutting back considerably on even those foods as part of the overall process of learning to eat in a healthier new way—and unlearning old eating habits.

As you go through your first few weeks without sugar, you may have cravings—sometimes very strong cravings—for the sugary, high-carb foods you've left behind. It's a common experience for people starting out on the controlled-carb path. Most people are able to master the cravings with a few simple strategies. Look back at Chapter 17 for some good carb-craving busters. To quell the specific need for something sweet, try either a drink sweetened with your favorite sugar substitute (tea and decaf coffee are good appetite quenchers) or, if you really feel yourself in danger of straying, opt for a low-carb treat. Try a small amount of sugar-free gelatin with real whipped heavy cream (you can sweeten it with a substitute sweetener). If you simply must have chocolate, your best bet is a low-carb protein bar. Be aware, however, that eating low-carb sweets instead of high-carb ones won't necessarily help you break your carb addiction.

The good news is that these intense early cravings are temporary. As you progress on the ABSCP, you'll find that your sugar cravings will quickly diminish or even vanish. Once you've gotten your blood sugar under control by following the program, you'll probably find that you've gotten your sweet tooth under control as well. People who follow the Atkins Nutritional Approach (ANA) or the ABSCP, generally find that most cravings vanish by the end of the first week. They lose their taste for sugary foods—cookies and candy seem unbearably sweet and even small portions of the acceptably sweetened products are more than enough.

For those rare cases where sugar cravings continue to be a problem, supplements of the amino acid L-glutamine can help. Dr. Atkins often recommended one or two tablets 30 minutes before meals.

HIDDEN SUGAR

Think those cookies sweetened with concentrated fruit juice instead of white sugar are somehow "healthier" for you? Think again. Sugar is sugar, whether it is called fructose, sucrose, glucose, or lactose. Ditto for words like *syrup* or *concentrate*. Every teaspoon of sugar contains 4 grams of carbohydrates and has a glycemic index rating of 100. That means the sugar you consume, especially when it's in liquid form such as soda pop, turns into sugar in your bloodstream almost as soon as you swallow it.[2]

Similarly, don't fall for misleading food labels. Beware of words like *no sugar added* or *contains only natural sugars*. Always check the label. The product may still contain a lot of carbs in the form of some sort of natural sugar that can upset your insulin/blood sugar levels and start the roller coaster again.

Be aware of serving sizes, too. Products that claim to be low in sugar are—but the portion size might be unrealistically small. You could end up eating a lot more carbs than you realize. The bottom line is this: Eat no foods with any ingredients listed in "Spot the Sugar."

SPOT THE SUGAR

Food manufacturers have a lot of different ways to sneak sugar into their products under another name. If you spot any of these words on the ingredients list, the product contains added sugar:

Brown sugar
Brown syrup
Cane juice
Corn sweetener
Corn syrup
Corn syrup solids
Crystallized cane juice
Dextrose
Evaporated cane juice
Fructose
Fruit juice concentrate
Fruit syrups
Galactose
Glucose

(continued)

Glucose-derived syrup
Golden syrup
High-fructose corn syrup
Honey
Invert sugar
Lactose
Levulose
Malt
Maltose
Malt syrup
Maple sugar
Maple syrup
Molasses
Rapadura
Raw sugar
Rice syrup
Sucrose (table sugar—not to be confused with sucralose, a substitute
   sweetener marketed as Splenda)
Sweetened carob powder
Treacle
Turbinado

No matter what it's called, added sugar is unacceptable on any phase
of the ANA or ABSCP—especially for those of you with impaired in-
sulin/blood sugar metabolism.

JUST ANOTHER CARBOHYDRATE?

For many years, people with diabetes were told not to eat sugar because it would raise their blood sugar. In 1993, however, the American
Diabetes Association (ADA) modified its stance, based on a lack of
any real scientific evidence that small amounts of sugar in the diet—
as long as it was part of a regular meal plan and eaten along with

other foods—raised blood sugar. In other words, sugar was now to be treated as "just another carbohydrate" in the official diabetic diet.

There's a big problem with that approach. It's true that a teaspoon of table sugar contains only 4 grams of carbohydrates, and that simply eating a spoonful of sugar as part of a larger meal is unlikely to have much effect on your blood sugar. Unfortunately, it's pretty unlikely that you'll have just a teaspoon of sugar. If you're like most Americans, your diet contains the equivalent of about 20 teaspoons of pure sugar every day (not counting the natural sugars in fruits and other foods). That works out to 80 grams of nutritionally empty carbohydrates every day. A lot of that sugar is contained in high-carb baked goods made with bleached flour and manufactured trans fats. The rest might come from candy and soft drinks, products that are about equal in their abundance of carbs and lack of nutrition. A typical 12-ounce can of cola contains about 9 teaspoons of sugar in the form of high-fructose corn syrup, about the same amount of sugar found in a candy bar.

Realistically, if you know you're "allowed" to eat sugar on your ADA-approved diabetic diet, you will. And if you're a sugar addict, even a small amount will get you started again. Even if you are not addicted, why waste your carb grams on sugar, when you could be using those same carb grams to enjoy foods that are much more nutritionally valuable and will allow you to be more comfortably in control of your blood sugar? Once you are in control, your chances of long-term success will improve dramatically.

SUITABLE ALTERNATIVES

Today's substitute sweeteners are very useful tools in the controlled-carb approach. They let people enjoy sweet flavors without adding significant carbs to the diet and without raising blood sugar in most people. You still have to watch out for other carbohydrates, however. For example, controlled-carb ice creams, including the Atkins brand, do not include added sugar, but they do contain naturally occurring sugars in the form of lactose. Moreover, most cookies made with artificial sweeteners are still loaded with carbs from bleached white flour—and they're often full of trans fats as well. But for making low-carb sweet treats such as puddings, cheesecake, and gelatin desserts, and for use at the table instead of sugar, substitute sweeteners are ideal.

WHICH SWEETENER TO USE?

So many different sweeteners are available today that the array on the grocery shelves can be a little confusing. To a certain extent, your choice of sweetener depends on what you want to do with it. Some sweeteners, such as aspartame, lose their sweet taste when heated, so you wouldn't use them in cooked foods. Beyond that, follow your personal preferences. Some people can detect an aftertaste from some sweeteners, while others don't notice it; you may also be concerned about possible health effects from certain substitute sweeteners. Try the following different sweeteners until you find the ones you like:

- *Sucralose* (Splenda). The only noncaloric sweetener made from sugar, sucralose is 600 times sweeter than sucrose (table sugar). It is highly stable and doesn't break down in heat, so it is widely used in cooking and baking.
- *Acesulfame K* (acesulfame potassium) (Sweet One, Sunett). A noncaloric sweetener that is about 200 times sweeter than sucrose, acesulfame K holds up to heat and can be used in cooking and baking.
- *Saccharin* (Sweet'n Low). A noncaloric sweetener that has been in use for nearly a century and is about 300 times sweeter than sugar, saccharin turns bitter when heated and should not be used in cooking and baking. In 2000, the FDA removed saccharin from the list of carcinogenic products, citing the lack of evidence that it causes cancer in humans. Products containing saccharin no longer have to carry a warning label, although many still do.
- *Stevia.* Extracted from the leaves of a plant called *Stevia rebaudiana*, stevia is about 300 times sweeter than sucrose. Although stevia is safe and has been widely used around the world since its discovery in 1931, in the United States it can be sold only as a dietary supplement. It can be found in any natural foods store.

- *Aspartame* (NutraSweet, Equal). A low-calorie sweetener that is about 180 times sweeter than sucrose, aspartame is used very widely in sugar-free beverages and foods. It breaks down when heated, so it cannot be used in cooking or baking. Atkins Nutritionals does not use aspartame in its products.

All of the preceding sweeteners are often described as intense because they are so much sweeter than sugar. Very small amounts are needed, but even so they do add small amounts of carbohydrates to the products that contain them. FDA regulations allow food manufacturers to say a product has no carbs when it has less than 1 gram of carbohydrate per serving—but even fractions of grams can add up. We recommend that you count each packet of sweetener as 1 gram of Net Carbs so that you do not exceed your carb threshold.

SUGAR ALCOHOLS

Sugar alcohols don't contain alcohol in the conventional sense of rubbing alcohol or alcohol you can drink. Sugar alcohols, also known as polyols, are carbohydrate-based caloric sweeteners; if it ends in -*ol*, it's a sugar alcohol. The most commonly used sugar alcohols in low-carb foods are mannitol, sorbitol, xylitol, lactitol, and maltitol. Isomalt and hydrogenated starch hydrolysates (HSH) are also sugar alcohols. (Although glycerol and glycerin are not sugar alcohols, they also have minimal impact on blood sugar.)

Sugar alcohols are found naturally in many foods. Mannitol, for instance, is found in carrots, pineapples, olives, asparagus, and sweet potatoes. Sorbitol is in many fruits and vegetables. Xylitol is also found in fruits and vegetables—as well as mushrooms and even corncobs.

Sugar alcohols aren't as sweet as sugar, and they contain only about one-half to one-third the calories. What makes sugar alcohols so useful as sweeteners is that the carbs in some of the sugar alcohols are absorbed very slowly by your body—so slowly that they don't really have an impact on your blood sugar. In others, such as lactitol and xylitol, there is little or no conversion to glucose.[3] Most of the carbs from sugar alcohols will pass out of your body before they're absorbed, so sugar alcohols don't add much to your daily carb count. On the glycemic index, sugar alcohols are extremely low. Xylitol, for instance, is ranked at 7—compare that with table sugar, which is ranked at 100.

Sugar alcohols don't raise blood sugar in most people, but there are exceptions. Some people seem to be sensitive to sugar alcohols, especially mannitol, and do get a rise in their blood sugar after eating foods containing them, especially if they eat large amounts. Sugar alcohols in large amounts (more than 25 grams a day) can also cause gas and cramping or have a laxative effect in some people. Xylitol and lactitol are generally the worst culprits in these cases; maltitol and erythritol are the least likely to cause problems. In some people, sugar alcohols may elevate blood sugar. If you are diabetic, be sure to check your blood sugar approximately 90 minutes after eating foods that contain sugar alcohols. If there is an abnormal increase in your blood sugar, discontinue such foods. You can try reintroducing them when your metabolism improves.

SUGAR ALCOHOLS AND FOOD LABELS

Chemists don't classify sugar alcohols as carbohydrates, but the Food and Drug Administration does. That's because the law says that after the fat, protein, ash (minerals), and water are removed from a product, what's left is carbohydrate and has to be listed as such on the food label. There's logic but not a lot of common sense behind this, because sugar alcohols aren't really metabolized and don't usually have an impact on your blood sugar. To comply with the FDA, the manufacturers of controlled-carb products that contain sugar alcohols have to list them as total carbs on the food facts label, just as they do for fiber. When calculating the Net Carbs of a food, simply subtract the grams of fiber and sugar alcohols.

An interesting fact: The sugar alcohol xylitol inhibits the growth of bacteria in the mouth, so products that contain it, such as chewing gum and breath mints, are allowed to claim that they can help prevent tooth decay.

In low-carb products, sugar alcohols not only add sweetness, they also add bulk and texture and help the products retain moisture. Sugar alcohols hold up well to heat, so they can be used in commercial cooking and baking. They are not marketed for home use.

FRUCTOSE: THE DIABETES CULPRIT?

Back in 1975, the annual per capita consumption of refined sugars (as opposed to natural sugars) in the United States was about 117 pounds a year. Of that, almost all was sucrose, or table sugar. Twenty years later, the annual per capita consumption of refined sugars in the United States had zoomed to 149 pounds a year. Of that, 66 pounds was sucrose; the other 83 pounds was in the form of high-fructose corn syrup.[4] This inexpensive sweetener is very widely used in soft drinks, baked goods, candy, and other sugary foods. It's possible that this huge increase in the amount of fructose in the average American's diet is one of the major culprits behind both the obesity and diabetes epidemics.

When you consume fructose—by swallowing 12 ounces of a soft drink sweetened with high-fructose corn syrup, for example—your blood sugar, of course, goes up. Technically, fructose doesn't immediately stimulate your pancreas to release insulin, but the breakdown products of fructose do stimulate insulin release. We know from human and animal studies that consuming a high-fructose diet leads to increased appetite, increased body weight, and increased fat—and we know from animal studies that fructose brings on insulin resistance and high blood pressure. At the same time, fructose can raise your blood lipids by making your liver produce more triglycerides and possibly by increasing insulin resistance in other cells in your body. If your cholesterol is high to begin with, or if you have the metabolic syndrome, prediabetes, or diabetes, this could cause your total cholesterol, your triglycerides, and your LDL cholesterol to go even higher.[5]

When you follow the Atkins Blood Sugar Control Program you give up all those foods sweetened with high-fructose corn syrup, so fructose will be less of a problem for you. Fructose is naturally found in fruit, but in combination with fiber, pectin, and other substances;

therefore whole fruit is less likely to have these negative effects. Even so, you need to be aware of the carbohydrates in the fruit you consume. Even low-GI fruits such as strawberries have carbs—be very aware of portion size. If you're having trouble getting your blood sugar down, you may need to eliminate fruit from your diet completely. Once your blood sugar is under control, however, you can slowly reintroduce fruit in moderation, depending on your individual metabolic response. (See Chapter 16 for more on this.)

Dr. Atkins would often encounter patients who told him they were willing to try his approach, but just couldn't live without chocolate, or ice cream, or some other sugary treat. He would remind them that there are plenty of good low-carb versions of these favorites, but would also ask them to give up these foods, at least during the first few weeks. When the patients returned, they almost always told him how they no longer missed sweet foods. And in the next breath, they would tell him how much more energy they now had. It always gave him great pleasure to point out the connection between the two. By eliminating sugar and controlling their carbs, these fortunate folks had gotten off the blood sugar roller coaster. Instead of struggling with energy ups and downs, they now had stable blood sugar, which gave them a steady supply of energy. They did it—so can you.

WHAT'S YOUR SWEETENER IQ?

1. How many carb grams are in 1 teaspoon of table sugar?
   a. 9
   b. 4
   c. 6
   d. 1
2. Which of the following ingredients are disguises for sugar?
   a. corn sweetener
   b. dextrose
   c. fruit juice concentrate
   d. malt syrup
   e. molasses

3. Which of the following are acceptable substitute sweeteners?
   a. maple syrup
   b. sucralose
   c. saccharin
   d. sweetened carob powder

Answers

1. b. 2. all of them. 3. b, c.

Chapter 19

DRINK TO YOUR HEALTH

When you first begin controlling your carbs, your focus is understandably going to be on what you can and can't eat. Don't forget, however, that you'll likely need to make some changes in what you drink. If you're not a big water drinker, it's time to develop a relationship with the office water cooler. It's all too easy to forget that the liquid carbs count just as much as the solids. On the Atkins Blood Sugar Control Program (ABSCP), you also need to give careful thought to the pros and cons of drinking alcohol.

STAY LIQUID

Most medical authorities agree: For good health, you should drink at least 64 ounces of water each day. That's eight 8-ounce glasses, or 2 quarts, or about 2 liters. (However, individuals diagnosed with renal function decline need to follow the advice of their physician with regard to water intake.) That might sound like a lot, but it really isn't, especially when you spread it out over the day. Bear in mind that a typical can of soda pop or other beverage contains 12 ounces, and that today's supersized beverages often contain 20 ounces or more. These beverages do not count toward your 2 liters a day; water is still the best drink of all and diet sodas should be only a small part of your daily fluid intake.

Getting plenty of fluids keeps your system hydrated and flushes waste products from your body efficiently. Regardless of your dietary approach, if you drink less than you should, you may experience constipation and an increased risk of kidney stones.

There's another problem with not drinking enough: It may increase your food intake. That's because it's common to confuse thirst with hunger, especially if both sensations happen at the same time. Instead of drinking, you eat. That fools you into thinking your thirst has been quenched, even though you haven't taken in any fluids. Next time you feel hungry between meals, try drinking something instead, or having a drink along with a small protein/fat snack such as some nuts or a piece of cheese. You may be surprised to see how quickly your hunger goes away. Likewise, having something to drink before you eat a main meal may help you avoid overeating. The liquid fills you up a bit so that your meal satisfies you faster. For some reason, hot drinks seem to work better than cold ones—try a cup of hot tea or herbal tea or some hot broth about half an hour before suppertime.

By the time your body signals that it's time for some fluid, you're already a little dried out. Also, as you get older, your sense of thirst generally gets less acute, and it's easier to become dehydrated. You also need to drink more in both hot *and* cold weather. Hot weather makes you lose fluid by sweating; in cold weather, the air is usually dry, which pulls moisture from your body.

THIRST IS A DANGER SIGNAL

Increased thirst, increased hunger, and increased urination are all classic symptoms of diabetes. If you notice these symptoms, even if you've already been diagnosed with diabetes, check with your doctor immediately. (See Chapter 6, Diagnosis: Diabetes.)

WATER, PURE AND SIMPLE

What's the best thing to drink when you're following the ABSCP? Water. Convenient and carb-free, water is the way to go. Bottled water, mineral water, and filtered water are good choices. If you prefer something with a bit of flavor, look for no-carb flavored water and flavored seltzers; you can also add a squirt of lemon or lime juice or some sugar-free flavored syrup to your water or club soda.

Fruit juice, despite its reputation for being "healthy," is actually high in carbohydrates and low in fiber. Whether they're made only with pure fruit juice or contain some juice and additional high-fructose corn syrup, fruit juices are higher on the glycemic index than whole fruit.[1] Whole fruit is a better choice if your carb threshold allows you to include fruit, because the fiber content slows down the absorption of fructose.[2-4] Once your palate adjusts to your new eating style, you will be amazed by how sweet fruit juice tastes.

NOT MILK?

When you choose your beverages, remember that an 8-ounce glass of whole milk has more than 11 grams of carbohydrates, mostly in the form of lactose, or milk sugar. It's not acceptable on Induction. For active kids and teenagers who can add more carbs to their diet, however, using up some carbs each day on a glass or two of full-fat milk is fine—the protein and calcium in the milk are important nutrients. If you want the taste of milk without all the carbs, try one of the new reduced-carb dairy beverages, which have about 3 grams of Net Carbs per cup. Those few grams of carbs are in the form of lactose, however. If you're very lactose intolerant, you still might not be able to drink these beverages.

You'll still be getting dietary calcium when you follow the ABSCP, because you'll be eating a lot of green vegetables, along with cheese and nuts. (One ounce of almonds has 80 mg of calcium and about 4 grams of Net Carbs.) Leafy green vegetables, such as kale, Swiss chard, collard greens, and broccoli, are excellent sources of calcium. Unlike milk, they also contain the other vitamins, minerals, and flavonoids that are essential for helping your body absorb calcium and use it to build your bones.

You may have heard something about calcium in greens not being absorbed as easily. The calcium in some greens is bound up to some extent by other natural substances such as phytates and oxalates. Some dark leafy greens, such as beet greens, spinach, and Swiss chard, are high in oxalate. Individuals with a predisposition to form calcium oxalate kidney stones should consult with their physicians. The calcium in broccoli, however, is easily absorbed. Cheese is a great source of calcium—and it's definitely an indulgence you can enjoy during all phases of Atkins. One ounce of Cheddar cheese has 204 mg of calcium. Some emerging research also suggests that the calcium and protein in dairy products may have a potential benefit for weight loss.[5]

CAFFEINE AND YOUR BLOOD SUGAR

Coffee and tea are the world's most popular beverages, and that means caffeine is perhaps the world's most widely used drug. Caffeine is perfectly legal, of course—in fact, caffeine is the only drug that can legally be added to foods in the United States. You may find that caffeine can cause a slight, temporary rise in your blood pressure; it may also interfere with your sleep. Excessive caffeine also seems to have an effect on blood sugar and insulin—so, especially at the beginning of the ABSCP, you may want to switch entirely to decaffeinated beverages. (See Caffeine and Insulin on page 238.)

Tea is a better source of caffeine than coffee because it also contains a lot of valuable antioxidants and other substances, such as vitamin K, which can benefit your health. We discourage excessive caffeine intake, but 1 or 2 cups of green tea or black tea a day may well be beneficial. However, if you have blood sugar abnormalities or diabetes, you may find that you are more sensitive to caffeine and may need to limit it.

CAFFEINE AND INSULIN

A study in 1993 confirmed what Dr. Atkins had long observed in many of his patients with unstable blood sugar: Caffeine in large quantities can make you feel hungry, even if your blood sugar is normal. The amount of caffeine used in the study was 400 mg, or about the amount found in 4 cups of strong brewed coffee.[6]

Two studies in 2002 suggested that caffeine can decrease insulin sensitivity. In the first study, 12 healthy volunteers were given either a caffeine-loading dose or a placebo and their insulin response was measured. When they got the caffeine, their insulin sensitivity decreased by about 15 percent. The amount given was equal to a "moderate" caffeine intake. The authors noted that the decrease in insulin sensitivity was roughly the same as the improvement in insulin sensitivity that is obtained from drugs used to control blood sugar, such as metformin.[7] The second study looked at the effects of caffeine on how well skeletal muscles took up glucose—another way of looking at the effect of caffeine on insulin resistance. Seven healthy volunteers were given doses of caffeine and then they exercised for an hour; their blood was tested for insulin levels before and after. The researchers concluded that caffeine decreased the ability of the muscles to take up glucose, although exercise can reduce the effect of caffeine.[8]

Do the studies indicating that caffeine increases insulin resistance mean you should give up your morning coffee? Not necessarily—unless you are unusually sensitive to caffeine, but it does mean you should have no more than 1 or 2 cups of caffeinated coffee a day, taken with meals.

When you get up in the morning, your blood sugar may well be on the low side, because you haven't eaten anything during all the hours you were asleep. But if you have a breakfast of only java, or coffee with a sweet roll, you'll probably spike your blood sugar too high. A few hours later, your blood sugar could crash and send you on a seek-and-devour mission for carbs and more coffee. Following the ABSCP, however, you start the day with a good breakfast containing protein, fat, and a small amount of allowable carbohydrates along with your morning cup of coffee. That keeps your blood sugar steady and maintains it on an even keel for several hours. You'll then find it much easier to resist the doughnuts in the break room later in the morning.

If you can bite the bullet and substitute decaf for regular coffee, you may find that your carbohydrate cravings decrease. If you're a confirmed caffeine addict, taper off slowly by combining caffeinated and decaffeinated coffee and then gradually increasing the amount of decaf over a week or so. (Watch out for flavored coffee drinks, even if they are decaf. They often contain added carbs and trans fats. Choose sugar-free, milk-free versions.) Although tea has far less caffeine than coffee (only about 50 mg in 8 ounces of brewed tea), you may also experience mild withdrawal symptoms if you go cold turkey—follow the same combination approach, using decaffeinated tea.

Most colas and some other soft drinks contain caffeine—in fact, some have added caffeine for an extra jolt. If you want to consume soft drinks, choose the sugar-free, caffeine-free versions. And be aware that those caffeine-laden energy drinks in the little cans are full of carbs.

Some herbal teas, such as maté and guarana, and tea mixtures also contain caffeine. Most herbal teas are caffeine-free, however, and make a good alternative to caffeinated coffee and tea. Caffeine also occurs naturally in chocolate, although the amounts are minimal— about 20 mg in an ounce of dark chocolate.

TEA AND YOUR HEALTH

Tea—either black tea, the kind most commonly consumed in the United States, or green tea—can have a very positive effect on your health. Numerous studies of large groups of people have consistently shown that those who drink the most tea also have the lowest risk of heart disease. In a study of men and women in the Boston area, for example, the participants who drank at least 1 cup of tea a day had a 44 percent lower risk of a heart attack than those who drank no tea.[9]

When it comes to controlling blood sugar, it's also possible that tea can be helpful. In a study in Taiwan in 2003, twenty people with diabetes who were taking an antihyperglycemic drug were randomly assigned also to drink either 1,500 ml (about 6 cups) of oolong tea (a type of tea that is halfway between black and green) or an equal

RESEARCH REPORT: THE HEALTH BENEFITS OF TEA

A daily cup or two of brewed black or green tea could be beneficial to your overall health—and might even help speed up weight loss. One health benefit is that tea can help keep your bones strong as you age. A study of over 1,200 older British women found that those who drank tea had higher bone mineral density levels in their spines and hips than those who drank no tea at all. Because higher bone mineral density generally means a lower risk of fracture (from falling, for example), it appears that tea had a definite protective effect for these women.[10]

What about tea and weight loss? There is some suggestive evidence that green tea could increase your metabolic rate and slightly help speed up weight loss. A recent study of ten healthy young men showed that when they took capsules containing green tea extract, they had an increase in their energy expenditure that was greater than when they took capsules containing caffeine or fiber. In other words, the green tea extract made their metabolism run faster so they burned more fat. The study is a small one, done on healthy young men in a highly controlled setting. Even so, it shows that it's not the caffeine in tea that causes the metabolic increase. The researchers believe the effect comes from the catechins, a group of natural chemicals found in tea.[11]

amount of plain water every day for 30 days. They then switched off and repeated the process. The researchers found that after 30 days of tea drinking, the participants had markedly lower blood sugar levels. There was no change after 30 days of drinking plain water.[12] It's probably the catechins and other chemicals called polyphenols in tea—not the caffeine—that have the beneficial effect.

Given all the other beneficial effects of tea, Dr. Atkins recommended drinking 1 to 2 cups of brewed green tea each day. This type of tea has the most catechins and polyphenols and the least caffeine, with only about 30 mg to 40 mg per 6-ounce cup. There's no reason not to sweeten the tea with your favorite sugar substitute if you like. Let the tea steep for at least three minutes in boiling water to get the most benefit from the leaves.

TO IMBIBE OR NOT?

The question of whether you should drink alcoholic beverages is a complex one without an easy answer. Some recent research suggests that moderate alcohol consumption in the form of red wine may decrease your risk of diabetes and possibly decrease oxidative stress.[13] Even so, the researchers are always quick to point out that the benefits of alcohol are very minor relative to other steps such as losing weight and exercising more.

Alcohol in Moderation

Once your insulin/blood sugar metabolism has normalized and other markers, such as high blood pressure, have gone down, you can enjoy a glass of wine or other low-carb alcoholic beverage, but we strongly recommend that you limit your alcohol consumption to no more than one drink a day—and preferably less. (And remember, Induction is an alcohol-free zone.) To minimize the effects of alcohol, always have it with a meal that contains protein and dietary fat. A drink is one standard unit of alcohol: 12 ounces of beer, 1.5 ounces of distilled spirits (gin, rum, vodka, whiskey, scotch, bourbon), or 4 ounces of wine.

Drawbacks of Alcohol

People with blood sugar problems need to be aware of alcohol's drawbacks:

- Alcohol can interfere with weight loss, because your body will burn the alcohol before it burns fat.[14]
- If you are in ketosis, you may experience a decreased tolerance for alcohol.

- If you have unstable blood sugar, the metabolic syndrome, or diabetes, drinking on an empty stomach or having more than one or two drinks could trigger symptoms. In clinical practice, people with diabetes, especially those with Type 1, are cautioned on the use of alcohol.[15]
- Excessive alcohol intake can worsen some health problems caused by diabetes, such as high triglycerides, neuropathy, and high blood pressure.[16]
- Excessive alcohol can distort the results of the glycated hemoglobin blood test and make them seem higher than they are. (Check Chapter 6 for more information on this test.)[17]

The bottom line is this: Only if your blood sugar is under control can you consume a moderate amount of alcohol (one drink or less a day) and then only as part of a full meal.

WHAT'S YOUR FLUID IQ?

1. How many ounces of water should you drink each day?
   a. 16
   b. 32
   c. 64
   d. 128
2. Which of these beverages contain caffeine?
   a. coffee
   b. tea
   c. orange juice
   d. maté
   e. ginger ale
3. Green and black tea may:
   a. help speed weight loss
   b. strengthen bones
   c. help prevent heart attacks
   d. all of the above
   e. none of the above

4. A standard serving of wine is:
   a. 1 ounce
   b. 4 ounces
   c. 8 ounces
   d. ¼ of a bottle

Answers
1. c, 2. a, b, d, 3. d, 4. b.

Chapter 20

GETTING EXTRA HELP: SUPPLEMENTS FOR BLOOD SUGAR CONTROL

Let's be clear from the start: Dr. Atkins did not have any magic pills that will solve your insulin/blood sugar problems and simultaneously make you lose weight. No supplement can substitute for the permanent dietary changes that are integral to getting your blood sugar under control and losing weight. Nor has anyone invented a supplement that replaces the need for exercise.

Nonetheless, certain supplementary nutrients can help counteract some of the damaging effects of high blood sugar; others can play a supporting role in your blood sugar control campaign. Because of the state of your health or because of poor eating habits up to now, you may also be low in some important vitamins and minerals and may need supplements to ensure that you're getting basic, optimal nutrition. In this chapter, we'll focus on the value of specific nutrients for conditions related to abnormal blood sugar and obesity. Chapter 21 will look at supplements for high blood pressure and heart health.

WHY RECOMMEND SUPPLEMENTS?

Most, but not all, of the supplements discussed in this chapter are common vitamins and minerals that you've heard of throughout your

RESEARCH REPORT: ONE A DAY

Does taking a daily multivitamin/mineral supplement really improve health?[1] Unquestionably. Here's one good example of how: A study in 2003 looked at whether people who took a daily multivitamin/mineral had fewer infections than people who didn't. Researchers divided 130 adults into two groups. One group took a daily multisupplement for a year; the other group took a placebo. Neither the participants nor the researchers knew who was getting the real pill and who was getting the dummy. Over the course of the year, 43 percent of those who took the supplement had an infectious illness such as a cold or flu; 73 percent of the people who took the placebo got sick. Particularly revealing is that among the 51 participants with diabetes, 93 percent of the placebo takers got sick, but only 17 percent of the supplement takers did. The research showed that the benefit of supplements for diabetics was significant, unlike the nondiabetics, where the data revealed no difference between the treatment group and the placebo group. However, as a practitioner of complementary medicine, Dr. Atkins routinely used a good-quality multivitamin supplement as the foundation for the nutrient arm of his therapies.[2]

life. A few others are valuable substances that have been shown to be very helpful for people with blood sugar problems and associated risks. Although some are not yet in the medical mainstream, there is research to back them up.

Dr. Atkins first began prescribing supplements to his patients in the 1970s, both for therapeutic purposes and to optimize health. He often recommended higher doses than the government's minimal RDA (recommended dietary allowance), now known as DRI (dietary reference intake). However, beyond the DRI, Dr. Atkins believed strongly that supplements can play an important role in optimizing health and minimizing exposure to needless drug therapy. He was also convinced that we can no longer rely on obtaining an adequate supply of many nutrients from our foods.

First, it's difficult to find vegetables that are grown in nutrient-rich soil; overfarming and chemical treatments have depleted the soil in which most of our produce is grown. Second, the loss of vitamins from processing, transportation, and cooking is significant. You're just not getting the fresh, nutrient-abundant vegetables our preindustrialized ancestors did. When you consider these factors, you can understand Dr. Atkins' interest in enhancing nutrition with vitamin and mineral supplements.

Added to that is the fact that many of you with evidence of insulin/blood sugar problems already have suffered years of nutritional deficits as a result of the oxidative stress of a high-carbohydrate diet (we'll discuss this in more detail later in this chapter).[3] Although it might be possible to overcome this accumulated deficit with diet alone, we want you to regain your health as rapidly as possible, which means supplements are needed. After you read this chapter, we think you'll agree.

DEFINITIONS AND DIFFERENCES

A vitamin is an organic substance that your body needs but can't manufacture. Minerals are inorganic substances such as calcium and magnesium. Some minerals are essential, meaning that you must have them, even if only in very small amounts. You must get vitamins and minerals from the foods you eat and, if necessary, from supplements.

Vitamins and minerals are crucial for the smooth operation of the thousands of chemical processes that are constantly taking place in your body. You need a constant and adequate supply of all of them to create enzymes, hormones, neurotransmitters, and all the other complex substances that make your body run efficiently.

A genuine deficiency of any vitamin or mineral is very rare in individuals who live in developed countries. You're highly unlikely to get scurvy, the disease caused by a lack of vitamin C, for instance. The typical Western diet, however, often ends up low in vitamins and minerals because high-carb refined and heavily processed foods often crowd out fresh vegetables, nuts and seeds, berries and other fruits, beans, and whole grains. When you switch from the standard American diet

(SAD) to the Atkins Blood Sugar Control Program (ABSCP), your intake of vitamins and minerals from food automatically soars.

The foundation of any supplement program is a good-quality multivitamin/mineral. Unless your physician has prescribed iron supplements for you, choose a multivitamin that is iron-free, because elevated iron levels have been statistically associated in some studies with an increased incidence of Type 2 diabetes.[4] Your multivitamin should also contain no artificial colors, flavors, hydrogenated oils, corn or wheat (to which many people are sensitive), salt, sugar, starch, or gluten. As an example, a complete list of the nutrients in the Atkins Basic 3 multivitamin appears below. When supplements are needed for a particular purpose, they should be considered as an addition to, not as a replacement for, a multivitamin.

ATKINS BASIC 3 INGREDIENTS

SUPPLEMENT	AMOUNT PER SERVING
Vitamin A (as retinyl acetate and 60% from natural carotenoids)	10,000 IU
Vitamin C (as ascorbic acid)	300 mg
Vitamin D (as cholecalciferol)	200 IU
Vitamin E (as d-alpha-tocopheryl succinate)	150 IU
Thiamin (as thiamin HCl)	25 mg
Riboflavin	25 mg
Niacin (as niacinamide)	20 mg
Vitamin B$_6$ (as pyridoxine HCl)	25 mg
Folate (as folic acid)	400 mcg
Vitamin B$_{12}$ (as cyanocobalamin)	25 mcg
Biotin	300 mcg
Pantothenic acid (as D-calcium pantothenate)	60 mg
Calcium (as dicalcium phosphate, calcium ascorbate, and calcium citrate)	250 mg
Phosphorus (as dicalcium phosphate)	190 mg

(continued)

ATKINS BASIC 3 INGREDIENTS

SUPPLEMENT	AMOUNT PER SERVING
Magnesium (as magnesium oxide and glycinate)	125 mg
Zinc (as zinc citrate)	15 mg
Selenium (as sodium selenate)	70 mcg
Copper (as copper glycinate)	2 mg
Manganese (as manganese glycinate)	5 mg
Chromium (as chromium dinicotinate glycinate)	120 mcg
Molybdenum (as molybdenum glycinate)	75 mcg
Potassium (as potassium citrate)	297 mg
Boron (as calcium chelate)	0.2 mg
Vanadium (as vanadium BMOV)	40 mcg
Fruit and Vegetable Phytonutrient Concentrates: pineapple, broccoli, carrots, apple, orange, tomato, Brussels sprouts, cauliflower, beet, blueberry, celery, grape, grapefruit, kale, lemon, lime, plum, raspberry, strawberry, watermelon, radish, cantaloupe, cherry, leek, onion, papaya, peach, pear	200 mg
Soluble and Insoluble Fiber Base: vegetable cellulose, guar gum, and citrus pectin	300 mg
Absorb-Best: plant-source enzymes (acid-stable protease [from pineapple] and lipoprotein lipase), choleretic herbs (gentian root, orange peel), and Bioperine standardized black pepper extract	75 mg

THE ANTIOXIDANT CONNECTION

Even with a better diet, your intake of some important vitamins and minerals may still be on the low side for your needs. Why? Because high blood sugar, high insulin levels, and insulin resistance all cause your body to produce large amounts of free radicals. Your body is normally well supplied with antioxidants—enzymes and other substances that neutralize free radicals. But when your free-radical production is sky-high and your body can't make enough antioxidants to keep up, it is in a state of what's called oxidative stress. When free radicals aren't neutralized quickly, they end up doing significant damage to cells in your body, increasing your need for antioxidants. At the same time, in a process called glycation, the extra sugar in your blood can damage cells.

Damage from free radicals and glycation can contribute to the cycle of worsening diabetes. The current thinking about how this cycle works is this: Insulin resistance causes high levels of glucose in your blood, which causes glycation. Your pancreas pours out insulin to deal with the high blood sugar, resulting in hyperinsulinemia, which in turn causes excessive free-radical production. The oxidative stress of the free radicals can worsen insulin resistance by reducing the number of insulin receptors in your cell walls and impairing their ability to respond to insulin. The free radicals and glycation reduce the amount of insulin your pancreas can put out by damaging the beta cells. What happens then? More insulin resistance, more demand for insulin from damaged pancreatic beta cells, more glucose in your bloodstream— which in turn leads to more glycation and free radicals . . . we're sure you get the picture.

Oxidative stress can also do a lot of damage to your blood vessels and nerve endings, which results in most of the complications of diabetes, such as kidney disease, eye disease, neuropathy, and even the need for amputation. Oxidative stress is also thought to play a big role in creating the atherosclerotic plaques that can clog arteries and cause a heart attack or stroke.[5] (See Chapter 21 for more on this.)

The best way to avoid all those extra free radicals is to cut the carbs in your diet, lose weight, and be more active. Until you do, and even after you have done so, supplements can give you the extra antioxidants you need to neutralize those free radicals quickly, before they can do their damage.

Another reason supplements are important for people with blood sugar problems: Drugs taken for elevated blood sugar and other chronic conditions can interfere with the absorption of vitamins and minerals from food. Supplements can help make up the shortfall.

Important note: Supplements that help stabilize your blood sugar could have an effect on the blood sugar medications you're taking, as well as those you may be taking for other conditions, such as high blood pressure. We suggest that you work with a nutritionally oriented physician who understands and supports the application of the ABSCP and can help you decide which supplements (and dosages) are best for you. (See page 134 for help in finding this type of physician.) Before taking these or any other supplements, discuss a strategy with your doctor about how you will reduce or change your medications as your blood sugar and other values improve. Dosage ranges may differ from those used in other books by Dr. Atkins because they are specific to the issues discussed in this book. For other medical conditions or for patients with multiple conditions, he might as well have prescribed higher doses.

ANTIOXIDANT SUPPLEMENTS

Vitamins

Two vitamins are particularly important for fighting off free radicals: vitamin C and vitamin E. Overall, people with diabetes tend to have low levels of vitamin C, even when they get adequate amounts of it in their diet.[6] It's possible that hyperglycemia is the cause. Unfortunately, people with blood sugar problems need more vitamin C, not less, because vitamin C helps improve insulin action.[7] It appears that a good insurance policy for everyone, especially diabetics, is adding vitamin C to the supplement program. Vitamin C also helps improve the ability of blood vessels to open up and let blood flow through them easily.[8,9] Multiple studies have shown that vitamin C can help bring down high blood pressure and prevent heart disease. And in general, a diet rich in vitamin C lowers risk of death from all causes, including heart attack and stroke.[10,11]

Vitamin C. The DRI for vitamin C is 90 mg for men and 75 mg for women.[12] Getting that much and more from your diet is very easy. Vitamin C is found in all fresh vegetables and fruits (there's even some in meat, poultry, fish, and dairy products—and a small amount in legumes and grains). You'll be eating a lot of those foods on the ABSCP, so you'll easily meet and surpass the daily minimum. For example, there's 58 mg of vitamin C in ½ cup of cooked broccoli and 48 mg in ½ cup of cooked Brussels sprouts. If your daily carbohydrate total allows moderate amounts of low-glycemic fruits, you can get additional vitamin C that way. For example, there are 45 mg of vitamin C in ½ cup of strawberries.

Dr. Atkins felt that everyone should supplement with at least 1,000 mg of vitamin C every day, but if you have insulin/blood sugar imbalances, the minimum should be 2,000 mg (2 grams). Vitamin C is water-soluble, which means you don't really store it in your body—any excess simply washes out of your system. To keep your vitamin C levels up throughout the day, take half your dose in the morning and the other half in the evening. Large doses of vitamin C can cause diarrhea in some people. It is not likely to occur at this dose, but if this happens to you, cut back.

Vitamin E. Vitamin E supplements offer protection against oxidative stress in diabetics and probably improve metabolic control.[13] Another valuable benefit of vitamin E is its ability to lower inflammation levels, which are generally much higher than normal in people with diabetes.[14] Lowering inflammation is thought to help prevent heart disease by reducing free-radical levels and preventing the growth of plaque inside artery walls.

The DRI for vitamin E is 15 mg, or 22 IU (you may see it listed either way), which can be easily obtained from food, especially if you eat a lot of vegetables, nuts, and seeds.[15] But the value of vitamin E in preventing diabetes and other problems kicks in only at higher levels. We suggest taking 400 IU to 800 IU daily. (Please note: It has been observed in clinical practice that a few individuals experience elevated blood pressure while taking vitamin E; if your blood pressure goes up while taking a high dose, cut back.) If you have a tendency to get leg cramps, take your vitamin E at night. Many of Dr. Atkins' patients told him that taking it before bedtime helps relieve leg cramps.

Choose a brand of vitamin E that contains natural mixed tocopherols with selenium—this trace mineral works synergistically with vitamin E, enhancing its effectiveness as an antioxidant. If you cannot find vitamin E with selenium, be sure it is included in one of your other supplements.

Please note: If you're already taking a daily aspirin or other drugs to thin your blood, or if you have high blood pressure, discuss vitamin E supplements with your doctor first.

The B Family

All eight members of the B vitamin family are crucial for helping your body metabolize food and turn it into energy. That's especially important for people with the metabolic syndrome, prediabetes, or diabetes because you may use up these vitamins faster than do people with normal blood sugar. For that reason alone, Dr. Atkins recommended taking a daily supplement that contains, at a minimum, 100 percent of the DRIs for all of the Bs. If needed, in individual cases, he would use far more. We'll explain in the next chapter why some of the B vitamins are important for preventing heart disease.

Lipoic Acid for Neuropathy

Lipoic acid (also sometimes called alpha lipoic acid or thioctic acid) isn't technically a vitamin because you produce some of this powerful natural antioxidant in your body. It's a close relative of the B vitamins, though, so we'll discuss its value for treating diabetic neuropathy, a painful complication of diabetes. Neuropathy causes severe pain, tingling, and numbness, often in the legs; it's the result of damage to the nerve endings from years of high blood sugar levels and free radicals run amok.

Doctors in Europe have been prescribing lipoic acid for diabetic neuropathy for years—as did Dr. Atkins. Despite the fact that many studies over the years have shown its effectiveness, it's only recently that more American physicians have begun to use lipoic acid in treating neuropathy. The most recent study, reported in 2003, was a double-blind, randomized, placebo-controlled study that compared the effects of daily doses of 600 mg of intravenous lipoic acid on patients with similar degrees of diabetic neuropathy. Sixty of the patients got the lipoic acid; 60 got a placebo. After 14 treatments, the lipoic acid group showed remarkable improvement in pain and function, with no side effects. The placebo group didn't improve.[16]

Most studies of lipoic acid have used an intravenous dose or a combination of intravenous and oral doses. Dr. Atkins found that patients with milder neuropathies show improvement with oral treatment alone; more severe cases may need intravenous treatment under a doctor's care. For oral treatment, he recommended 600 mg a day in divided doses. If your condition is persistent, you may need to use lipoic acid for a minimum of three months before expecting to see symptoms diminish.

Biotin and Inositol

A member of the B family, biotin is an interesting vitamin because you don't get it from food, although some foods, such as egg yolks and nuts, contain biotin. Instead, bacteria in your small intestine manufacture it for you. The DRI for biotin is 30 mcg. Biotin, like the other B vitamins, is important for keeping your nerves functioning properly and for converting the fats and proteins you eat into energy. Large doses of biotin may be helpful in lowering your blood sugar by improving insulin sensitivity.[17-19] Moreover, like lipoic acid, biotin can also help relieve the symptoms of diabetic neuropathy.[20]

For milder cases of unstable blood sugar and diabetes, a good dosage range is 2,000 mcg to 4,000 mcg per day in divided doses. For people with severe diabetes, especially those requiring insulin, Dr. Atkins recommended a dose of 7,500 mcg (once a day) to 15,000 mcg (in divided doses).

Inositol is a sort of cousin to the B vitamins. As with biotin, bacteria in your small intestine manufacture it, so it's almost impossible to be deficient under normal conditions. Inositol is a critical part of a molecule used to communicate insulin's action inside the cell.[21] High levels of insulin exhaust the cellular stores of this nutrient faster than your body can supply it. Inositol also plays a role in the management of stress and blood pressure.[22] This nutrient, in a form called myo-inositol, is found in foods such as nuts and beans. Inositol is a common ingredient in blood sugar support formulations and, for this purpose, the dosage ranges from 500 mg to 1,000 mg daily.

BLOOD SUGAR SUPPLEMENTS

Chromium

This trace mineral is essential for helping insulin work properly in your body. If you have a low level of chromium, as many people do, it might be making your blood sugar problems worse. By the same token, raising your chromium level may help improve your insulin resistance.

Exactly how much chromium you need each day isn't really known, but an adequate intake range for adults is anywhere from 50 mcg to 200 mcg. Even though you need such a tiny amount, numerous surveys show that dietary intake of chromium is inadequate.[23]

Chromium works in concert with insulin as part of your natural mechanism for controlling blood sugar. Researchers still aren't sure exactly how, but it's probably because your body needs chromium to produce glucose tolerance factor (GTF), a compound that helps regulate insulin levels. GTF helps keep your blood sugar steady and may also help increase insulin sensitivity, lower blood sugar, and control your appetite.[24]

A number of studies support the use of supplemental chromium for people with prediabetes and diabetes. One published in 1997, for example, looked at the effects of chromium supplements on 180 people with Type 2 diabetes. For four months, 60 people were given 100 mcg of chromium picolinate twice a day; 60 received 500 mcg of chromium picolinate twice a day; and 60 got a placebo twice a day. The subjects continued with their usual diet and medications during this time. At the end of two months, the group taking 500 mcg twice a day had significant improvements in blood sugar levels. At the end of four months, both the 500 mcg and 100 mcg groups showed significant improvements, but there was no improvement in the placebo group. As a bonus, the people in the chromium groups also showed improved blood cholesterol levels.[25]

Other studies suggest that your need for extra chromium is related to how severe your glucose intolerance is. For those with only mild glucose intolerance, an extra 200 mcg seems to be enough; people with more severe cases need larger doses, and certainly more is needed by those who are already diabetics.[26]

Tiny amounts of chromium are found naturally in a variety of foods, including beef, cheese, dark green leafy vegetables, mushrooms, clams, lobsters, scallops, and barley. There's only about 20 mcg of chromium in a cup of broccoli, however, so it would be hard to get 200 mcg of chromium a day just from your food—you need a supplement in order to get a therapeutic dose. Your body absorbs chromium best from chromium picolinate or chromium polynicotinate. (Some recent test tube studies seem to suggest that very large doses of chromium picolinate could cause DNA damage.[27] The doses used were extremely large, however—far larger than the doses used in the studies mentioned earlier, and far larger than any dose you would ever take. And of course, what happens to hamster ovary cells in a test tube is a very long way from what would happen in your body.) Overall, there's plenty of good evidence for the safety of chromium supplements in doses of up to 1,000 mcg (1 mg) a day. Dr. Atkins usually suggested a maximum of 1,000 mcg a day for patients with Type 2 diabetes and between 400 mcg and 800 mcg a day for patients with the metabolic syndrome or prediabetes, always divided into three doses.

Magnesium

Many people with diabetes have low levels of this important trace mineral, even when they get adequate amounts from their food. Similarly, people who have low magnesium levels, even though they're eating a normally adequate amount, have a high likelihood of getting diabetes—in fact, low magnesium levels are considered a strong independent predictor of diabetes.[28] Magnesium is also a very important mineral for heart health (see Chapter 21 for more information).

Because magnesium plays an important part in the complex chemical processes that regulate your insulin and blood sugar sensitivity, having low levels of it could make high blood sugar and insulin resistance worse. But does bringing your magnesium level up to normal help? In the case of high blood sugar, maybe—the studies are inconclusive. Some say yes; others say no. In the case of insulin resistance, however, the evidence for magnesium is a little stronger.[29] There's also some evidence that improving your magnesium levels could help prevent some complications of diabetes, particularly kidney disease, retinopathy, and neuropathy.[30]

When you eat plenty of nuts, as you do when you follow the ABSCP, you get a lot of dietary magnesium, but the amount may not be sufficient to raise your magnesium level if you have Type 2 diabetes. Although it can be hard to find, Dr. Atkins preferred to use the supplement magnesium orotate because it contains a small dose of elemental magnesium that is absorbed very well. It is also less likely to cause gastrointestinal side effects. However, many vitamin stores and natural foods stores don't carry this form of magnesium. Magnesium citrate, magnesium gluconate, and magnesium taurate are more easily found.

Some magnesium supplements can cause diarrhea and, in some cases, low blood pressure. Start with a small amount and gradually increase to no more than 350 mg a day of elemental magnesium in divided doses. If you have kidney disease, magnesium supplementation may not be appropriate. Do not take magnesium supplements before discussing it first with your doctor.

Calcium

You probably already know that calcium is crucial for maintaining strong bones, but you may not know that this mineral also stimulates your pancreas to produce insulin. Again, it's a complex process—too involved to discuss here—but having optimal levels of calcium in your diet helps the process run smoothly. When supplementing with calcium, you should be sure to maintain the proper balance of magnesium and phosphorus.

If you take the drug metformin (Glucophage) to help treat insulin resistance, you may need to take calcium supplements. Metformin can decrease the absorption of folic acid and vitamin B_{12}. Supplementing with 1,200 mg a day of calcium can counteract this problem.[31]

The DRI for calcium is 1,000 mg for adults between the ages of 19 and 50, and 1,200 mg for older individuals.[32] But for all the reasons mentioned earlier, you probably need to take in at least 1,200 mg. As a bonus, the level of calcium in your diet from dairy sources may also help with weight loss.[33] Although the cheese, nuts, and green leafy vegetables you'll be eating as part of the ABSCP will give you plenty of dietary calcium, food alone may not be enough to provide this therapeutic level. Dr. Atkins recommended calcium supplements to virtually all his patients. Keep your total calcium intake from food and supplements to no more than 2,000 mg daily. You can't absorb any more than that, and, although it's very rare, taking more than 2,000 mg a day for a long time could actually cause an overload of calcium in your bloodstream.

Zinc

For reasons researchers don't understand yet, people with Type 2 diabetes tend to have very low levels of the trace mineral zinc. Because zinc is needed to make a variety of antioxidant enzymes in your body, and because people with the metabolic syndrome, prediabetes, and diabetes usually have high levels of oxidative stress, you need to have plenty of available zinc.[34] Zinc is also needed to help your pancreas manufacture insulin and to help insulin transport glucose into your cells.[35] Aside from oysters, which are very high in zinc, zinc isn't very abundant in food; it's also hard to absorb zinc from food. If you're low on zinc, it's difficult to raise your level through diet alone—supplements are almost always needed. Generally recommended is a dose ranging from 30 mg to 50 mg daily. It is common for zinc to be found in blood sugar formulations. For an individual with severe diabetes, Dr. Atkins would add additional supplementation of up to 100 mg per day.

Iron

A hereditary disorder of iron metabolism called hemochromatosis can cause Type 2 diabetes in anywhere from 50 percent to 80 percent of people with the problem. What happens is that high levels of iron accumulate in the pancreas (and other parts of the body) and damage the beta cells that produce insulin. Some recent research suggests that high iron levels play a role in diabetes, even among people who don't have hemochromatosis. But it's too soon to say exactly what that means.[36, 37] In the meantime, just to be on the safe side, we suggest that you choose a daily multivitamin/mineral supplement that doesn't contain iron. (Of course, if you have iron-deficiency anemia or are pregnant, follow your doctor's instructions about iron supplements.)

Coenzyme Q$_{10}$

Also known as CoQ_{10} or ubiquinone, this substance is produced by your body and plays a vital part in producing energy for the tiny mitochondria found in all your cells. If these little power plants don't work properly, one of the consequences can be insulin resistance. We know from a recent study in Australia that CoQ_{10} supplements can help improve blood pressure and blood sugar control in people with Type 2 diabetes.[38] Dr. Atkins usually prescribed a minimum dose of 100 mg daily, taken three times a day. (For important information on the role of CoQ_{10} in heart health, see Chapter 21.)

AMINO ACIDS

As we discussed in Chapter 13, amino acids are the building blocks for the thousands of proteins your body needs to function properly. A few of those amino acids are particularly important for the proteins that control insulin production and sensitivity. An interesting study in 2003 showed that amino acids can stimulate the pancreas to produce more insulin, even in people who have diminished insulin production as a result of having had Type 2 diabetes for a long time.[39]

The research on how amino acids can help blood sugar is evolving.[40] Dr. Atkins recommended the amino acid carnitine for many of his patients. You need carnitine to transport fats into the mitochondria so they can be burned for energy. The more carnitine you have, the more efficient that transport will be—and if you take carnitine supplements, you may burn fat a little faster.[41]

For people with diabetes, carnitine can be useful for more than weight loss. The results of a study in Italy in 1999 showed that it can help improve insulin sensitivity as well.[42] Typical daily dosages range from 1,500 mg to 3,000 mg.

Important note: Valuable as amino acids can be, you should not try them on your own. Health care professionals differ in their opinions on the use of individual amino acids for therapeutic effect. Work

HERBS FOR BLOOD SUGAR

A number of herbs have been recommended for helping control blood sugar, such as fenugreek, cinnamon, garlic, turmeric, gymnema sylvestre (a plant from India), and banaba (a plant from the Philippines). Dr. Atkins did not recommend using herbs as your primary therapy for diabetes; however, they can be useful to enhance the effect of other blood-sugar-supporting nutrients and are often included in blood-sugar-regulating supplement formulations.

with a nutritionally oriented physician to discuss what's best for you and to monitor your progress.

For ease in designing your supplement regimen, Atkins Nutritionals makes supplements that support the needs of those with blood sugar imbalances and also addresses cardiovascular health. Turn to page 247 for the formulation of Atkins Basic 3 and to page 267 for the Essential Oils Formula, to give you an idea of the ingredients and dosages of these two basic supplements. For information on specialized formulations, go to www.atkins.com/shop/supplements. Many of the dietary supplements discussed here in the context of blood sugar can also help your blood pressure and blood lipids. The next chapter explains how.

WHAT IS YOUR SUPPLEMENTS IQ?

How well do you know your supplements for blood sugar? Take this quiz to find out.

1. Vitamin C is:
   a. an important antioxidant   True ❑   False ❑
   b. often low in people with diabetes True ❑   False ❑
   c. found only in citrus fruits   True ❑   False ❑

2. Vitamin E is found in:
   a. fish
   b. red meat and poultry
   c. fruit
   d. nuts and seeds

3. Lipoic acid is helpful for treating:
   a. headaches
   b. diabetic neuropathy
   c. kidney disease
   d. high blood pressure

4. People with prediabetes and diabetes often have:
   a. low magnesium levels
   b. normal magnesium levels
   c. high magnesium levels
   d. excessive magnesium levels

5. Which foods are good dietary sources of calcium?
   a. dark green leafy vegetables
   b. tofu (bean curd)
   c. dairy products
   d. nuts
   e. all of the above

Answers

1. a, True; b, True; c, False. 2. d. 3. b. 4. a. 5. e.

Chapter 21

GETTING EXTRA HELP: SUPPLEMENTS FOR HEART HEALTH

For people on the path to diabetes, there are two equally frightening endpoints to try to avoid at all costs: full-blown diabetes, with complications such as blindness or amputation, and deadly heart disease. We've just reviewed in detail the extra help you can get from nutritional supplements that may give you the edge you need in controlling your blood sugar. Now let's look at supplements that can improve your heart health.

Most of these supplements are the same ones Dr. Atkins recommended for helping to balance your blood sugar. Remember, these are recommended in addition to a good-quality, iron-free multivitamin/mineral supplement. The combination can help you lower your blood pressure and improve your blood lipids—the two vital steps in improving your heart health.

We suggest that when planning a supplement program for improving your risk factors for heart disease, you work with a nutritionally oriented physician who understands and supports the application of the Atkins Blood Sugar Control Program (ABSCP). He or she will help you to decide which supplements—and dosages—are best for you. If you take medications, this is particularly important because certain supplements can react with or magnify the effects of certain drugs.

Important note: By making diet and lifestyle changes and adding supplements, you may be able to cut back on or even discontinue medications for high blood pressure and abnormal blood lipids. Some supplements could have an effect on medications you may be taking for other conditions. Before taking these or any supplements, discuss them with your doctor and plan ahead about how you will reduce or change your medications as your blood pressure and other values improve. As one example of many, Dorothy W. (see page 89), who had hypertension as a result of her underlying metabolic imbalance, was able to taper down to only a small dose of blood pressure medication once she made the lifestyle changes that are part of the ABSCP.

ANTIOXIDANTS FOR HEART HEALTH

For people who are at risk of heart disease—which includes anyone with the metabolic syndrome, prediabetes, or diabetes—Dr. Atkins recommended supplementing with several important antioxidant vitamins and minerals as well as some other nutrients. (Review Chapter 20 for an introduction to antioxidants.) Here are the supplements and dosages he recommended for boosting heart health.

Vitamin C

High levels of vitamin C help keep your blood vessels relaxed so that blood flows smoothly through them. And if you have the high blood pressure that usually accompanies blood sugar abnormalities, extra vitamin C can help bring it down.[1] The usual dosage is 1,000 mg to 2,000 mg a day in divided doses.

Vitamin E

The most valuable use of vitamin E for people with blood sugar abnormalities and diabetes may be in helping to protect your LDL cholesterol from oxidization by free radicals. According to one study, the large, buoyant LDL particles received more protection from oxidative stress than did the small dense, more dangerous LDL particles.[2] Remember, when an individual follows the Atkins approach, both HDL and LDL particle size shifts to predominantly larger, more buoyant particles.[3, 4] What all of this means is that it may decrease your tendency toward clogged arteries. Vitamin E makes your blood less "sticky," which helps prevent clots that cause heart attacks.[5] Dr. Atkins generally suggested 400 IU to 800 IU daily.

Important note: It has been observed in clinical practice that a few individuals experience elevated blood pressure while taking vitamin E. If your blood pressure goes up while taking a high dose, cut back.

B VITAMINS

Although you need all the B vitamins to keep your heart healthy, three of them are particularly important for heart health, especially for people with blood sugar problems. The first is folic acid, also known as folate. Folic acid could save your life.

The reason is a little complex. One of the normal by-products of metabolizing the amino acid methionine is a substance called homocysteine. Statistically speaking, a high level of homocysteine in your blood is associated with an increased risk of heart disease from clogged arteries. That can automatically raise the risk of death from heart disease for those individuals who have a tendency toward high homocysteine levels. If you have high homocysteine levels *and* diabetes, your risk is about 2.5 times greater.[6]

People with diabetes and elevated homocysteine are more likely to have complications such as kidney disease and eye problems.[7] Another study showed that lowering homocysteine improves blood sugar control.[8] The commonly used diabetes drug metformin (Glucophage), in some instances, may also raise your homocysteine level.[9]

Fortunately, you can take positive steps to bring your homocysteine level down if it's too high. (Your doctor can do a blood test to find out.) First, getting your blood sugar down almost always also brings down your homocysteine.[10] Second, folic acid supplements, along with vitamin B_6 (pyridoxine) and vitamin B_{12} (cobalamin), contribute to lowering homocysteine levels by helping your body form the enzymes that break it down.[11] To lower homocysteine, Dr. Atkins used 2,000 mcg to 4,000 mcg (2 mg to 4 mg) a day of folic acid, along with 50 mg of vitamin B_6 and 500 mcg to 1,000 mcg of vitamin B_{12}. To get your homocysteine under control with such doses, however, work with your doctor because follow-up blood monitoring for homocysteine will be needed until the optimum level is reached. Dr. Atkins' goal was a homocysteine blood level of 8 μmol/L or below. Another important reason to review this with your physician is that, in some women, additional folic acid can have a mild estrogenic effect, which may need to be monitored. These nutrients have been helpful for patients with neuropathies. A good example of the effectiveness of the use of B vitamins in lowering homocysteine levels was Martha N., who saw Dr. Atkins for weight management and to reduce some of the five medications she was taking, including those for elevated triglycerides—hers had been as high as 700. Interestingly, although she had a number of cardiovascular risk factors, she never had her homocysteine level tested. On her initial visit her homocysteine level was 20.6. After two months with additional supplementation of B_6, B_{12}, and folic acid, her level dropped to 8.8.

Another valuable B vitamin for heart health is niacin, also known as vitamin B_3. Long before statin drugs appeared on the scene, doctors used large doses of niacin to help bring down LDL cholesterol and triglycerides and to raise HDL cholesterol.[12] This treatment was improved by the development of a form of niacin called inositol hexanicotinate (IHN), which works well without the unpleasant flushing side effect that can result from large doses of niacin. If you want to try IHN to improve your lipid profile, you must work with a nutritionally oriented physician to find the right dose, monitor your progress, and check your liver function. Dr. Atkins usually prescribed 500 mg to 1,500 mg per day in divided doses.

One problem with niacin and IHN is that they might raise your blood sugar a bit if you have diabetes.[13] For patients with elevated blood sugars, Dr. Atkins usually prescribed a slightly lower dose of IHN and the higher dose range for chromium (check Chapter 20 for more information on this mineral). Blood sugar elevation does not happen to everyone, but be sure to monitor your blood sugar. The combination therapy he used is just as effective as a larger dose of IHN alone for improving cholesterol levels.

Pantethine, a form of the B vitamin pantothenic acid, can also be helpful for improving your lipid profile, particularly total cholesterol and LDL.[14] Pantethine can be very effective with minimal side effects. (Some patients get diarrhea, but this usually goes away if the dose is reduced.) Dr. Atkins found that his patients usually benefited most from taking two or three 450 mg capsules of mega-pantethine a day. If that formulation isn't available, take three to six tablets daily of a standard pantethine complex supplement.

MAGNESIUM

If you have the metabolic syndrome, prediabetes, or diabetes, your magnesium levels are likely to be low, as we explained in Chapter 20. That's not just bad for your blood sugar, however—it's also bad for your blood pressure and your heart. Low levels of magnesium can cause heart arrhythmias (irregular heartbeat) and may also make your blood "stickier" and more likely to form clots.[15, 16]

Magnesium can have a major impact on your blood pressure. When you're low on magnesium—as many people with hypertension are—the walls of your blood vessels tighten up, which raises your blood pressure. Magnesium helps the blood vessels relax, which brings your blood pressure down.[17] For treating high blood pressure, Dr. Atkins used 500 mg a day of magnesium orotate in three or four divided doses. He preferred this form of magnesium, as it is generally well absorbed. Alternatively, use magnesium taurate in doses of three to four a day.

Important note: If you have kidney disease, you must discuss magnesium supplements with your doctor before you try them.

TAURINE

The amino acid taurine is another valuable supplement for treating high blood pressure and helping your heart.[18] It acts as a natural diuretic, which helps your body excrete excess fluid.[19] That, in turn, lowers your blood pressure and puts less strain on your heart. Taurine has been shown to enhance immunity and protect against oxidative stress.[20] It's usually available in 500 mg tablets. The usual dose range is 1,500 mg to 3,000 mg a day in three divided doses.

Important note: Amino acids such as taurine can have powerful effects, especially in the presence of medications such as diuretics, and should be used only under the supervision of a nutritionally oriented physician. Health care professionals differ in their opinions on the use of individual amino acids for therapeutic effect.

ESSENTIAL FATTY ACIDS

Omega-3 fatty acids are extremely helpful for preventing heart disease (as discussed in Chapter 8) in people with diabetes, mostly by lowering their triglyceride levels and blood pressure. Eating cold-water fish twice a week gives you a lot of the benefits of the omega-3s, in addition to providing high-quality protein and some nice variety in your diet. Taking omega-3 capsules can boost that benefit—especially if you don't like eating fish. (Flaxseed oil is another source of omega-3.) There is solid evidence to show that supplemental omega-3 helps your blood pressure.[21] In addition to its blood-pressure-lowering effect, omega-3 supplementation was found to reduce triglycerides without adverse effects on glucose metabolism.[22–25]

To obtain all the omega-3 fatty acids, including eicosapentenoic acid (EPA) and docosahexanoic acid (DHA), which are found only in fish oil, we recommend taking a soft gel containing 600 mg total. Dosage can range from two to six soft gels per day. If triglycerides are significantly elevated or inflammation markers are high, the higher dose range may be needed until lab results fall to the optimum level. If you currently take any prescription medications to thin your blood, discuss omega-3 supplements with your doctor first.

It's important to balance your intake of omega-3 and omega-6 fatty acids. For supplements of omega-6 (also called gamma linolenic acid or GLA), Dr. Atkins used borage oil in 240 mg soft gels; the dose ranges from one to three capsules daily. Atkins Formula Essential Oils combines the essential fatty acids in the optimal balance. A table listing all of the nutrients in Atkins Essential Oils follows.

ESSENTIAL OILS FORMULA

SUPPLEMENT	AMOUNT PER SERVING
Vitamin E (from mixed tocopherols)	20 IU
Alpha linolenic acid (from flaxseed oil)	440 mg
Docosahexaenoic acid (from fish oil)	160 mg
Eicosapentanoic acid (from fish oil)	240 mg
Gamma linolenic acid (GLA) (from borage seed oil)	192 mg
Linoleic acid (from borage, flaxseed, and fish oils)	305 mg
Oleic acid (from borage, flaxseed, and fish oils)	405 mg

COENZYME Q_{10}

One of the worst things about statin drugs, the *de rigueur* prescription for people with high cholesterol, is that they interfere with your production of coenzyme Q_{10} (ubiquinone or CoQ_{10}). Because you need CoQ_{10} to create energy in your mitochondria, the tiny power plants found in all your cells, a shortage of it can lead to fatigue and muscle weakness. That's more than just a minor side effect—it can be a real problem when it comes to your heart, a powerful muscle that has more mitochondria per cell than any other part of your body. The last thing you want to take is a drug that weakens your heart, yet statin drugs are being liberally prescribed as a way to *help* your heart.[26] Dr. Atkins believed that this self-defeating paradox would soon be recognized, when people who have been taking statin drugs for years start showing the signs of heart failure, cardiomyopathy, arrhythmias, and other problems caused by insufficient amounts of CoQ_{10}. What the medical establishment will say then should be interesting to observe.

Even without statin drugs, your production of CoQ_{10} naturally drops off a bit as you get older. Dr. Atkins routinely prescribed CoQ_{10} for all of his patients who were at risk for heart disease. He also found CoQ_{10} to be effective for lowering high blood pressure. The usual dose is 100 mg three times per day; in some cases he recommended a higher dose.

For ease in designing your supplement regimen, Atkins makes supplements that support the needs of those with blood sugar imbalances and address blood sugar imbalances and cardiovascular health. You have already seen the formulations of Atkins Basic 3 (page 247) and Essential Oils Formula (page 267). For information on specialized formulations, go to www.atkins.com/shop.

You've learned about two of the major aspects of the Atkins Blood Sugar Control Program—diet and supplements. Now it's time to learn about the all-important third leg of the program: exercise.

WHAT'S YOUR HEART HEALTH SUPPLEMENT IQ?

How do different supplements help keep your heart healthy? Check your knowledge with this quiz.

1. Vitamin C helps your heart by:
   a. preventing scurvy
   b. improving digestion
   c. relaxing blood vessels
2. Vitamin E helps your heart by:
   a. preventing cholesterol oxidation
   b. building strong bones
   c. making your heart beat slower
3. Folic acid, vitamin B_6, and vitamin B_{12} are valuable for:
   a. lowering A1C levels
   b. lowering homocysteine
   c. lowering blood pressure
4. Niacin or IHN can help:
   a. lower cholesterol
   b. lower blood pressure
   c. lower blood sugar
5. Magnesium can help:
   a. lower cholesterol

    b. lower blood pressure

    c. manage blood sugar

6. Omega-3 fatty acids help your heart by:

    a. lowering triglycerides

    b. lowering blood pressure

    c. improving blood flow

7. Taurine helps the heart by:

    a. lowering blood pressure

    b. increasing loss of excess fluid

    c. decreasing oxidative stress

Answers

1. c. 2. a. 3. b. 4. a. 5. b and c. 6. a, b, and c. 7. a and b.

AN ALTERNATIVE TO DRUGS

When her doctor prescribed diabetes medication, April Greer vowed never to take it. By choosing to follow the Atkins Nutritional Approach instead, she kept her promise to herself—and is living proof that a low-carb lifestyle reaps healthy rewards.

NAME: **April Greer**
AGE: **34**
HEIGHT: **5 feet 3 inches**
WEIGHT BEFORE:
    237 pounds
WEIGHT NOW:
    137 pounds

For several months, I had been going to the doctor because of chronic bladder infections. One day he decided to run a urine test. It turned out that the sugar level in my urine was very high, which led him to investigate further. He found that my average blood sugar was 207. When he said, "You are a full-blown diabetic," his words triggered what would be my personal turning point.

My doctor prescribed diabetes medication, but I did not fill it because I didn't want to become dependent on pills. I knew that the typical treatment for Type 2 diabetes starts with pills and ends with shots. So I visited the Atkins Web site, and after reading the information, I wanted to start implementing the Atkins program that very minute. Truly, the last thing

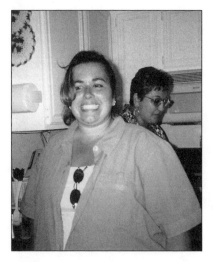

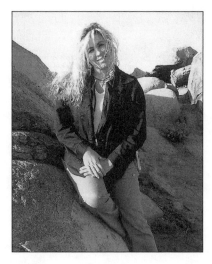

BEFORE   **AFTER**

on my mind was losing weight. My husband liked me the way I was. What I did think about was being able to play football with my sons, who are now six and nine years old. I also feared having organ troubles and maybe losing limbs if I couldn't get my diabetes under control.

From the beginning, I was very serious and careful about doing Atkins. I tested my blood sugar every morning and evening. During the first two weeks my blood sugar dropped from 207 to 148. At the end of six months I had lost 100 pounds and my fasting blood sugar stabilized at between 80 and 110. I no longer needed to test my blood sugar every day, which was a real victory.

Looking back, my diet had been a nutritional nightmare. For breakfast, I would have fast-food pancakes or French toast and orange juice; for lunch, takeout burritos or tacos; and pasta with bread was a typical dinner. Now I eat hard-boiled eggs at my desk or pick up some scrambled eggs with bacon or sausage. I still eat a fast-food lunch but I might order a chicken breast with no bun, plus a salad. If I'm pressed for time, I'll eat an Atkins Advantage bar. For dinner, we have chicken or fish or bunless hamburgers. Sometimes we'll have breakfast foods like eggs and bacon for dinner. We always have a green veggie. Broccoli has become my vegetable of choice.

I had always been a size 5 in high school, but after my first child I began to gain weight and eat for comfort. It was a very negative cycle: eat, sit, gain, feel tired and depressed, eat, sit, gain. . . . Eventually, I wore a size 22 and had to shop at plus-size stores. My husband really hated those "old lady" clothes. After I had lost about 50 pounds, I no longer wanted to just sit on the couch. I began swimming laps in our pool. At first, four laps left me huffing and puffing but I kept at it and still try to swim every day. Our family also began walking to the park together and playing touch football there regularly. Exercise really gives you an energy boost so the more you exercise, the more you want to exercise. This is important for me because I also have a full-time job as a broker for an international freight service that keeps me sitting at a desk.

A week ago I saw my doctor and he said, "Do you realize because of you I now recommend Atkins to all my diabetic patients?" I feel so proud of what I've accomplished and feel blessed to be taking no medication or shots. My kids used to look at old pictures of me and ask, "Mom, when are you going to be skinny again?" It hurt me and I hurt for them. Before, when a man would be ahead of me going into a restaurant or store, he'd look behind him, see me, and let the door slam in my face. Now I have three guys waiting *to hold the door open for me. I can't tell you what that does for your self-esteem. But what really matters most to me is that I have my health and I'll be around to enjoy it with my kids.*

Note: Your individual results may vary from those reported here. As stated previously, Atkins recommends initial laboratory evaluation and subsequent follow-up in conjunction with your health care provider.

Chapter 22

WALKING AWAY FROM DIABETES

Exercise isn't an option when it comes to helping improve your insulin sensitivity. It's mandatory. That it also helps you lose weight and improves your health in other ways is just another huge bonus.

THE EXERCISE ADVANTAGE

Exercise doesn't just reduce body fat; it increases the amount of muscle you have. Here's something we bet you didn't know: More muscle mass helps reshape your body, preserve your strength, and turbocharge your metabolism. The more muscle you have relative to your body weight, the more insulin sensitive you are. And because muscles burn glucose faster than fat can, the more muscle you have, the more energy you're able to expend. That's why exercise and controlling carb intake are the two integral components of the Atkins Blood Sugar Control Program (ABSCP).

Loss of muscle mass is an inevitable part of aging, especially in the absence of regular exercise. That's one reason your metabolic rate slows down, making it far easier to gain weight. But vast societal changes in the last century have conspired to make even young people fatter as we exercise less and eat more empty calories. The reliance on

ELEVEN REASONS TO WORK OUT

If exercise were a drug, factories wouldn't be able to make it fast enough. Here are 11 reasons to step it up:

1. To build and tone muscle
2. To improve insulin sensitivity
3. To raise your ACE (Atkins Carbohydrate Equilibrium)
4. To help maintain weight loss with a more liberal food plan
5. To help prevent diabetes if you don't already have it
6. To improve cardiovascular fitness and longevity
7. To help lower blood pressure
8. To help improve blood lipids and clotting factors
9. To help maintain balance and joint support to prevent falls
10. To maintain bone density
11. To improve energy levels, mood, and ability to deal with stress

machinery, particularly the automobile and household appliances such as vacuum cleaners and washing machines, has significantly diminished the amount of physical activity in most people's lives. To compound our increasingly inactive lifestyles over the past few decades, many people now spend work hours staring at a computer screen or standing in one spot on an assembly line, only to go home, where they crash in front of the "tube." Combine this couch-potato mentality with a diet heavy in carbohydrates and relatively low in protein (the recommendations of the USDA as expressed in the food guide pyramid), which signals your body to store fat instead of burning it, and you have a recipe for the current health crisis.

To buck the trend and avoid becoming a statistic in the epidemic of "diabesity," you should follow the blood sugar control program outlined in previous chapters and begin an exercise program. In tandem, they will shift into high gear those hormonal signals to burn fat.

EXERCISE HELPS PREVENT DIABETES

The protective effect of exercise against diabetes is powerful—and it's strongest in the people who are most at risk. Let's look at a very interesting study. Researchers reviewed the patterns of physical activity and other personal characteristics of nearly 6,000 male graduates of a major university over a 15-year period. Among the men who had several risk factors for diabetes at the start of the study—including a family history, being overweight, and high blood pressure—the ones who actually went on to develop diabetes by the end of the study were the ones who were the least physically active. The at-risk men who were the most physically active were far less likely to develop diabetes. In other words, the protective benefit of increased physical activity was strongest for the men who were at highest risk of diabetes.[1]

Similar results were found in a long-term study of more than 110,000 men and women in China. When the members of the group were screened for diabetes in 1986, the researchers found nearly 600 who already had impaired glucose tolerance, or prediabetes. The participants were randomly divided into four groups. One group was the control group, who made no dietary or exercise changes. Of the others, one group made only dietary changes based on the standard diabetes recommendations; one group made no dietary changes but added exercise; and one group added exercise and made dietary changes. After six years, nearly 68 percent of the control group had developed diabetes. In the diet-alone group, nearly 44 percent had developed diabetes; in the exercise-alone group, 41 percent had developed diabetes; and in the diet-and-exercise group, 46 percent had developed diabetes. Exercise alone was actually more helpful in preventing diabetes than the standard diabetes diet alone or the diet in combination with exercise.[2] This is no surprise. The standard carb-filled diet didn't allow people to do as well, even when they exercised to overcome the effects of all those carbohydrates.

EXERCISE AND YOUR BLOOD SUGAR

Researchers have known for decades that exercise helps to improve insulin resistance by making your muscles more responsive to the effects of insulin. So, if you have signs of the metabolic syndrome, prediabetes, or diabetes, your primary motivation for exercising is crystal clear. But exactly how much improvement can you expect? In an attempt to answer that question, researchers recently conducted a meta-analysis of clinical trials on the effect of exercise in patients with Type 2 diabetes. They looked at the results of 14 different studies using moderate exercise alone—the patients in the study didn't take any drugs to treat diabetes and they didn't change their way of eating. The result? Not a lot of weight loss, but significant improvement in blood sugar control as measured by the glycated hemoglobin (A1C) test. In fact, the improvement was enough to make a dent in the risk of diabetic complications.[3] And that was just with exercise alone! Just imagine what can happen when you combine the Atkins controlled-carbohydrate program with exercise.

THE RIGHT PROGRAM FOR YOU

Almost everyone can find an exercise plan that is safe and achievable, but we strongly advise you to consult your doctor before you begin. If you have been completely inactive or have a heart condition, it is *absolutely essential* to do this. You may need a stress test to check if you can exercise safely. These tests are usually easy to do, so don't hesitate to ask for one. You may be asked to exercise by walking on a treadmill or riding a stationary bike while hooked up to a heart monitor. Sometimes a doctor may also use a medication or a sound wave test (echocardiogram) to provide additional information about your heart function while exercising.

GETTING GOING

Once your physician has given you the green light, how should you begin? First, before making any fitness changes, you may want to wait

SPECIAL EXERCISE CONCERNS FOR PEOPLE WITH DIABETES

Some common complications of diabetes may impact your fitness choices. If you have diabetes, discuss your exercise plans with your doctor before you start.

Diabetic Retinopathy. If you have this eye condition, you may need to avoid activities that raise your blood pressure sharply, such as strenuous weight training, or those that involve a lot of pounding and jarring, such as jogging, running, and racquet sports. Brisk walking and working out on exercise machines such as the elliptical trainer and exercise bike are almost always acceptable.

Peripheral Neuropathy. A common complication of diabetes, peripheral neuropathy often causes a reduction or loss of sensation in the feet. Repetitive exercise involving the legs, such as long walks, jogging, running, using a treadmill, or doing step exercise, could cause hard-to-heal foot ulcerations and even bone fractures. You may have to stick to non-weight-bearing or *nonconcussive* exercise, such as swimming, water aerobics, riding a stationary bike, or using a rowing machine. Be sure to inspect your feet carefully on a regular basis for evidence of redness, blisters, or skin changes.

until you've established your new controlled-carbohydrate dietary program for at least two weeks. Allow your body time to adapt to your new way of eating. Then it will be ready to move on to the next component of your new lifestyle. Of course, those of you who are eager to step up your fitness level can certainly begin to be more active in general to prepare for the official start of your exercise regimen.

TWO TYPES OF EXERCISE

The kinds of exercise we are talking about can be divided into two basic types: one that improves cardiovascular fitness (aerobic) and one that builds and maintains muscle (resistance). Running, jogging, brisk walking, bicycling, in-line skating, and swimming are all aerobic exercise. Resistance exercise may raise your heart rate and respiration somewhat, but it mostly builds muscles. Weight training falls in this category, as do isometrics and the kind of circuit training that is popular at many health clubs and gyms. A good fitness plan includes both types of exercise. In the next chapter, we'll tell you about ways to incorporate both types to get the most out of your exercise program, both enhancing your cardiovascular health and preserving or gaining strength.

TAKE IT EASY

If you are heavy and not used to moving much, or if you're simply very out of condition, begin slowly, proceeding step-by-step to a more active lifestyle. This will reduce the likelihood of joint problems. Even if you are eager to see results, it is essential that you gradually increase activity to allow your muscles, joints, ligaments, and tendons time to adjust to a new level of use. Otherwise, you may injure yourself, sabotage your grand plan, and send yourself back onto the couch.

SETTING YOUR EXERCISE GOALS

Once you have made a firm commitment to exercise, the next step is to figure out how much is enough. A lot of researchers have looked at that question, and the answers pretty much come down to this:

1. At least half an hour of aerobic activity, such as brisk walking, at least three days a week. Four to six days is even better—as is longer duration. In fact, in recommendations made in 2002, the Surgeon General of the United States called for an hour of moderate-intensity physical activity every day. An alternative goal recommended by the Centers for Disease Control in conjunction with the American College of Sports Medicine is 30 minutes of "at least" moderate activity all or most days of the week.[4] You may not be able to start out at such a

level, but it should be your goal, since research suggests a relationship between increased exercise and improved health benefits.[5] Whatever activity you choose, it should raise your heart rate.

2. Do additional strength-training exercise at least twice a week. A good whole-body strengthening workout takes only about half an hour, although you may not have the stamina for this duration initially. On the days you do this type of workout, you can reduce the amount of aerobic activity proportionately. Do not work the same muscle groups two days in a row.

3. Give yourself a day off from exercise once a week, although if you grow to enjoy exercise, as many people do, it would be fine to take a walk on your "day off."

Do understand that you may not be able to achieve these goals initially—but that's not a reason to skip exercising altogether. Even a small amount of exercise is better than none at all, and most people can gradually increase their exercise level.

FIND YOUR TARGET HEART RATE

Just like any other muscle in your body, the heart gets stronger when it is worked. When you do aerobic exercise, you make your heart beat faster and harder. You don't want to overdo that, of course, so you need a way to determine just how much faster your heartbeat should get. There's a simple formula you can use to figure that out.

1. Begin by finding your resting heart rate. This is your heart rate when you are relaxing. Sit quietly for 15 minutes (read or watch television), then locate your pulse either on the thumb side of either wrist or on either side of your neck under the angle of your jaw. Using a watch or clock that counts seconds, count your heartbeat for ten seconds. Multiply that number by six to get the number of beats in a minute. For most people, the resting heartbeat is between 60 and 80 beats per minute. (In general, the fitter you are, the more slowly your heart beats when you're at rest.) Write the number down and label it "resting heart rate." As you get fitter, you'll see two things happen: Your

heart will return to its resting rate more quickly after exercise, and your resting heart rate may slow down a little.

2. Next, subtract your age from 220. Write the number down and label it "maximum heart rate." This step compensates for your age. If you're 50, for instance, your maximum heart rate would be 170 beats per minute ($220 - 50 = 170$).

Important note: You do not want to push yourself to your maximum heart rate.

3. Your starting heart rate goal during exercise is 60 percent of your maximum heart rate. So, take your maximum heart rate, as determined in step 2, and multiply it by 0.60. If your maximum heart rate is 170 beats a minute, then your exercise goal, which is called your target heart rate, is 102 beats a minute ($170 \times 0.60 = 102$). But bear in mind that everyone's heart rate is different, and your personal maximum heart rate could vary as much as 15 beats higher or lower than the formula. Use the numbers you get from the formula just as a guideline, not a firm target.

4. When you first start exercising, you should aim for a heart rate that is 60 percent of your maximum rate. As your fitness level increases, challenge yourself to gradually raise your exercise heart rate to 65 percent, then 70 percent or even more (up to 80 percent) of your maximum heart rate. Since your primary goal is to achieve fitness, not compete in the Olympics, the key is to build to a level that you can maintain comfortably while gaining optimum cardiovascular benefit for your time exercising. A reasonable long-range goal is a target heart rate of 70 to 80 percent of your maximum heart rate. Building to this slowly will prevent injury as well as burnout from exercising at a level that is "too hard." Some medications, such as beta-blockers for lowering high blood pressure, can limit how quickly your heart beats. Again, if you take any prescription medications, be sure to discuss your exercise plans with your doctor first.

5. Always remember that some exercise is better than no exercise, so don't feel discouraged if you can't exercise for long or can't comfortably raise your heart rate to the recommended level. Congratulate yourself for doing what you can!

Use the chart below to estimate your heart rate during exercise at the level that is right for your age and level of fitness.

TARGET HEART RATES FOR EXERCISE

PERCENT OF MAXIMUM HEART RATE	AGE					
	20	30	40	50	60	70
50%	100	95	90	85	80	75
60%	120	114	108	102	96	90
70%	140	133	126	119	112	105
80%	160	152	144	136	128	120

Your goal is to start your exercise program and work up to the point where your heart rate reaches your target minimum and stays there for 30 minutes three times a week. Eventually, you'll be able to exercise at your target maximum every day if you wish—you may also be able to stay at that level beyond 30 minutes.

CHOOSE ACTIVITIES YOU ENJOY

Exercise may be mandatory, but it should also be fun. Find an activity you like and can do without strain, a lot of advance planning, or a lot of expense. For many people, walking fills the bill, but there are plenty of other ways to get your exercise. All you have to do is find one—or more—you enjoy and do it. Dr. Atkins loved to play tennis, for instance, so he played as often as he could.

For those of you who are hard-core exercise haters, find the activity you hate the least. Give yourself rewards for small improvements. For instance, buy a book you've been wanting and read it while you walk on the treadmill. Treat yourself to a new CD with energetic music to keep you motivated while working out. Check out an exercise video from the library.

Some of the activities you used to enjoy—running or basketball, for instance—may now be off-limits to you because of excess weight or joint problems, such as arthritis of the knee. That's no excuse for not exercising. Swimming, water exercises, riding a stationary bike, using an elliptical training machine, and low-impact aerobics are generally easy on your joints. And as you lose weight and strengthen your body, you may well find that your aching joints improve and let you exercise in more varied ways. If you have inflammation in your joints, after following the ABSCP and taking supplemental essential fatty acids, you should find inflammation and aching is decreased, which will allow you to exercise more.

DRINK *BEFORE* YOU'RE THIRSTY

The very first thing you should do at the start of any exercise session is fill up your 1-liter water bottle, drink about a quarter of it, and keep it close by. When you're sweating and breathing hard, you lose fluid rapidly. By the time you get thirsty, you may already be a little dehydrated—even in cold weather, when you're not sweating that much. Drinking water before, during, and after your workout keeps you properly hydrated. The payoff is that you will be able to get through your workout more comfortably. When you have adequate hydration, your body can more quickly clear away lactic acid, the by-product of exercise metabolism that causes that aching sensation in your muscles. Becoming dehydrated makes it harder to exercise and produces no long-term benefit. This isn't about sweating off water, it is about safely burning fat, increasing muscle mass, and developing cardiovascular fitness so that you can live longer.

EXCUSES, EXCUSES

For every antiexercise excuse, there is a rebuttal:

"I hate to exercise." I can't tell you how often we've had a patient tell us, "I can't stand exercising. It's so boring." Our usual reply: Unless you get moving, life as an invalid, barely able to leave the house, will be a lot *more* boring. Besides, exercise can be fun if you make it fun. Instead of walking alone, for instance, use that time to walk with family members and friends. Your walk stops being a chore and turns into family quality time or a pleasant visit with a friend—and everyone benefits from the exercise.

"*I don't have time to exercise.*" Really? The average American watches four hours of television every day. You can easily manage to do a home aerobics workout or your weight-training routine while watching just one half-hour sitcom episode. It's certainly better than sitting there passively.

"*I really don't have time to exercise.*" If you are truly overburdened

STAYING MOTIVATED

There are some days when the very idea of exercising seems overwhelming. How can you overcome this and stay motivated? We suggest that you:

- Find a form of exercise that's both convenient and enjoyable. When exercise is a hassle or unpleasant, it doesn't get done.
- Many people find it helpful to plan to get exercise "out of the way" by working out first thing in the morning.
- Focus on the benefits of exercise—you know you'll feel better afterward, even if it's hard to get started.
- Plan to walk or exercise for just five minutes. Chances are good that once you get started, you'll keep going for the full session.
- Find an exercise buddy. Walking and working out are more fun with some company, and you're more likely to do it if you know someone is counting on you.
- Join a gym. Once you've paid to join, you'll want to get your money's worth.
- Sign up for exercise classes. When you've got a class schedule to keep, you're more likely to go.
- Listen to your body. You may feel uninterested because you're getting sick, are overtired, or have been exercising too much recently. Of course, you shouldn't exercise if you're ill, injured, or exhausted. It's okay to take a day off now and then just to give yourself a break, but if you skip more than a couple of days, you'll likely find it hard to get back into the exercise groove again.

with things that must be done, it may be time to reconsider your priorities, because your exercise *must* be done as well. If you have to cut back on something else to be able to exercise, then do so—your health should be up there on your list of top priorities. And don't forget that with a little imagination, you can almost always manage to work more exercise into your day (see Staying Motivated on page 283).

"*I'm so heavy that I'm embarrassed to go to a gym.*" If you are uncomfortable exercising in public you can do so quite effectively in the privacy of your own home. Moreover, exercise programs (including

TEN WAYS TO SNEAK IN SOME EXERCISE

Anything that gets you moving—even housework—counts as exercise. Studies have also shown that three 10-minute sessions of exercise per day are almost as effective as one 30-minute session.[6] Especially on days when you just can't work in an exercise session, try these simple ways to add some movement to your daily life:

1. Take the stairs instead of the elevator or escalator.
2. Park at the far end of the parking lot if you can do so safely.
3. Walk or bike to nearby locations, such as shops or the library, instead of driving.
4. Get off the bus or train one stop earlier and walk the rest of the way.
5. Take the dog for longer walks—you'll both benefit.
6. Leave the shopping cart at the store entrance and carry your bags to your car.
7. Take short walks at the office during breaks and at lunchtime.
8. Do some arm exercises with a light barbell while you talk on the phone.
9. Use a cordless or cell phone and walk around the house while you talk.
10. Do chair exercises when you have a few minutes at work or when you're watching television.

water aerobics) designed especially for overweight people are now available in many communities, often through local hospitals, community centers, and health clubs. Look for such a program; you'll probably find one nearby. Instead of being embarrassed, you may end up finding yourself an exercise buddy with the same goals as yours.

WHAT'S YOUR EXERCISE IQ?

1. Which forms of exercise below are aerobic?
   a. yoga
   b. walking
   c. weight training
   d. swimming
   e. bike riding
   f. elliptical trainer
2. Your goal is to exercise how often?
   a. almost every day for 30 minutes
   b. twice a week for 30 minutes
   c. twice a week for 1 hour
   d. every other day for 20 minutes
3. Your goal when you exercise is to raise your heart rate to:
   a. 90 percent of maximum
   b. 50 percent of maximum
   c. between 60 and 80 percent of maximum
   d. no more than 50 percent of maximum
4. Bonus question for women:
   Which of the following statements are true about exercise for women?
   a. Exercise causes bulging muscles.   True ❏   False ❏
   b. Exercise causes hot flashes.   True ❏   False ❏
   c. Exercise strengthens bones.   True ❏   False ❏
   d. Exercise can tone your muscles.   True ❏   False ❏
   e. Exercise improves your balance.   True ❏   False ❏

Answers
1. b, d, e, f. 2. a. 3. c. 4. a. false; b. false; c. true; d. true; e. true.

Chapter 23

YOUR PERSONAL EXERCISE PROGRAM

No exercise program is one-size-fits-all, although some basic principles do apply to everyone. This chapter will show you how to get started on a walking program and also how to do some basic weight training and other exercises. We've set it up so that you can design an individualized regimen that works for you. Of course, as we've stressed before, check with your physician before you begin.

TAKE A WALK

Of all the many ways you can exercise, walking tops the list. It's the ideal form of low-impact aerobic exercise. It gives you a good workout, you certainly know how to do it, you can do it just about anywhere, and all it takes in the way of equipment is a pair of comfortable shoes. It's the ultimate "no excuses" exercise.

Begin just by walking as far as you can. Push yourself a little bit, but not to the point of feeling exhausted. For beginners, the goal is to walk for at least a half hour at a comfortable pace, but if you're very unfit, you might not be able to walk for that long; and even if you can, you might not get very far. Walking just a short distance for a short time is still a good start. Remember the old Chinese saying "A journey of a thousand miles begins with a single step."

There's a natural tendency to be overly enthusiastic when you first start an exercise program, but it's important to take the time to allow your body to adjust. Slow and steady is the way to protect your joints as you begin to reverse years of inactivity, restore muscle mass, and re-balance your body chemistry. There is no benefit in being so enthusiastic that you hurt yourself. It is also important to remember that those at greatest risk of developing serious cardiac complications associated with exercise are people who have been sedentary and begin with too much zeal.[1] You're changing your habits for life—taking it slowly for a few weeks to avoid injury will get you good results in the long run.

A good rule of thumb is to increase your walking distance and frequency gradually but steadily. Start by walking three times a week. For many people, increasing distance (and or time) by 10 percent a week prevents overuse injuries and allows your mind and body to adjust to the increased activity. It may seem slow, but if you stick with it, you'll be up to a walk of 30 minutes' duration pretty quickly. If you can only walk slowly to the corner of your street and back the first week, aim for twice the distance the next week. When you've reached the point of walking for 30 minutes, the next stage is to try to walk just as long, but a little faster. Your eventual goal is to walk nonstop at least every other day (preferably every day) for at least 30 minutes at a time at a brisk pace. What's a brisk pace? Use a heart monitor or take your pulse every five minutes or so to verify that you're exercising at your target heart rate (see Chapter 22). A more informal way is to use the talk-sing test. If you can carry on a conversation without gasping for breath, but don't have enough breath to sing, your pace is about right.

As you continue with your walking program, you'll find that you can go longer and longer with your heart rate around the target number. The time it takes after exercise for you to return to your resting heart rate will get shorter, and your resting heart rate may also decrease. Both shortened recovery time and a slower resting heart rate are signs that your exercise program is working, because they are indicators that your heart muscle is getting stronger and doesn't have to work as hard to pump your blood.

RESEARCH REPORT: WALKING TO PREVENT DIABETES

We know that exercise helps prevent diabetes, but do you have to exercise strenuously? Not necessarily—brisk walking is almost as effective as more vigorous forms of exercise, such as jogging. When researchers looked at the activity levels of the women in the Nurses' Health Study over an eight-year period, they found that overall, the more physically active a woman was, the less likely she was to develop diabetes. Compared with the women who were least active, the most active women had about half the risk. When the researchers adjusted the numbers to take body mass index (BMI) into account, there was still a strong benefit from physical activity. Even among the heaviest women, the ones who exercised the most—by walking or doing some other form of physical activity—cut their risk of diabetes by about 25 percent compared with the women who exercised the least.[2] Just think how much more improvement these women could have experienced if they had used the ABSCP! Dr. Atkins knew, from years of seeing patients, that Type 2 diabetes can almost always be avoided!

WALKING ALTERNATIVES

If you don't want to walk or if it's not convenient, there are lots of good aerobic alternatives. You can swim or ride a bike; at the health club, you can take an aerobics class or work out on aerobic equipment, such as the stair-stepper, elliptical trainer, or treadmill. If you'd rather stay home, you can ride an exercise bike, do stepping exercises (if your leg joints are up to it), or exercise to a video tape—there are even walking tapes that give you the equivalent of a mile's walk right in your own living room.

Walking might not be right for you if you have problems with your back, hips, knees, or feet. Never fear—there are plenty of other enjoyable aerobic exercises you can still do. Low-impact aerobics, water aerobics, swimming, biking, riding an exercise bike (consider a re-

WALK SAFELY

Some commonsense precautions will help keep your walks safe and comfortable:

- Wear comfortable, properly fitted walking shoes with cushioned, athletic socks. Check the shoes often and replace them when they show signs of wear, especially on the soles.
- Try to walk on level surfaces, such as dirt paths, running tracks, smooth sidewalks, or flat, grassy areas. Walking on uneven surfaces, such as rough fields, could cause foot and joint injuries.
- Choose a safe place to walk. When walking at night, choose a well-lit route and wear a reflective vest for extra visibility. Tell someone where you're going and when you plan to be back. Carry your ID and a cell phone if possible.
- Be aware of traffic. Stay on the sidewalk whenever possible; if not, face into the traffic.
- Dress for the weather. Particularly in cold weather, dress in layers so you can remove them as you warm up. Wear a hat in both hot and cold weather. In very hot or very cold weather, or on high-ozone days, consider walking indoors at a shopping mall or on a treadmill.

cumbent bike for added comfort), and using an elliptical trainer are all good options. Today there's a wonderful world of exercise equipment that anyone, even someone who is very unfit or very overweight, can use. Just about every community has a place for just about anyone to exercise safely, often at little or no cost. You'll find swimming pools, aerobic classes, and exercise equipment at health clubs, YMCAs, community centers, private exercise studios, and fitness centers at local hospitals. Some insurance companies cover fitness programs if they are prescribed by a physician.

EVERY STEP COUNTS: A GADGET TO GET YOU GOING

A newly popular way to work more physical activity into your life is to track your daily steps with a pedometer, a small, inexpensive gadget that clips to your waist and detects and records the motion of your steps. The average healthy adult takes some 6,000 to 8,500 steps a day—wear your pedometer for a week without changing your activities to find your personal average. Depending on how much you move around in the course of a typical day, to achieve 10,000 steps a day—about 4½ to 5 miles—you may only need to take a 30-minute walk. People who are less active will have to walk longer or find other ways to add more motion to their daily activities. The pedometer lets you see how close you come to achieving your goal. Keeping a chart can also help you track your progress.

CHAIR EXERCISES

If you still think all this talk about exercise is not meant for you because you're very unfit or have trouble moving around, listen up: You can still exercise! Dr. Atkins generally recommended chair exercises in such cases, although anyone can certainly do them—they're an excellent way to sneak in some exercise while sitting in your cubicle at work. We could suggest a dozen different exercises, but only have space here for a few. A good personal trainer can help you learn more, and there are plenty of books, videos, and Web sites that can give you additional suggestions. Just make sure your chair is up to it!

Arm Raises

Sit in a sturdy chair (without wheels, of course) with your feet flat on the floor. Stretch your arms out to either side at shoulder height with your palms facing out. To the count of five, slowly raise your arms above your head until your fingertips meet. Hold for a count of five,

GOOD PAIN AND BAD PAIN

As you begin your exercise program, it's perfectly normal to feel a little stiff and sore. After all, you're moving muscles and joints that haven't been used very much recently. There's a difference between the "good" pain that comes with being more active and the "bad" pain that signals an injury. Here's how to tell the two apart:

Good pain: A slight dull ache or soreness in a muscle or a slight stiffness around a joint that goes away after a couple of days, or even after a good soak in a warm tub. This sort of pain gradually diminishes as your fitness level increases.

Bad pain: Sharp or sudden pain that keeps hurting after you stop the activity. This could indicate a joint problem or an injury. If the pain is severe or persists, or if the joint is red or swollen, see your doctor.

and then slowly lower your arms to shoulder height. Repeat at least four more times.

Knee Extensions

Sit in a sturdy chair with your feet flat on the floor. Keeping your feet together, to the count of five, slowly extend your legs until your calves are parallel to the floor—or as parallel as you can get them for now. Hold for a count of five, then slowly lower your feet again to the floor. Repeat at least four more times. If it's too hard for you to do both legs together, do them one at a time.

Marching in Place

Sit in a sturdy chair with your feet flat on the floor. Alternating legs, "march" in place at a walking pace. Continue for at least three minutes or for as long as you are comfortable.

DANGER SIGNS!

The moderate exercise recommended here is unlikely to cause problems, especially if your doctor has cleared you to do it. Even so, be alert to the danger signs. If you experience any of the following, stop exercising immediately and seek medical care:

- pain or pressure in the chest, shoulder, arm, jaw, or neck area
- dizziness, lightheadedness, feeling faint
- severe shortness of breath, wheezing, coughing, or difficulty breathing
- nausea
- excessive sweating (not from exercise or a hot flash)
- visual disturbances, such as seeing flashes of light or blurred vision

WEIGHT TRAINING

In the next phase of your program, you will maintain your aerobic exercise every other day for at least 30 minutes at the level that keeps your heart rate at around your calculated target number. You will then begin to add weight training (also known as resistance training) to your plan. Your goal will be to do your weight routine on the days between your aerobic exercise—or two or three times a week for about 30 minutes at each session. You'll be exercising almost every day.

GETTING STARTED

Despite the ads you see on TV for expensive, complicated equipment, weight training can be very simple and inexpensive. You can even start with cans of soup instead of weights, but we recommend starting with inexpensive 1- or 2-pound dumbbells or strap-on adjustable wrist and ankle weights. You can buy these in any sporting goods department or store. You may need to start with just a ½-pound weight and move up gradually to heavier weights as you get stronger.

STRETCH FIRST!

The first few minutes of any exercise session should be spent on some gentle stretching exercises. This allows your body to prepare for exercise and avoids joint and ligament damage.

Take note: If you have physical challenges that would make the exercises mentioned here difficult, discuss your exercise plan with your doctor or a physical therapist.

Start by stretching the muscles in the backs of your lower legs (calves). Stand facing a wall, about 12 inches away. Place your palms on the wall at shoulder height. Keeping your feet flat on the floor, slowly and gently do a "push-up" against the wall. Hold the stretch for 10 to 15 seconds and let your muscles stretch out naturally—don't bounce—then repeat. You should feel mild tension but no pain from the stretch. To feel more of a stretch, stand farther back from the wall. The muscles in the backs of your legs are the ones that tighten up the most from sitting, so they require the most stretching. It is also beneficial to stretch the muscles in the back of the thigh, the hamstrings. An easy way to do this is to extend both legs while sitting in a chair, bending forward at the hips with the back straight.

Next, stretch the muscles in your shoulders, middle back, and arms. Stand with your feet apart at shoulder width. Interlace your fingers and turn your hands palms out. Extend your arms out in front of you at shoulder height. Hold for 10 to 15 seconds, relax, and repeat.

If you don't have back problems, use this stretch for your middle back. Stand with your feet apart at shoulder width and your knees slightly bent. Place your hands on your hips. Gently twist your upper body to the left at the waist until you feel a gentle stretch. Hold for 10 to 15 seconds, relax, and repeat. Repeat twice more, twisting gently to the right.

Here's a good stretch for your arms: Throw a bath towel over an open door. Stand facing the edge of the door. Hold on to the ends of the towel with one hand on each side of the door. Now pull down on the towel with one arm, as if you were pulling it off the door. Your other arm will be lifted up as you pull down. Do this, alternating arms each time, five to ten times, to gently warm up your arm and shoulder muscles.

By beginning your workout slowly, you will stretch the muscles in the rest of your body; as you warm up, increase the pace.

READY, SET, LIFT

To get the most from weight-training exercise, it should be done slowly and repetitively. Lift your weights to a slow count of three or four, pause at the top of the motion, and then lower the weights to a slow count of three or four. Breathe out slowly as you lift the weight up and breathe in as you lower it—don't hold your breath! Repeat each exercise five times (this is known as doing five "reps") to start. Each group of reps is a set. To get the most out of this experience, start with a weight that can be lifted 10 to 20 times. By starting with an easy weight, you can practice good technique and also begin developing muscular endurance while building strength. Rest for a minute or two between each set and between different exercises. When an exercise starts to get too easy, you can increase the weight, remembering to move up in increments that allow you to continue with at least ten reps at a time. By changing only the weight or number of reps at any one time, you can minimize the stress on muscles and tendons and hopefully avoid injuries.

There are many different weight-training exercises, each designed to help strengthen a particular group of muscles, such as the quadriceps in your upper thigh. Here are five exercises that would make up a very basic starting program. (For more suggestions, visit www.atkins.com.) To take your weight training further—and we hope you will—we strongly recommend working with a personal trainer, if this option is available to you.

Biceps Curl

This exercise strengthens your biceps, the muscle in the front of your upper arm (the muscle that bulges when Popeye eats his spinach).

Stand with your feet apart at shoulder width. Grasp a dumbbell in each hand and hang your arms at your sides with your palms facing outward, away from your body. Holding your elbows in close to your sides, curl (lift) both dumbbells up toward your shoulders. Lower and repeat. You can alternate arms.

Triceps Curl

This exercise strengthens your triceps and the muscle in the back of your upper arm, and it can help add definition in this frequent trouble spot. You only need one dumbbell for this exercise.

Stand with your feet apart at shoulder width. Grasp the dumbbell vertically and hold it with both hands above and slightly behind your head. Keeping your upper arms close to your head, lower the dumbbell behind your head until your forearms touch your biceps. Raise the dumbbell up again and repeat. Alternately, to put less stress on the elbow joint and shoulder, consider doing overhead extensions. Simply hold the dumbbell at shoulder height and elevate it above your head. Repeat on the other side.

Upward Row

This exercise strengthens your trapezius (the large upper-back muscle), your deltoids (the shoulder muscles), and your biceps (front arm muscles).

Stand with your feet apart at shoulder width. Hold a dumbbell in each hand. Place your arms in front of your thighs, with your palms facing your thighs. Lift the dumbbells up until your hands are under your chin and your elbows are at shoulder height and pointing out to the sides. Lower and repeat.

Side Hip Raise

This exercise strengthens the muscles of your thighs and your hips. These muscles help you stand up easily and also help you keep your balance. You'll need your ankle weights (you can do it without weights at first) and a sturdy chair to do this exercise.

Stand behind a sturdy chair and place your hands lightly on the back for balance. Slowly lift your foot straight out to the side until it is about six inches off the ground. Return and repeat. Do one set and then switch to the other leg. Be careful to keep your body upright as you do the exercise; don't lean to the side.

Leg Swings

This exercise strengthens the muscles on the inside of your thighs. You'll need your ankle weights (you can do it without weights at first) and a sturdy chair to do this exercise.

Stand sideways to the chair back, with your left hand resting lightly on the back for balance. Slowly swing your right leg forward until your heel is about six inches off the ground; then slowly swing your leg back until your toes are about six inches off the ground. Return to a standing position and repeat. Do one set and switch to the left leg. You'll have to turn around and put your right hand on the chair back.

To complete your weight training, consider performing some toe stands. The weight you lift in this exercise is your own body. For this one, once again, you'll need a sturdy, nonrolling chair.

Stand behind the back of the chair with your feet slightly apart. Rest both hands lightly on the back for balance. Slowly raise yourself up on your toes, pause for a moment, and then slowly lower yourself back down until your feet are flat on the floor. Repeat five to ten times.

Now that you've finished your exercises, don't forget to cool down— repeat a couple of your favorite stretches (especially leg stretches) or take an easy walk.

SHOULD YOU JOIN A HEALTH CLUB?

Joining a health club is a great way to get in shape. The clubs offer exercise equipment that's too big and expensive to have at home, along with classes and expert help from a personal trainer on designing your workout. Many health clubs now offer classes just for people who are overweight or very out of condition. Also, the range of activities at a health club lets you find the ones you particularly enjoy. Another advantage is the camaraderie that comes from working out with other people. Finding some good exercise buddies helps keep you motivated.

If you're thinking of joining a health club, here's what to look for:

- Pick a club with a location that's convenient. If you have to go out of your way to get there, you may stop going.
- Inspect the facilities. Make sure the locker rooms and workout areas are clean, all equipment is in good working order, and there are enough exercise machines.
- Look at the hours. If you like to work out early in the morning, will the club be open then? Is the schedule of classes convenient for you? Does the club offer child care (if that is a consideration)?
- Check out the atmosphere. Look for a gym that seems relaxed and friendly, with a variety of classes for people at all levels of fitness. Visit at a busy time and note how many people there are your age and at your fitness level.
- Before you sign up for an expensive yearlong membership, purchase a day pass or a short trial membership to make sure the club is the right one for you.
- If you want to work with a trainer—and we recommend that you do—make sure he or she is someone you are comfortable with before you sign up.

THE NEXT STEP

After you have established both your weight and aerobic programs, you can advance further. Use the principles of interval training and cross-training to continue your improvement.

Interval training means alternating periods of regular exercise with periods of more intense exercise. In your walking program, for instance, you would add interval training by exercising harder for two minutes out of every ten that you walk. Start by warming up as usual. Increase to your usual brisk pace for eight minutes, and then walk as fast as you safely can for two minutes. Return to your usual pace for another eight minutes, and add the speed burst again for two minutes, and so on for the duration of your walk. When you can do five minutes of fast walking for every ten minutes of exercise, it's time for congratulations! You're doing great! In fact, you can now start thinking about cross-training—adding other activities to your exercise program for variety and to work additional muscles. You may now well be able to return to activities you used to enjoy or try some new ones. Proceed cautiously, of course, and with the advice of a personal trainer if at all possible.

TRACK YOUR PROGRESS

Keeping track of your progress is a great way to help you stick with your exercise program. Use these sample exercise log sheets to record your daily activity. (You can copy them or use them as a template for designing your own log.) After you've been exercising regularly for a few months, you'll be amazed at how far you've come along.

AEROBIC PROGRAM

Date	Start Time	End Time	Duration	Distance	Comments
____	_____	_____	_____	_____	_____
____	_____	_____	_____	_____	_____
____	_____	_____	_____	_____	_____
____	_____	_____	_____	_____	_____
____	_____	_____	_____	_____	_____
____	_____	_____	_____	_____	_____

WEIGHT-TRAINING PROGRAM

Date: _____	Weight	Reps/Sets
Biceps Curl	_____	_____
Triceps Curl	_____	_____
Upward Row	_____	_____
Side Hip Raise	_____	_____
Leg Swings	_____	_____

Chapter 24

IT'S NOT JUST BABY FAT

As sad and overwhelming as it is to hear that more than half of American adults are overweight or obese, it's truly shocking to hear the current statistics on children. One in three children born in the year 2000 is destined to get diabetes as an adult.[1] Childhood overweight and obesity has become an epidemic. More than 15 percent of American kids ages 6 to 19 are now overweight. Incidence of overweight and obesity among this age group has nearly tripled in the last 20 years.[2]

Carrying excess weight sets the stage for serious health problems that begin early and last a lifetime—a lifetime that may well be shorter than it should be. In fact, so many kids today are so seriously overweight that we are looking at the first generation that may have a shorter life span than their parents. Morever, as we'll discuss in the next chapter, there has been a staggering rise in the number of children with Type 2 diabetes. Without mincing words, this is a crisis for our nation and a personal tragedy for these youngsters and their families.

Fortunately, there is a bright side: Overweight kids have youth on their side. When they control their carb intake and increase their activity level, the results can be amazing. Dr. Atkins found it tremendously satisfying to see a child who was once overweight, sedentary, and withdrawn come back to his office a few months later slimmer and brimming with energy. Formerly overweight children who undergo this transformation are happier as well. Being the butt of jokes and victim of bullying, as many overweight kids are, is enormously painful. As a side benefit, when children lose weight, the parents usually end up slimmer, too—treating childhood obesity and preventing diabetes must be a family affair.

A PROBLEM OF GLOBAL SCALE

Unfortunately, the United States is leading the pack—and the epidemic is spreading, with Europeans, Asians, and other peoples quickly catching up.[3] What has caused this explosive growth in childhood overweight and obesity? In recent years, two major factors have contributed: a diet heavy in nutrient-depleted, high-carbohydrate snack foods and sugary drinks (including fruit juice and soda), and a lack of physical activity. As these factors combine with genetics, we have the recipe for a disaster.

The two trends feed each other, only aggravating the situation. Instead of playing outdoors, kids watch television, play video games, or surf the Web as they fill up on carb-packed snack foods. Even when parents make an effort to buy snacks that seem healthy, the "multigrain" cereal bars, fruit snacks, and "real cheese" crackers are just well-disguised junk food made with sugar, hydrogenated oils, and bleached flour. At the same time, more than half of all commercials on children's television shows hawk snacks, breakfast cereals, and drinks full of sugar, and, of course, high-carb fast food. It's the rare parent who can resist the pleas to satisfy these demands. A larger number of commercials for snacks actually leads to increased consumption of these foods, according to a recent study.[4]

Even worse, those same foods are the daily fare your youngsters eat in school. Your child can be served a school lunch of chicken nuggets coated with high-carb batter and deep-fried in unhealthy hydrogenated oil—along with a pile of potato chips, a slice of tomato, and a leaf of iceberg lettuce—as well as canned fruit cocktail in heavy syrup and a heavily sweetened drink. The irony is that this dreadful fare is considered a healthy, well-balanced meal by the federal government's dietary standards.[5]

302 ATKINS DIABETES REVOLUTION

At the same time, the typical school is full of vending machines selling candy, sugary snack foods, and sweetened drinks as a way to raise desperately needed money for school activities. And even as schools are signing contracts that force them to serve your children high-sugar drinks in the cafeteria, they are cutting back on physical education classes, recess time, and after-school sports—even though the money from the contracts is often supposedly dedicated to sports and other after-school programs! Not only are your kids bulking up (and getting dental cavities) from the food and drinks they're served in school, they're often not getting any sort of supervised exercise. This is the worst sort of vicious cycle—and it's very hard for most parents to counteract its effects. Even if your child is still of normal weight, seemingly healthy, and not displaying any behavioral problems, that does not mean that he or she cannot benefit from cutting down on sugar and other refined carbohydrates.

LIQUID CANDY

Of all the things kids shouldn't be consuming, sugary drinks top the list. Fruit juice may sound healthy, but it's really not much more than pure sugar in the form of fructose, without any of the fiber and other nutrients from whole fruit. (It takes eight to ten oranges to produce one glass of orange juice.) Recently, a number of supposedly healthy milk-based drinks have become popular, but they too are crammed with added sugar. The worst of the worst, though, is most carbonated beverages. A typical can of what nutritionists call "liquid candy" is so heavily sweetened with high-fructose corn syrup that it contains the equivalent of up to 10 teaspoons of sugar,[6] to say nothing of the caffeine in many of them, which is associated with headaches, irritability, and sleeplessness.[7] The average teen today gets about 8 percent of his or her daily calories from soda and other sweetened soft drinks; teenage boys are very heavy consumers of soda, often drinking three or more cans a day. There's a direct link between soft-drink consumption and weight gain. For every 12-ounce can of soda a youngster drinks each day, the risk of weight gain and becoming obese goes up.[8]

The weight gain from soda is bad enough, but these drinks also displace other, more nutritious foods. Today, many teens fall short of the recommended intake DRI of one or more of the following nutrients: vitamins A, B_6, C, and E and the minerals calcium, iron, and zinc.[9] This is especially dangerous, as young bodies need these nutrients in the proper amounts to continue normal growth and development.[10]

SKIP THE BUBBLY FOR HEALTHY BONES

Even sugar-free soda isn't a good beverage choice for kids—or adults. Fizzy drinks, especially colas, contain phosphorus, which can interfere with the skeleton's ability to absorb calcium. Kids already aren't getting enough calcium because soda displaces milk and other calcium-rich foods from their diet; the last thing they need is a chemical that interferes with the absorption of what calcium they do get. The result of all this is weaker bones. A recent study of ninth- and tenth-grade girls showed that those who drank the most soft drinks were three times more likely to have a bone fracture than those who drank the least. Among physically active girls, the ones who drank the most colas were five times more likely to have a bone fracture than those who drank the least.[11] It appears that not only are obesity and diabetes a major concern for this generation of children, they also face an increased likelihood of osteoporosis.

WHY NOT WATER?

What should youngsters be drinking instead of soda or juice? Plain water is always the simplest and best choice, and nothing quenches thirst better. The best recent teen trend: It seems that carrying around a water bottle has become a fashion accessory. However, sticking to just water while their peers are having soda can be a challenge for many kids.

Caffeine-free sodas made with substitute sweeteners such as Splenda are a reasonable alternative, but only in limited amounts—you want to help your child get over the idea that every drink should be sweet. Flavored seltzer, or seltzer with a splash of sugar-free syrup, is a good compromise. If your child has no blood sugar or weight problems, vegetable juices are acceptable, but all fruit juices have the potential to cause insulin/blood sugar problems and contribute to weight gain. Occasionally—for instance, when you are away from home—you might allow your child to have a small portion of fruit juice (with the lowest-carb count, please). But such drinks should always be accompanied by food containing protein and fat to keep the sugar from being dumped into the bloodstream too quickly.

The same is true of milk, which contains 11 grams of carbs per 8-ounce glass, primarily sugar in the form of lactose. It is best to drink full-fat milk as part of a meal or with a protein snack. If weight or insulin/blood sugar problems exist, consider limiting milk to one 8-ounce glass a day, depending on blood sugar response. If your child wants more milk, try one of the new reduced-carb dairy beverage products. Look for one with at least 10 grams of protein and about 3 grams Net Carbs per 8-ounce glass. You probably needn't worry about calcium—if *you're* following the Atkins Nutritional Approach (ANA) or the Atkins Blood Sugar Control Program (ABSCP)—since your child will probably be getting plenty of calcium from the greater amounts of cheese and vegetables you are serving. Of course, your child will almost certainly eat more carbohydrates than you do.

SOY FOODS FOR KIDS

Parents sometimes serve kids soymilk instead of milk, but some cautions apply here. Unless it's unsweetened soymilk (which contains anywhere from 1 to 4 grams of Net Carbs per 8 ounces), this may not make much of a difference in terms of carb count. Youngsters may not like the taste of unsweetened soymilk, however. Sweetened soymilk, which is sometimes labeled a little misleadingly as "plain" (meaning unflavored) soymilk, has added sugar to cover the taste; 8 ounces contains about 12 grams of Net Carbs. Flavored soymilks have even more. There are about 28 Net Carb grams in 8 ounces of chocolate-flavored soymilk. Avoid sweetened and flavored products altogether.

There are other reasons to be cautious about soy. Some children are allergic to it (though soy is recommended as an alternative for kids who are allergic to milk). Soy also contains phytoestrogens, natural chemicals that can weakly mimic the action of the female sex hormone estrogen. To avoid any hormonal effects from soymilk and other soy products such as tofu (bean curd), Dr. Atkins recommended limiting youngsters to two servings a day.

THE SNACK TRAP

According to data from the third Continuing Survey of Food Intakes by Individuals (CSFII),[12] 82 percent of children aged six to eleven reported eating at least one snack a day—and those snacks made up some 20 percent of their daily calories. In order of frequency, the snacks were:

1. soft drinks
2. salty snacks, such as potato chips, corn chips, and popcorn
3. cookies
4. nonchocolate candy
5. artificially flavored fruit beverages
6. whole milk and chocolate milk
7. 2 percent milk
8. white bread
9. chocolate candy
10. cake
11. ice cream
12. fruit

As you can see, the type of snacks most children eat explains in large part why so many of them struggle with their weight. With the exception of whole milk, the only nonprocessed food on the list is fruit, coming in at a distant twelfth. With these two exceptions, all the other foods on the list are not just high in carbs but low in nutritional value. Most are also made with unhealthful hydrogenated or partially hydrogenated oils. The same survey also showed that more than half of all elementary-school-age children ate no fruit on any given day.

A PALATE MAKEOVER

Over and over Dr. Atkins saw children who cut down on their intake of high-carb foods quickly lose their taste for sweets and salty snacks. That doesn't mean they don't still enjoy these foods, it simply means that they aren't beset with cravings for them. When the kids do eat such snacks, as long as they are combined with protein and/or fat, they're more able to moderate their intake and the food is unlikely to trigger their cravings. Because there are now so many good low-carb substitute foods, kids who need to control their carbs can still enjoy occasional candy bars, ice cream, and even chips—as long as they select a quality low-carb brand. If you'd like to make your own low-carb treats, check the abundance of recipes on www.atkins.com and in any of the good low-carb cookbooks now available, including *Dr. Atkins' Quick & Easy New Diet Cookbook.* Also turn to page 402 for a small selection of additional recipes.

The same survey indicates that the top five sources of calories for the typical American youngster are, in order, whole and chocolate milk, pizza, soft drinks, low-fat milk, and cold breakfast cereal, a particularly high source of sugar. Three out of ten kids eat less than one serving of vegetables a day.[13] These appalling statistics go a long way to explaining why so many children today are overweight. Their diets consist primarily of low-quality carbohydrates.

THE TV TRAP

A lot of junk food is consumed in front of the television. But snacks aside, TV viewing alone is associated with childhood obesity. In a study of sixth and seventh graders in California, more TV meant higher weight. Of the youngsters who watched less than two hours of television each night, 26.2 percent had a BMI (body mass index) at or above the 85th percentile, while among those who watched three or more hours of television each night, 47.1 percent had BMIs at or

HOW TO USE LOW-CARB PRODUCTS APPROPRIATELY

The growth of the low-carb replacement foods offers choices to people who miss traditional high-carb foods or are looking for ingredients that cut carbs without sacrificing taste. Low-carb bread makes it easy for kids to take sandwiches to school. Pancake mix is a great breakfast alternative. Shakes and protein bars can make a satisfying occasional after-school snack. But all low-carb products need to be used in moderation. They are not a substitute for whole foods. Make sure your child is eating enough meat, fish, eggs, and other sources of protein and healthy fats as well as vegetables, nuts, seeds, fruit, and whole grains, before he or she fills up on low-carb convenience foods. This advice applies to adults as well.

above the 85th percentile.[14] Of course, even 26.2 percent of a group of kids shouldn't be that heavy, but we know from other studies that less TV viewing is associated with a lower weight. Many people, regardless of age, go on automatic pilot when they are in front of the tube, eating mindlessly, regardless of whether they feel hungry or full.

YOUNGSTERS NEED TO MOVE

TV isn't the only culprit. Today half of all high school students aren't taking phys ed class, mostly because their schools no longer require it or no longer even offer it. Currently, only Illinois requires *any* phys ed! Suburban neighborhoods without sidewalks, appropriate parental worries about the risks of unsupervised activity, and many other factors all conspire to keep kids indoors and sedentary; yet physical activity is crucial for their health. Regular physical activity helps build and maintain healthy muscles, bones, and joints. It helps control weight, reduce fat, and build lean body mass. It also helps children burn off excess energy and has been shown to help reduce feelings of depression and anxiety. Activities that decrease stress hormone production,

BLOOD SUGAR AND BEHAVIOR

You hear a lot about ADD in kids, but have you ever heard anyone talk about blood sugar problems in children? Kids with unstable blood sugar can suffer from mood swings, irritability, depression, and difficulty concentrating—which in turn can lead to serious problems with schoolwork and mental health. Dr. Atkins felt that these symptoms are often confused with learning disabilities and attention deficit hyperactivity disorder (ADHD). (In addition to nutritional deficits caused by poor diet, other environmental factors can contribute to these conditions.) The "treatment" is to medicate them with stimulants and/or antidepressants. (Some antidepressant drugs cause weight gain, which worsens the situation on all fronts.) Would you believe that Prozac is now being given even to preschoolers!

In Dr. Atkins' experience, a high-carb diet and a lack of exercise can

as exercise does, are important in our stress-laden society—even for children. As a bonus, when kids are physically strong and don't feel restless, depressed, or anxious, they do better in school and have fewer behavioral problems.

IS YOUR CHILD OVERWEIGHT?

With children, it's a bit more complicated to decipher how overweight someone is. We can use the basic idea of the BMI to figure out if a child is overweight or not, but we have to adjust the numbers to account for the child's age and gender, and for the fact that there is a wide range of normal growth rates. The BMI charts for children aged 2 to 20 give a BMI number based on weight and height, but then use a curve to show how the child's BMI-for-age compares with that of all other children of the same age and gender. So, if a girl has a BMI-for-age that puts her in the 60th percentile, that means that compared with other girls of the same age, 60 percent have a lower BMI. A BMI-for-age that is lead to blood sugar imbalances that affect brain chemistry. These "behavioral problems" often dissipate once the underlying blood sugar problem is finally diagnosed and treated, and in some cases drugs are no longer needed.

In children with mental health issues, the ABSCP can be the foundation of their treatment program—of course, under the guidance of a physician. Stable blood sugar often helps a "hyperactive" kid stay calmer and more focused on schoolwork; it also helps stabilize mood. And once blood sugar is under control, kids lose their cravings for carbs and start to lose weight, which is the most effective treatment of all for depression caused by low self-esteem, poor body image, parental nagging, and the relentless teasing of other kids. Some psychiatrists have found the use of supplemental oils helpful for depression, as did Dr. Atkins. If additional medications are needed, then the sound nutritional base of the ABSCP will enhance the child's health.

below the 5th percentile would indicate that a child is underweight. A BMI-for-age in the 85th to 94th percentile for a child's age and gender would mean that the child is at risk of being overweight. A BMI-for-age in the 95th percentile or above means that the child *is* overweight. (Note that the term *obesity* is not used in this context.)

To put that into numbers, the normal weight for a 13-year-old boy who stands five feet three inches tall would be anywhere from 88 to 123 pounds. The normal range is so wide—35 pounds—because among boys that age there's a broad range of normal physical development. Some boys will already be near their adult height and weight, while others are just reaching puberty. That same boy would be in the 85th to 94th percentile and at risk for being overweight if he weighed between 124 and 141 pounds, and he would be at the 95th percentile and overweight at 142 pounds. In some cases, the BMI-for-age charts can be a little misleading. A teen who is very strong and muscular, for instance, could seem to be at risk for overweight even though he or she is actually very fit and healthy. Similarly, a child with very poor health might seem to be in the midrange for his or her age, but should actually weigh more. For almost all kids, though, the BMI-for-age charts give a good idea of where their weight should be within a fairly broad range.

The great advantage of the BMI-for-age chart is that it can be used continually from age 2 until adulthood, so you can see where a child stands in terms of weight as he or she develops from toddler to young adult. (For more on BMI charts, go to www.cdc.gov/nchs/data/nhanes/databriefs/growthch.pdf.)

As a parent, you may not be able to be objective about your child's weight. There's a natural tendency to think those excess pounds are just baby fat or chubbiness, and to think that the child will somehow grow out of it. Other parents worry needlessly that their children may be overweight because of their own struggles with weight. The BMI-for-age charts are completely objective, however, and give you a more accurate idea of whether your child is overweight, and if so, by how much.

IT'S NOT JUST IN THE GENES

Overweight kids grow up to be overweight adults. About a third of all adults who are obese or overweight were that way by the time they reached age 20. According to a recent study, being at or above the 95th percentile of BMI-for-age at age 12 is practically a guarantee of being overweight as an adult. A 12-year-old girl with a BMI of 25 or more would be in the 95th percentile of BMI-for-age and would have an 80 percent or better chance of being overweight as an adult. If she's still in the 95th percentile of BMI-for-age at age 20, she has a better than 99 percent chance of a lifetime of obesity.[15]

Weight problems tend to be a family affair. That's not surprising, as the parents supply not just the genes but the meals and the attitudes toward food for their offspring. After all, youngsters don't drive themselves to fast-food restaurants—at least not until they are teenagers. The odds that an overweight child will grow up to be an overweight adult increase if one or both parents are overweight as well. In fact, even for kids under age 10 who aren't obese, if their parents are, this more than doubles their risk of adult obesity.[16] And when overweight kids become overweight adults, they tend to be dangerously heavy. A study published in 2003 found that those who were overweight at ages 12 or 13 were five times more likely to be severely obese as adults than those who were not overweight at these ages.[17]

Of course, this is a matter of genetics interacting with environment. If a child has parents who have the metabolic syndrome, then the child will be genetically "set up" to have the same body chemistry. Feed this child the typical high-carbohydrate American diet and watch his or her waistline expand and youthful arteries begin to clog. Often, the parents are on the couch watching TV and eating the same snacks next to the child. And then there are doting grandparents and other relatives who may press sweets and other poor-quality treats on a child as demonstrations of their love. Finally, there are caretakers who may use high-carb snacks to encourage good behavior. In sum, this scenario is a recipe for fattening American youth!

HEALTH RISKS OF CHILDHOOD OBESITY

More and more studies reveal that the origins of adult heart disease lie in being overweight as a child. A British study that went on for 57 years showed a direct link between being overweight as a child and dying from heart disease as an adult. Over the course of the study, the participants who were heaviest as children were 1.5 times more likely to die from any cause and twice as likely to die from heart disease as those who were normal weight as children.[18] More frighteningly, a 37-year follow-up study of 227,000 Norwegian teens found that among the men whose BMI-for-age in adolescence was above the 95th percentile, the death rate was 80 percent higher than that for the men who were of normal weight. Among the women, the death rate was 100 percent higher.[19] Another study showed that arterial plaque can start forming in early childhood.[20]

Because overweight and obese kids already show many of the classic risk factors for heart disease, it's not surprising that they develop it at a much earlier age, often in their thirties and forties. In a study of 1,366 Taiwanese 12- to 16-year-olds, 70 percent of the boys who were obese already had one risk factor for heart disease, and 25 percent of them had two or more risk factors.[21]

THE CONSEQUENCES OF CHILDHOOD OBESITY

Children who weigh too much get a head start on chronic diseases that ordinarily only develop much later in life. To take just one example, up to 20 percent of obese kids have hypertension.[22]

A recent estimate based on NHANES III data says that among all kids ages 12 to 19, about 4.2 percent already have the metabolic syndrome. And among overweight adolescents, a staggering 28.7 percent already have it! That means that about 910,000 American teens are already at risk of heart disease, diabetes, and premature death.[23]

The problem is even more severe in minority communities. Among overweight Latino children, nine out of ten have at least one risk factor for heart disease and Type 2 diabetes, and three out of ten have three or more risk factors for the metabolic syndrome.[24]

Impaired glucose tolerance is now common among obese kids. In one study at Yale University, 25 percent of obese children ages 4 to 10 were glucose intolerant; 21 percent of obese teens were glucose intolerant. And in the course of the study, the researchers found that 4 percent of the teens already had diabetes and didn't know it![25]

Heart disease and diabetes aren't the only health problems overweight youth face. Such was the case with 10-year-old Samantha B., who came to Dr. Atkins suffering from allergies, sinus problems, almost daily migraines, palpitations, gas, and bloating. With a large appetite for carbohydrate foods, Samantha weighed 134.8 pounds at four feet three inches tall, giving her a BMI-for-age-and-gender of 36.5, which placed her at the 95th percentile, making her overweight. Rather than putting her on a strict Induction-phase regimen, Dr. Atkins cut her carbohydrate intake just enough to stabilize her blood sugar and control her appetite. After four weeks Samantha's headaches had diminished in frequency and intensity, and her parents related that her moods and energy level were much better. After eight months her weight was stable at 120 pounds, and she had no headaches and a significant decrease in gastrointestinal problems. Dr. Atkins felt that so long as she continues to control her carbohydrate intake at an appropriate level to meet her nutritional needs, she should grow into the excess weight she still carries.

Overweight children are also more likely to suffer from asthma due, in part, to the increase in inflammatory chemicals caused by elevated levels of insulin.[26] They also often end up having bone and joint problems for the same reasons.[27] Overweight girls tend to reach puberty and begin menstruating at a younger age. This means that they stop growing sooner than other girls—and end up as short, overweight adults.[28] They're also likely to suffer from polycystic ovary syndrome (PCOS).[29] The underlying metabolic imbalance, combined with a probable genetic component that causes PCOS, makes these girls much more likely to become diabetic as they get older.[30]

Children's mental health can suffer as much as their physical health. Obese kids are at greater risk for emotional problems and low self-esteem, and can become isolated and depressed, especially if they're teased about their weight. The flip side of this is that behavioral problems, such as being hyperactive or depressed, can lead to obesity. A study in 2003 showed that normal-weight kids diagnosed with a behavioral problem were five times more likely to become overweight over the next two years than youngsters without a problem.[31]

Why do these children gain weight? Dr. Atkins believed it's because they're "medicating" themselves with high-carb foods as a way to deal with stress and unhappiness—yet the very foods they use to comfort themselves only make the problems worse. And, according to a recent study, severely obese children (and their parents) rated their obesity as affecting their quality of life to the same extent as that experienced by children going through chemotherapy for cancer.[32]

CONTROLLING CARBS HELPS CHILDREN

The Atkins approach is beneficial to overweight kids, just as it is for overweight adults. (To make sure they're getting proper nutrition and to monitor their progress, anyone under the age of 18 should do the weight-loss phases of the Atkins program only under the supervision of a physician.) Dr. Atkins knew that it works for youngsters because he helped hundreds of them lose weight. Not only does a controlled-carb program help overweight kids slim down or at least stop gaining weight, it helps restore their blood lipids to normal and cuts their risk of early heart disease.

In one study, a group of 16 overweight teens followed a controlled-carb approach for 12 weeks; a control group of 14 overweight teens followed a low-fat diet for the same time. At the end of the period, the controlled-carb teens had lost more weight than the low-fat teens—and triglyceride levels had plummeted.[33]

A FAMILY AFFAIR

When a whole family starts cutting back on unhealthy carbs, everyone benefits, even those who don't need to lose weight and/or stabilize their blood sugar. When you are more sensitized to the value of protein and fats along with healthy carbs, both parents and children will be more likely to eat regular meals and fewer unhealthy snacks, more fresh vegetables and low-glycemic fruits, better-quality carbohydrates overall, and a lot less junk food.

Breakfast comes by its name rightfully. It is important to send children off to school with the foods that get their chemistry off to a healthy, stable start after a long night's fast. Having a high-protein breakfast means that they won't be hungry or craving sugary foods a couple of hours later, and their behavior and schoolwork should improve, often to a remarkable degree. So serve up some eggs and cheese to get the day off to a good start, adding foods such as fruit, full-fat milk, and whole grains as your child's individual metabolism and activity level allow.

On the Atkins family plan—by which we mean that every person is cutting back on carbs to some degree—everyone ends up a lot fitter, too. If you are doing Atkins properly, you are exercising regularly, and your children will see you as a role model. Kids, like adults, benefit greatly from adding a minimum of half an hour a day of physical activity. Of course, this has to be fun or they won't participate. After-school activities aren't always an option, so try to find ways to help your child build more activity into daily life—you'll get more exercise that way, too. Make sure to include physical activity in weekend plans; even a rousing indoor game of catch with a foam ball is enough to get a youngster moving and enjoying it. Exercise videos can be fun if everyone participates. Maybe your child can teach you the latest dance

SCHOOL FOOD

How can you protect your children from the bad nutritional influences they encounter every day at school? Fight back by sending them off to school fueled with a good breakfast—and armed with healthy snacks like an apple to be eaten along with nuts or string cheese, and a good, low-carb lunch such as chicken salad on whole grain bread. Let your kids buy the school lunch or a treat now and then (if you limit kids too much, they can end up getting teased or feeling resentful). Remember, you can't control everything your children eat—you certainly aren't going to keep them from visiting their friends and going to birthday parties—so work on controlling what you can. If you can just cut most of the junk food out of your children's diet and continue to serve high-quality, low-carb meals at home, you'll start seeing progress by decreasing cravings and controlling appetite better, stopping further excessive weight gain, or even encouraging some weight loss.

steps, and both of you can get a good laugh. The important thing is to set a good example by being active yourself and finding ways for the whole family to join in.

WHAT TO EXPECT

In a child, the warning signs of trouble ahead are pretty clear: inappropriate weight gain, cravings for carbohydrate foods, a family history of overweight, and the beginnings of the metabolic syndrome (see Chapter 4). If that describes your child, the steps you need to take are also clear:

- Remove enough unhealthy carbs from meals and snacks to stop any more weight gain. In other words, cut back on junk foods and foods like French fries and cookies that have minimal nutritional content.

- Introduce healthful foods early in life; that way, children develop a taste for them.
- Replace those unhealthy carbs with protein, natural fats, and vegetables. This will help decrease excessive hunger and cravings and introduce the child to a healthier way of eating.
- Don't fixate on the scale—what you want is fat loss, not weight loss, which is why increasing a child's activity is also key. Judge progress by how clothing fits, not by pounds dropped.
- For younger kids who aren't close to puberty (they're not yet showing signs of physical sexual development), the goal is simply to stabilize the child's weight and prevent further gain. Usually as the child grows, he or she will simply "grow into" a normal weight. In extreme cases, physicians may recommend active weight loss, which should be medically supervised.

Likewise, for kids who are already overweight and moving toward obesity, are approaching puberty, or have advanced signs of the metabolic syndrome, you may want to consider a medically supervised program. The child needs to control carbs enough to stabilize his or her abnormal blood sugar, lose inches, and maintain long-term appetite control. That may take some fine-tuning, and supplements may be necessary to ensure that your child is getting the maximum nutritional benefit from the program.

JUST TRY IT, YOU'LL LIKE IT

When Dr. Atkins would explain to overweight children and their families what they had to do to make the necessary dietary and lifestyle changes, he often heard a chorus of concern about how difficult it would be. He suggested that they just give it a try for a month or so to see how it went. When he saw them again, the tune had almost always changed for the better. The youngsters and their families would tell him that the first week or so did take some getting used to, but that in the end the changes weren't so disruptive or difficult at all. And after that, it was easy to stick with the program, because everyone, not just the overweight child, was now eating better, exercising more, and feeling better both physically and mentally—and eating foods they liked.

IS MY CHILD AT RISK?

Agree or disagree with the following statements to see if your child is at risk for obesity.

1. I am overweight.	Yes ❑	No ❑
2. Other close family members are overweight.	Yes ❑	No ❑
3. My child's BMI-for-age is at or above the 85th percentile.	Yes ❑	No ❑
4. My child is physically active less than 30 minutes each day.	Yes ❑	No ❑
5. My child drinks more than one can of soda each day.	Yes ❑	No ❑
6. My child eats a lot of sugary and salty snack foods.	Yes ❑	No ❑
7. My child often eats fast food.	Yes ❑	No ❑
8. The doctor says my child has high blood pressure.	Yes ❑	No ❑
9. The doctor says my child has high blood sugar.	Yes ❑	No ❑
10. The doctor says my child has high cholesterol/high triglycerides.	Yes ❑	No ❑

Scoring: If you answered yes three or more times, your child may well be on a path to being overweight or obese if he or she is not already.

BOUNCING BABY JOY

Having almost developed gestational diabetes with her second pregnancy, unable to lose "baby fat" after the birth, and with a family history of Type 2 diabetes, Traci Reason was headed for trouble. But today, she's committed to setting a good example for her kids.

NAME: Traci Reason
AGE: 35
HEIGHT: 5 feet 9 inches
WEIGHT BEFORE: 237 pounds
WEIGHT NOW: 133 pounds

TOTAL CHOLESTEROL BEFORE: 230
TOTAL CHOLESTEROL AFTER: 173
LDL CHOLESTEROL BEFORE: 143
LDL CHOLESTEROL AFTER: 102
HDL CHOLESTEROL BEFORE: 55
HDL CHOLESTEROL AFTER: 55
TRIGLYCERIDES BEFORE: 160
TRIGLYCERIDES AFTER: 79

So many women never lose their pregnancy weight. With all the hard work of a new baby, we sometimes gain even more weight after the birth. That's what happened to me. I had two children 22 months apart; I had barely recovered from my first child when I became pregnant with my second. After my second baby girl was born almost four years ago, I was also struggling with depression.

I had never weighed more than 150 pounds in my life. But I weighed 225 when I delivered on March 15, 2000. I started doing Atkins for a short time and got myself down to 185, but within a year I was up to 237. After that, I refused to weigh myself.

Because my maternal grandmother has Type 2 diabetes, and because I had borderline gestational diabetes with my second pregnancy, my mother was very concerned about my health. But I wasn't. I kept telling myself, "I'm not like everybody else. Give me another piece of pie."

In the meantime, my heart was pounding in my chest and I'd get red-faced and winded just by walking up or down the stairs. I was sweating at night. My back hurt because I had a compressed disk that was straining from the weight. My knees and ankles ached. I could not pick up my children and couldn't play on the floor with them because I couldn't get back up. Every day it was a struggle just to get through the day. "Tomorrow, I'm going to do something about my weight," I'd say to myself as I

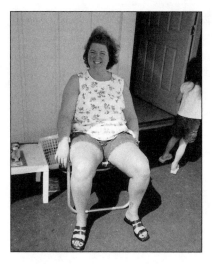

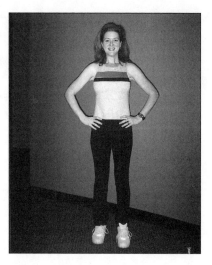

BEFORE   **AFTER**

plopped down in front of the television set with a bag of chips and a cup of soda.

On February 28, 2003, I had gone three days without taking a shower. My husband, an airline pilot, was away on a trip. Toys were strewn everywhere because I couldn't bend down to pick them up. And, suddenly, I got sick and tired of being sick and tired. Determined to succeed this time, I bought Atkins for Life *and started Induction. For six months, I stuck to 20 grams of carbs a day or fewer. By mid-July, I had lost more than 60 pounds. A blood test in August showed my total cholesterol had dropped from 230 to 173, and my triglycerides from 160 to 79. When I saw those numbers, they meant more to me than the number of pounds I had shed.*

I began walking daily and taking my girls to the playground. I was living life again after coming close to death at age 34. I lost 104 pounds using the Atkins Nutritional Approach, and went from a size 22 to a size 4. Today, I'm working out three days a week at the local gym, weight training, and running three miles on a treadmill. My marriage is healthier than it ever was before. I feel better than I did when I was 26 years old!

My ACE these days is 40 carbs. I still stick to a no-eating-after-six rule. I eat lots of chicken, shrimp with low-carb cocktail sauce, and pork ten-

derloin. My husband is a wonderful cook and loves to make Rib-eye Steak with Red Wine Sauce from www.atkins.com.

I'm so happy to be able to go outside with my daughters. We gave them a trampoline for Christmas, and now I'm out there bouncing with them whenever we get the chance! I'm showing them by my example how to live a healthy lifestyle—how to eat right, get exercise—that's what it's all about. It's not about vanity. It's about longevity and quality of life. There's no better gift I can give my family.

Note: Your individual results may vary from those reported here. As stated previously, Atkins recommends initial laboratory evaluation and subsequent follow-up in conjunction with your health care provider.

Chapter 25

TYPE 2 DIABETES AND YOUR CHILD

Not many years ago, Type 2 diabetes was an old people's disease. The only children with diabetes Dr. Atkins saw in his medical practice were those who had Type 1. But by the 1990s, a very disturbing trend had taken root. A virtual stream of overweight youngsters, most in their early teens, began showing up at The Atkins Center for weight loss. After doing blood work, Dr. Atkins ended up diagnosing all too many of them with the metabolic syndrome or Type 2 diabetes. It was as shocking as it was depressing: A few of these kids hadn't even hit puberty yet!

IT'S AN EPIDEMIC

It's a small step from having the metabolic syndrome or impaired glucose tolerance when you're only 10 (in some cases, even younger) to having Type 2 diabetes by the time you're 14. And it's a progression that far too many children are now experiencing. The diabetes problem among juveniles isn't just in this country. In Japan, for instance, the incidence has been rising almost as fast. The same is true in Europe, Australia, Asia—and around the globe.[1]

We can say that the epidemic of Type 2 diabetes in kids was born back in the early 1980s, when researchers noticed a surge in reported cases among Native American populations. The surge soon became a tidal wave. Before 1994, Type 2 diabetes was found in only 5 percent of youngsters newly diagnosed with diabetes; the rest had Type 1 diabetes, which almost always occurs in childhood. Although we don't yet have accurate statistics, today some estimates say that 45 percent or more of all new cases of diabetes in children are Type 2.[2] In one study of children in Cincinnati, the incidence of diabetes rose ten times in a little more than a decade, from less than 1 case per 100,000 kids in 1982 to 7.2 cases per 100,000 kids in 1994.[3]

The diabetes epidemic hits minority communities especially hard. Research has shown that more than 4 out of 1,000 Native American teenagers have diabetes. In one study of African American and Caucasian children aged 10 to 19, Type 2 diabetes accounted for 33 percent of all cases of diabetes.[4] And just as so many adults with Type 2 diabetes go undiagnosed for years, so do many kids. The real numbers are probably higher.

GETTING HARD TO TELL

The fasting blood sugar (FBS) cutoff level for either kind of diabetes in children is the same as for adults: a fasting blood sugar of 126 mg/dL or higher, or a postprandial blood sugar of 200 mg/dL or higher. That's almost the only thing the two types of diabetes have in common.[5]

Type 1 diabetes is a very serious autoimmune disease caused by the failure of the pancreas to produce insulin. It usually comes on suddenly, and the treatment is lifelong insulin administration and careful dietary management. Type 2 diabetes is no less serious but at the start the pancreas still produces insulin and symptoms develop gradually. Type 2 diabetes in kids is almost always preventable and can usually be stopped or reversed with weight loss and dietary changes. Sometimes, though, it's hard for a doctor to tell whether a child has Type 1 or Type 2 diabetes. (Although the focus of this book is Type 2, because in children it can be harder to differentiate, some discussion of Type 1 is necessary.) Recently, it has gotten harder to make the diagnosis.

It used to be that if a child was overweight, the chances were very good that he or she had Type 2 diabetes. Today, however, kids with Type 1 diabetes are just as likely to be overweight as youngsters in the general population—as many as 24 percent may be overweight when they start showing symptoms.[6] Being overweight may be an accelerating factor for developing Type 1 diabetes, because heavy kids develop the disease at an earlier age than those who aren't overweight. This could be at least part of the explanation for the increased incidence of Type 1 diabetes over the past several decades.[7] Particularly if there is a family history of Type 1 diabetes, parents must not be complacent about their children's weight gain. Of course, a family history of Type 2 means parents should *also* be concerned about preventing obesity.

On top of that, if a child with Type 1 diabetes is also obese, he or she could have "double diabetes"—insulin resistance from being obese as well as an inability to produce insulin from having Type 1.[8] This can cause some confusion, but in almost all cases, children with Type 1 diabetes have the classic symptoms of excessive thirst, hunger, and urination along with weight loss and sugar in the urine. If further confirmation is needed, blood tests can provide it. Kids with Type 1 diabetes also usually show specific types of autoimmune antibodies in their blood. In addition, testing for the presence of c-peptide in the blood reveals how much, if any, insulin the pancreas is producing. If the level is very low, indicating little or no insulin production, the diagnosis is usually Type 1. (It's necessary to run all the tests, however, because in some cases, children with Type 2 diabetes also have very little insulin production.)[9] For youngsters with diabetes, Dr. Atkins usually did a two-hour postprandial (after a meal) test of insulin and glucose to get a better idea of how well they could still produce insulin.

When the diagnosis in a child or teenager is Type 2 diabetes, the Atkins approach to evaluating the problem is very similar to that for adults. He did the same blood tests discussed in Chapter 6. However, depending on the child's age and ability to cooperate with testing, the five-hour glucose tolerance test might be terminated early. He always attempted to get the FBS (fasting blood sugar) and insulin as well as one-hour and two-hour blood sugar and insulin values. If the FBS was already high, he found that the two-hour postprandial test was sufficient to determine how much insulin the child was producing and his or her degree of hyperinsulinemia.

THE FACTS ON TYPE 1

Type 1 diabetes is the most common severe chronic disease of childhood. In the United States, about 1.7 out of every 1,000 kids under the age of 19 have it.[10] The symptoms are generally pretty clear: The child is suddenly very hungry and thirsty, has to urinate a lot, and may lose weight even though he or she is eating a lot of food. When the child's urine is tested at the doctor's office, it usually contains sugar and ketones. Most children who develop Type 1 get it as they reach puberty, generally around age 10 to 12 in girls and age 12 to 14 in boys. The disease can strike at any age, however, and even very young children can get it. Type 1 diabetes tends to run in families—siblings of someone with Type 1 diabetes may have a 30 times greater risk of getting Type 1 than the general population.[11] The identical twin of a child with Type 1 has a 35 percent higher risk of developing the disease.[12]

TYPE 1 DIABETES AND DOING ATKINS

Youngsters who have Type 1 diabetes have a lifelong condition that requires very careful management. The Atkins Blood Sugar Control Program (ABSCP) can help, particularly in one very important way: A controlled-carb food plan can assist in preventing dangerous episodes of both hypoglycemia and hyperglycemia. The Atkins approach helps keep the entry of glucose into the bloodstream steady, avoiding glucose spikes and sharp drops. Although kids with Type 1 must continue to take their life-saving insulin, on the ABSCP they can often achieve good blood sugar control with less insulin.

It is mandatory, however, that children with Type 1 who are following the Atkins approach do it only under the close supervision of a doctor experienced in its use. The program can be so effective in quickly lowering blood sugar and insulin requirements that accidental insulin overdose could occur.

HOW TO KNOW IF IT'S TYPE 2

The signs and symptoms of Type 2 diabetes are less clear-cut than those of Type 1, and they develop more slowly. The primary sign is obesity—80 percent or more of kids with diabetes are seriously overweight or obese at the time of diagnosis.[13] Unlike those with Type 1 diabetes, they usually haven't lost weight. They commonly don't experience increased thirst, increased hunger, or increased urination. Often the first hint that they have a problem comes from a routine urine test that shows a lot of spilled glucose, or when they see a physician for another problem.

Another common indicator, found in 67 percent of kids with Type 2 diabetes, is acanthosis nigricans (uh-kan-THO-sis NIH-grih-kans).[14] These are patches of dark, velvety skin that are usually found on the neck, in the armpit region, and in other areas where the skin folds or rubs together. Acanthosis nigricans, which can occur at any age, can be a sign of hyperinsulinemia, the precursor to diabetes.[15]

Although very young children can get full-blown Type 2 diabetes, most are older than age 10 and are in middle to late puberty when they develop the disease. This is partly because insulin resistance naturally increases during puberty.[16] When insulin resistance from obesity amplifies puberty's natural increase in insulin resistance, the result can be Type 2 diabetes, especially if there's also a family history of the disease. Almost all kids with Type 2 have at least one parent or close relative who became diabetic as an adult—and often the family history of diabetes goes back two or even three generations. Ethnicity plays a big role as well. Kids whose heritage is African American, Hispanic, Asian American, Pacific Islander, or Native American are all at much greater risk of Type 2 diabetes. For this reason, if you have a family history of Type 2 diabetes, it is crucial to keep your children's insulin levels in check with carbohydrate control prior to puberty if possible.[17]

TYPE 2'S GREATER DANGERS

One of the most distressing things about Type 2 diabetes in young people is that it so quickly leads to serious complications—even more so than Type 1. Because of this, it is essential that we recognize the warning signs leading to diabetes at the earliest stage possible and intervene swiftly.

One recent Swedish study of kidney disease in young people with diabetes was especially chilling. The study looked at 469 people who were diagnosed with diabetes between the ages of 15 and 34. Of the group, most had Type 1; only 43 had Type 2. Over a nine-year period, 5.6 percent of the people with Type 1 diabetes and 16 percent of the people with Type 2 diabetes developed kidney disease.[18]

Another study of the same group of patients showed a similar situation with diabetic retinopathy, an eye disease that can lead to blindness. Fifteen percent of the people with Type 2 diabetes had severe retinopathy, while only 5 percent of the people with Type 1 diabetes had retinopathy, and most of those with Type 1 had a milder form.[19]

Both these studies show how dire the consequences of Type 2 diabetes are when it occurs in young people. In most cases of chronic disease, being young provides some protection. Overall, in cases of early-onset Type 2 diabetes, this protection is simply lost. Compared with people who develop diabetes in later middle age, young people with diabetes are 80 percent more likely to end up needing insulin.[20] The risk of having a heart attack is also much higher. Older adults with diabetes have just under four times the risk of having a heart attack as someone their age without diabetes; young people with diabetes have 14 times the risk of having a heart attack as someone their age without diabetes.[21]

The complications don't stop there. A long-term follow-up study of First Nations (native Canadians) children looked at a group of 51 patients who were diagnosed with Type 2 diabetes in 1986; at the time, all were under age 17. When they were contacted 15 years later, two had died while on kidney dialysis, three were currently on dialysis (one of them had become blind), and another had had a toe amputation. Of 56 pregnancies among the patients, only 35 resulted in live births.[22]

Kids with Type 2 diabetes often end up taking the sorts of medications we usually associate with older adults. It's not uncommon to find 15-year-olds taking metformin (Glucophage) for their blood sugar, along with one or more drugs for high blood pressure and a statin drug for high cholesterol. Although metformin may be helpful for some kids and is probably safe for them—on occasion, Dr. Atkins did prescribe it—most of the other drugs these kids are taking have never been tested on children. (Some statins are FDA-approved for children beginning at age 12. Dr. Atkins never used these.) Diet, exercise, and supplements (if needed) may preclude the use of medications. Lifestyle changes are always a better approach.

TREATING KIDS THE ATKINS WAY

The ABSCP is particularly effective for treating kids and teens with diabetes. They—and their parents—don't have to follow a complicated exchange system. There's no calorie counting, portion measuring, or anxiety about the fat content of a food. Moreover, youngsters never have to feel hungry or stigmatized. They do have to learn to live without the junk food they've grown accustomed to—even "addicted" to—but this turns out to be a fairly easy transition. By making sure that kids get adequate protein and dietary fat, and by substituting better carb foods, such as low-carb bread with sugar-free peanut butter instead of potato chips, for example, the junk food habit can be tamed. And once these kids start eating the Atkins way, they simply stop being hungry all the time.

HOW MANY CARBS?

In general, kids with Type 2 diabetes will get their blood sugar under control, stabilize their weight, and even start to lose weight by controlling the quality and quantity of carbohydrates and by exercising more. But because Type 2 diabetes is a serious disease, you must discuss these changes with your child's doctor first. Work closely with him or her to track the child's progress and to be sure that your son or daughter is achieving normal growth and development milestones.

Medical supervision is even more important for kids taking diabetes medication of any sort. As the blood sugar normalizes, the medication dosage will probably need to be reduced or even eliminated to avoid hypoglycemia. Other medications for blood pressure, blood lipids, and anything else will also probably need to be changed or eliminated as these conditions normalize. Just as for adults, plan this strategy with the child's physician before dietary changes are instituted. Discuss with your doctor how often to monitor blood sugar levels and blood pressure, when to change medication doses, and when to report back to him or her.

In cases of severe obesity, very high blood sugar, or very high blood lipids in kids, Dr. Atkins usually recommended going to the Induction level of just 20 grams of Net Carbs a day. This must always be done under careful medical supervision with a doctor who understands the Atkins approach.

Goals when treating a child with Type 2 diabetes are similar to those of adults. The first concern is to reduce carbohydrates enough to control insulin and blood sugar levels. As the blood sugar stabilizes, hunger and cravings significantly improve. And as blood sugar and insulin abnormalities improve, so will lipid and blood pressure values. As his or her metabolism approaches normal, the child will probably lose fat and inches around the middle. For children who are very obese, normalization of their metabolism must still be the goal. As a result, weight loss often occurs.

Teens who are nearing puberty need their insulin and blood sugar levels supervised by a practitioner familiar with the ABSCP. As we mentioned earlier, obesity during the early teen years can lead to accelerated puberty and shorter stature than would otherwise have been the case. For this reason, helping a teen control his or her metabolism can play a role in ensuring proper growth to attain proper height.[23]

Measure progress in kids with Type 2 diabetes not by the scale but by other success markers that are far more revealing: better blood sugar control, improved blood pressure and blood lipids, and good appetite control. Frequent weigh-ins and too much emphasis on quick weight loss can lead to frustration and even eating disorders. Do not weigh your child more often than once every two weeks.

For both kids and adults, the loss of inches is far more rewarding and motivating than the loss of pounds. Remember that growing kids may lose fat even while gaining weight. Rather than recording your child's weight, record his or her waist and upper-arm measurements.

For a more tangible demonstration of how inches are being lost, have the child try on the same piece of clothing once every couple of weeks. Jeans that start out uncomfortably tight may well quickly become too loose, even if the scale is dropping only slowly. Provide encouragement and support for sticking with the program rather than for losing pounds or inches. Helping your child keep a chart of blood sugar values is a great way to illustrate progress, too.

THE OTHER HALF: EXERCISE

The foundation of the ABSCP is the control of carbohydrates to prevent diabetes. However, the dietary plan is only part of the ABSCP. As with adults, aerobic exercise of at least half an hour a day is mandatory. (Check back to Chapter 24 for more on exercise; the recommendations there apply to kids with diabetes as well.) Any activity that gets your child moving and that he or she enjoys is fine. We suggest keeping an activity record. A simple chart that tracks progress can be very motivating for a child, and it assures parents that the exercise is happening on a regular basis. Watch carefully for drops in blood sugar during and after exercise. This problem is most likely to occur in Type 1 diabetes. Eating protein about 30 minutes before exertion can help support the blood sugar levels during exercise.

As every parent knows, younger children and teens can be rebellious and moody. Your efforts to help with dietary changes can be seen by your child as controlling or interfering with his or her life. You can't expect perfect compliance with the program—especially if you're not setting a good example by ignoring your own health. Offer congratulations for every effort at improvement. Avoid nagging. Most kids with early-onset diabetes come from families where obesity and diabetes are long-standing problems and where many family members need to make lifestyle changes. Because the kids have seen their parents and other family members struggle with their weight problems without success, they may feel that there's little point in making the effort themselves. And it's almost impossible for a youngster to break free of bad eating habits if the rest of the family doesn't make an effort, too.

The best way to help your child with diabetes is to get the whole family to eat better, lose weight where necessary, and exercise more. That might mean major changes for everyone, but the reward of better health for each individual—and saving just one child from the ravages of diabetes—is worth the effort.

The only way to stop the epidemics of obesity and diabetes is to change the way we eat and live today—so that our children have healthy examples on which to model their own lives. It's never too early and never too late to recognize and renounce the American standard of unhealthy, high-carb eating combined with physical inactivity. The solution is in your hands. Why waste another minute?

At age 16 Amanda S. weighed 208 pounds and her waist measured 44 inches. Before she came to see me, she was well on her way to developing Type 2 diabetes, with a c-peptide level of 9.2 (almost twice the norm), signifying severe hyperinsulinism. Within six months of starting the ABSCP, Amanda's c-peptide level was normal at 4.5. After one year of controlling her carbohydrates, she weighed 142 pounds with a waist measurement of 35 inches. She reveled in the compliments she received from family and friends and had no difficulty maintaining the nutritional approach that made such a wonderful difference in her health. It was gratifying to see this young woman pull herself back from the brink of such a devastating illness and experience an enhanced quality of life.

—MARY VERNON

DOES YOUR CHILD HAVE DIABETES?

Just as many adults have Type 2 diabetes and don't know it, so too do many kids. Agree or disagree with the following statements to see if your child is at risk of diabetes.

1. **My child is overweight.** Yes ☐ No ☐
2. **Other close blood relatives have diabetes.** Yes ☐ No ☐
3. **My child's genetic heritage is African American, Hispanic, Asian American, Native American, or Pacific Islander.** Yes ☐ No ☐

4. My child doesn't get much exercise.   Yes ❏   No ❏

5. My child is hungry all the time.   Yes ❏   No ❏

6. My child is always eating junk food.   Yes ❏   No ❏

7. My child drinks a lot of sugary drinks.   Yes ❏   No ❏

8. The doctor says my child has high
   blood pressure.   Yes ❏   No ❏

9. The doctor says my child has high
   blood lipids.   Yes ❏   No ❏

10. The doctor says my child has high
    blood sugar.   Yes ❏   No ❏

Scoring: If you answered yes to just three or more statements, your child may be at risk for Type 2 diabetes or may already have it. Discuss these issues with your child's doctor.

Part Three

Living the Program

Chapter 26

MEAL PLANS

In this chapter, we provide you with meal plans at three different levels of Net Carb intake, starting with 20 grams and building to 40 and 60 grams; the next chapter presents recipes specially developed for this book. Your individual tolerance for carbohydrates may be lower, higher, or somewhere in the middle, but these meal plans are designed to give you an idea of the range of foods you can include at various levels. Carb counts for individual foods are those that appear in *Dr. Atkins' New Carb Gram Counter* (2002). The Net Carb level is indicated at the top of each meal plan and there is a subtotaled carb count for each meal. At the bottom of the plan, the total number of grams of Net Carbs for the day appears. There is a 10 percent spread in either direction for a given day, but they average out to the appropriate level. To a certain extent the numbers are approximations.

INDIVIDUALIZING MEAL PLANS

You can be assured that even at 20 grams of Net Carbs, each meal plan contains a minimum of five servings a day of vegetables and fruits. Remember, avocados, tomatoes, and olives are technically fruits. Understand that these meal plans are suggestions. They are not written in stone. We encourage you to make your own substitutions based on personal tastes, budget, and seasonality of produce. If you find that an ingredient listed on a meal plan is not one of your favorites, you can swap it for an equal portion of a similar vegetable—greens beans for asparagus, for example. (For an extensive list of acceptable vegetables in Induction, turn to pages 456–457.) Likewise, if you do not care for a recipe, substitute one with a comparable carb count.

To individualize these meal plans, use the following tools, where you will find other comparable food selections:

- The Atkins Glycemic Ranking (Appendix 4, page 467)
- The Carbohydrate Ladder (Appendix 2, page 462)
- The Power of Five, which lists 5-gram carb servings of many foods (Appendix 3, page 464)

Although the plans include the dishes from recipes in Chapter 27, you can also find numerous recipes at www.atkins.com and in books authored by Dr. Atkins.

BEYOND THE ATKINS NUTRITIONAL APPROACH

The Atkins Blood Sugar Control Program (ABSCP) differs from the Atkins Nutritional Approach (ANA) in important aspects that must be considered when moving from one phase to another or designing your lifetime way of eating. Depending upon the degree of imbalance in your blood sugar/insulin mechanism, the ability of your body to respond to a lowering of carbohydrates and other factors as detailed in this book, these meal plans can be added to, mixed, and matched. (If your tolerance for carbs changes as a result of aging, hormonal changes, or a decrease in your activity level, you may need to modify your meal plans in the future to maintain your health and well-being.) You are succeeding as long as the quantity and quality of carbs allow you to address your weight, control hunger, and maintain optimum lab values.

HELPFUL HINTS

Keep these guidelines in mind to be sure you are following the program correctly:

- Don't skip meals, especially breakfast.
- Each meal should include a sufficient amount of protein to satisfy your appetite.
- Eat until you are satisfied—but not stuffed.
- Be aware of the number of grams of Net Carbs you eat each day (use a carb gram counter).
- In addition to counting your daily carbs, it is important to spread them throughout the day.
- If you are hungry between meals, have a snack comprised of protein and fat, especially with fruit or vegetables. (Never eat pure carbohydrate foods alone as a snack.)
- We have provided for an evening snack, but if you are hungry between meals, you can have the snack earlier in the day.
- You can even add another snack, so long as it is composed primarily of protein and fat. Be sure to count the carbs.
- Pay attention to serving sizes on labels to avoid mistakenly overconsuming carbs.
- Read nutrition labels and avoid food with added sugars, bleached white flour, and manufactured trans fats (hydrogenated or partially hydrogenated oils).
- The longer you are on the program, the more likely it is that your hunger will be under control and you may no longer need snacks.

PROTEIN POINTERS

Except for recipes in Chapter 27, we leave protein sizes to your discretion: You can eat them until you are satisfied but not stuffed. When the meal plan calls for a pork chop or a breast of chicken, for example, we do not give a weight; you may choose to have two chops or two pieces of chicken. Keep in mind, however, that following the Atkins Blood Sugar Control Program is not a license to gorge. Unless otherwise indicated, tuna and other protein salads contain just mayonnaise and are listed as containing 0 gram of Net Carbs. Add extra grams of carbs for celery, onions, and other vegetable additions. As you increase your intake of carbs, you will naturally find you need slightly less protein and fat.

Meats such as sausages and beef jerky should be nitrate-free and without added sugars or fillers. Try to purchase brands with no carbohydrate content. Ham refers to boiled or baked, not honey-baked, which is made with sugar.

When we list an item such as a beef burger, you can grill it, broil it, or pan-fry it, whichever you prefer. Be sure not to char meat, which can form carcinogens.

DAIRY DO'S AND DON'TS

Cheeses vary in carb content. We often list a certain cheese. Feel free to make substitutions so long as the replacement contains a similar number of grams of Net Carbs. In any case, do not exceed more than 4 ounces of cheese each day. All dairy products and products such as mayonnaise should be full-fat products, which means they are the lowest in carbs. Do not use any low-fat products, such as cheese, cottage cheese, mayonnaise, and yogurt, which are almost inevitably higher in carbohydrates. Instead of commercially prepared whipped cream, which usually contains sugar and sometimes added trans fats, use heavy cream and whip it yourself.

Dairy beverages are a new food category made from milk but with significantly reduced-carb content. One brand is Hood Carb Countdown (which is Atkins-approved) and contains only 3 grams of Net Carbs per cup.

FATS, OILS, AND DRESSINGS

As with protein, we do not limit fat intake. You can dress your vegetables with olive oil or butter, but not margarine, which typically contains hydrogenated oils, known as trans fats. There are nonhydrogenated brands of margarine available. You are more likely to find them in natural foods stores. Although you do not have to skimp on fats and oils, there is no reason to drench your foods in them. The same applies to mayonnaise. A serving of salad dressing is 2 tablespoons. Commercial salad dressings should be labeled as low-carb or have at most 2 grams of Net Carbs and no added sugar or corn syrup. A safe bet is always vinaigrette made from (nonbalsamic) vinegar or lemon juice and olive oil.

VEGETABLES AND FRUITS

You need to carefully follow the portion sizes supplied for carbohydrate foods. In the case of salads, a small salad is equivalent to 1 cup; a large salad to 2 cups. Salad vegetables are measured raw. Other vegetables are measured cooked unless otherwise indicated. Cooking methods are suggested, but feel free to prepare them your favorite way. Vegetables can be steamed, sautéed, roasted, or grilled.

When fruit is listed, assume it is fresh, unless otherwise specified. If you are using canned fruit, be sure it is packed in water or juice (discard it), not syrup. If you use frozen fruit, be sure it contains no sugar.

While it is best to eat whole fruits and vegetables, tomato juice is low enough in carbohydrate to merit occasional use, so long as it is in the context of a meal where it is balanced by protein and fat. Do not drink juice alone as a snack. We also allow cranberry juice that is not sweetened with sugar. Presently we are aware of only one product that is sweetened with Splenda, which is listed by brand name to avoid confusion. If you prefer not to drink juice, simply substitute a fruit of equal carb content.

All grains and legume portions sizes are measured cooked, rather than dry.

THE STAFF OF LIFE

At the level of 60 grams of Net Carbs a day, you can occasionally have a portion of whole grain bread. Make sure that it contains only whole wheat or other whole grains and no sugar, honey, or other caloric sweetener. In the last couple of years, there has been tremendous growth in the number of controlled-carb breads on the market, including those manufactured by Atkins Nutritionals. Atkins bread contains 3 grams of Net Carbs per slice and a single slice is acceptable in Induction. When we list low-carb bread with a gram count of 3 Net Carbs, use Atkins bread or another brand with the same number of grams of Net Carbs.

DRINK UP

Although we have listed a few lower glycemic beverages, such as shakes and tomato juice (which is not acceptable at the 20-gram level), beverages such as water, tea, and coffee do not appear. It is best to avoid caffeine if you are sensitive to it. At most, have only one serving a day. Also limit "diet" soft drinks. Be sure to drink a minimum of eight 8-ounce glasses of water a day. (For information on all other fluids, see Chapter 19, Drink to Your Health).

SWEETENERS

Sweeteners are not listed unless they are a component of a recipe. We strongly discourage the use of more than 3 packets a day, especially in the Induction phase, for two reasons. You have to count 1 gram of Net Carbs per packet of acceptable sweetener (see page 459) and it is important to wean yourself away from the need to make all beverages excessively sweet. Gelatin desserts must be sugar-free. Our recommendation is Jolly Rancher brand, which can be found in the dairy section and is sweetened with Splenda.

BRAND NAMES

In most cases, we do not use brand names, unless it is necessary to avoid confusion. We do list a few Atkins brand foods, when we are unaware of others with the same carb counts. Otherwise, such as in the case of bread, where there are Atkins products and others with the same carb count, the mention is generic, but be sure to find a brand with the right carb count. Low-carb pancakes vary from one manufacturer to another, so be guided by the designated carb count, not the number of pancakes.

A GROWING FOOD CATEGORY

There are numerous low-carb foods now available that make it easier than ever to follow the ABSCP. However, it is not necessary to use them to be successful on the program. Many people find it satisfying and more enjoyable to concentrate on eating a wide variety of whole foods. Low-carb foods can be abused, just as low-fat foods have been. They must never be used as a substitute for eating a wide variety of fresh, whole foods. Instead, regard some of these products as handy when traveling or in a situation when proper food choices are unavailable. They can also add occasional variety.

The quality of low-carb foods can vary. Be sure that any new addition does not stop progress or provoke symptoms. If you are already a diabetic, be sure that a new food, especially one containing sugar alcohols, does not increase blood sugar or cause cravings. For some, even a sweet taste from an artificial sweetener will re-create cravings and can reestablish sugar addiction. Foods containing manufactured trans fats are to be avoided, even if they are low in carbs.

To attain your goals long term, it will be helpful to recognize and then unlearn the food habits that have sabotaged your efforts in the past. Overeating, emotional eating, and using food—even low-carb foods—as a reward can become obstacles to success. Begin to make food choices based upon health, not habit.

RECIPES

Recipes begin on page 402 in the next chapter. Hundreds of other recipes are available at www.atkins.com. When a meal plan (see pages 342–401) includes a recipe, we have indicated it with boldface type. You will notice that certain recipes have increasing carb-gram counts for the higher carb levels. That is because the recipe has variations that allow for greater variety in the form of additional carbohydrate ingredients. If you find it necessary to remain at 20 or 40 grams of Net Carbs, be careful to not mistakenly use a higher carb version.

MEAL PLAN—DAY 1

	20 GRAMS OF NET CARBS		40 GRAMS OF NET CARBS		60 GRAMS OF NET CARBS	
BREAKFAST	Egg stacks:		Egg stacks:		Egg stacks:	
	2 poached eggs	1	2 poached eggs	1	2 poached eggs	1
	2 slices Canadian bacon	0.5	2 slices Canadian bacon	0.5	2 slices Canadian bacon	0.5
	2 slices mozzarella cheese	2	2 slices mozzarella cheese	2	2 slices mozzarella cheese	2
	2 slices tomato	1.5	2 slices tomato	1.5	2 slices tomato	1.5
			½ medium orange	6	1 medium orange	12
SUBTOTAL		5		11		17
LUNCH	Chef's salad:		Chef's salad:		Chef's salad:	
	Smoked turkey strips	0	Smoked turkey strips	0	Smoked turkey strips	0
	1 oz. shredded cheese	0.5	1 oz. shredded cheese	0.5	1 oz. shredded cheese	0.5
	1 hard-boiled egg	0.5	1 hard-boiled egg	0.5	1 hard-boiled egg	0.5
	¼ cup cucumber slices	0.5	¼ cup cucumber slices	0.5	¼ cup cucumber slices	0.5

	2 cups lettuce greens with vinaigrette	2	2 cups lettuce greens with vinaigrette	2	2 cups lettuce greens with vinaigrette	2
			½ cup tomato juice	5	6 black olives	1
					¾ cup sugar-free tomato soup	12
SUBTOTAL		3.5		8.5		16.5
DINNER	Salmon en Papillote with Tomato-Basil Relish	4	Salmon en Papillote with Tomato-Basil Relish	4	Salmon en Papillote with Tomato-Basil Relish	4
	8 fresh asparagus spears	3	8 fresh asparagus spears	3	8 fresh asparagus spears	3
	Small red leaf lettuce and radish salad with vinaigrette	2	Large red leaf lettuce and radish salad with vinaigrette	4	Large red leaf lettuce and radish salad with vinaigrette	4
	½ cup sugar-free gelatin	0			2 tbsp. toasted pine nuts	2
			½ cup blueberries	8	½ cup blueberries	8
SUBTOTAL		9		19		21
SNACK	Large celery stalk	1	Large celery stalk	1	Large celery stalk	1
	1 tbsp. herb cream cheese	1	1 tbsp. herb cream cheese	1	1 tbsp. herb cream cheese	1
TOTAL		19.5		40.5		56.5

MEAL PLAN—DAY 2

	20 GRAMS OF NET CARBS		40 GRAMS OF NET CARBS		60 GRAMS OF NET CARBS	
BREAKFAST	Mushroom and cheese omelet made with 1 slice cheese and ⅓ cup cooked mushrooms	4	Mushroom and cheese omelet made with 1 slice cheese and ⅓ cup cooked mushrooms	4	Mushroom and cheese omelet made with 1 slice cheese and ⅓ cup cooked mushrooms	4
	2 tbsp. salsa	1	2 tbsp. salsa	1	2 tbsp. salsa	1
	2 turkey breakfast sausages	0	2 turkey breakfast sausages	0	2 turkey breakfast sausages	0
	1 slice low-carb toast	3	½ grapefruit	8.5	½ grapefruit	8.5
					1 slice low-carb toast	3
SUBTOTAL		8		13.5		16.5
LUNCH	Grilled Chicken and Avocado Salad with Sweet Mustard Vinaigrette and Olives	4	Grilled Chicken and Avocado Salad with Sweet Mustard Vinaigrette and Olives, Almonds, and Red Peppers	7	Grilled Chicken and Avocado Salad with Sweet Mustard Vinaigrette and Olives, Almonds, and Red Peppers	7
					3 Finn Crisp Rye Crispbreads	8
SUBTOTAL		4		7		15

	Meal 1		Meal 2		Meal 3	
DINNER	Broiled pork chop	0	Broiled pork chop	0	Broiled pork chop	0
	¾ cup sautéed spinach	2	¾ cup sautéed spinach	2	¾ cup sautéed spinach	2
	½ tomato broiled with 1 tbsp. Parmesan cheese	3.5	½ tomato broiled with 1 tbsp. Parmesan cheese	3.5	½ tomato broiled with 1 tbsp. Parmesan cheese	3.5
			⅓ cup baked butternut squash with butter	7	½ cup baked butternut squash with butter	10
SUBTOTAL		5.5		12.5		15.5
SNACK	Atkins Advantage shake	3	½ small peach	3.5	1 small peach	7
			½ cup ricotta cheese	3	½ cup ricotta cheese	3
TOTAL		20.5		39.5		57

MEAL PLAN—DAY 3

	20 GRAMS OF NET CARBS		40 GRAMS OF NET CARBS		60 GRAMS OF NET CARBS	
BREAKFAST	Atkins Advantage shake	3	½ cup cottage cheese	3	1 cup cottage cheese	6
			½ cup mixed berries	7	½ cup mixed berries	7
	1 slice low-carb toast topped with ham and 1 oz. melted cheese	4	1 slice low-carb toast topped with ham and 1 oz. melted cheese	4	1 slice low-carb toast topped with ham and 1 oz. melted cheese	4
SUBTOTAL		7		14		17
LUNCH	Beef burger	0	Beef burger	0	Beef burger	0
	1 large slice tomato and 1 large lettuce leaf	1	1 large slice tomato and large lettuce leaf	1	1 large slice tomato and large lettuce leaf	1
	Confetti Slaw	3	**Confetti Slaw**	4	**Confetti Slaw**	5
	½ cup steamed broccoli	2	1 cup steamed broccoli	4	1½ cups steamed broccoli	6
					½ cup Atkins Endulge ice cream	3
SUBTOTAL		6		9		15

	Roast chicken		Roast chicken		Roast chicken	
DINNER	Roast chicken	0	Roast chicken	0	Roast chicken	0
	⅔ cup herbed green beans	4	1 cup herbed green beans	5	½ cup herbed green beans	3
	Small butter lettuce salad with ranch dressing	2	Large butter lettuce salad with ranch dressing	4	½ cup carrots	5.5
			½ medium orange	6	Large butter lettuce salad with ranch dressing	4
SUBTOTAL		6		15		12.5
SNACK	1 hard-boiled egg	0.5	1 oz. mixed nuts	2	2 oz. mixed nuts	4
	6 black olives	1			¾ cup apple slices	10.5
TOTAL		20.5		40		59

MEAL PLAN—DAY 4

	20 GRAMS OF NET CARBS		40 GRAMS OF NET CARBS		60 GRAMS OF NET CARBS	
BREAKFAST	Vegetable Frittata	6.5	Vegetable Frittata	6.5	Vegetable Frittata	6.5
	2 slices tomato	1.5	2 slices tomato	1.5	2 slices tomato	1.5
			½ cup melon cubes	7	¾ cup melon cubes	10
SUBTOTAL		8		15		18
LUNCH	Tuna-celery salad	1	Tuna-celery salad sandwich on 1 slice low-carb bread	4	Tuna-celery salad sandwich on 1 slice low-carb bread	4
	Small lettuce salad with ½ cup green beans and vinaigrette	4	Large lettuce salad with ½ cup green beans and vinaigrette	6	Large lettuce salad with ¾ cup green beans and vinaigrette	7
	2 dill pickle spears	1			2 dill pickle spears	1
					½ pear	10
SUBTOTAL		6		10		22

	Option 1		Option 2		Option 3	
DINNER	Beef tenderloin	0	Beef tenderloin	0	Beef tenderloin	0
	½ cup raw mushrooms	2	½ cup raw mushrooms	2	½ cup raw mushrooms	2
	Large spinach salad	2	Large spinach salad	2	Large spinach salad	2
	2 tbsp. blue cheese	1	2 tbsp. blue cheese	1	2 tbsp. blue cheese	1
	Vinaigrette	0	Vinaigrette	0	1 tbsp. chopped pecans	1
			½ pear	10	Vinaigrette	0
					½ small sweet potato	12
SUBTOTAL		5		15		18
SNACK	1 cup consommé	1	1 cup consommé	1	1 cup consommé	1
	2 oz. string cheese	1	1 oz. string cheese	0.5	2 oz. string cheese	1
TOTAL		21		41.5		60

MEAL PLAN—DAY 5

	20 GRAMS OF NET CARBS		40 GRAMS OF NET CARBS		60 GRAMS OF NET CARBS	
BREAKFAST	2 scrambled eggs with	1	2 scrambled eggs with	1	2 scrambled eggs with	1
	2 tbsp. green onions	1	2 tbsp. green onions	1	2 tbsp. green onions	1
	2 slices bacon	0	2 slices bacon	0	2 slices bacon	0
	¼ Haas avocado, sliced	1	¼ Haas avocado, sliced	1	¼ Haas avocado, sliced	1
			1 slice low-carb toast	3	1 slice low-carb toast	3
			½ cup V-8 juice	6	½ cup V-8 juice	6
SUBTOTAL		3		12		12
LUNCH	Mexican Chicken Soup	3	Mexican Chicken Soup	6	Mexican Chicken Soup	6
	Large shredded iceberg salad with ½ cup chopped tomato and vinaigrette	4.5	Large shredded iceberg salad with ½ cup chopped tomato and vinaigrette	4.5	Large shredded iceberg salad with ½ cup chopped tomato and vinaigrette	4.5
					1 small corn tortilla	8
SUBTOTAL		7.5		10.5		18.5

	Day 1		Day 2		Day 3	
DINNER	Lamb chops	0	Lamb chops	0	Lamb chops	0
	1 cup sautéed zucchini	4	1 cup sautéed zucchini	4	1 cup sautéed zucchini	4
	Small arugula salad with vinaigrette	2	Small arugula salad with vinaigrette	2	1/3 cup cooked lentils	7
					Small arugula salad with vinaigrette	2
	1/2 cup sugar-free gelatin	0	**Ricotta Cream, Raspberries, and Almonds**	8.5	**Ricotta Cream, Boysenberries, and Almonds**	11
SUBTOTAL		6		14.5		24
SNACK	1 cup blanched broccoli and cauliflower florets	2.5	1 cup blanched broccoli and cauliflower florets	2.5	1 cup blanched broccoli and cauliflower florets	2.5
	1 oz. hard cheese	1	1 oz. hard cheese	1	2 oz. hard cheese	2
TOTAL		20		40.5		59

MEAL PLAN—DAY 6

	20 GRAMS OF NET CARBS		40 GRAMS OF NET CARBS		60 GRAMS OF NET CARBS	
BREAKFAST	Egg-celery salad	1.5	1 slice French toast made with low-carb bread; with sugar-free syrup	3.5	2 slices French toast made with low-carb bread; with sugar-free syrup	7
	1 slice low-carb toast	3	1 hard-boiled egg	0.5	¾ cup sliced strawberries	6
			½ cup sliced strawberries	4		
SUBTOTAL		4.5		8		13
LUNCH	1 cup chicken consommé	1	1 cup chicken consommé	1	1 cup chicken consommé	1
	Antipasto salad:		Antipasto salad:		Antipasto salad:	
	2 oz. each baked ham and provolone cheese	2	2 oz. each baked ham and provolone cheese	2	2 oz. each baked ham and provolone cheese	2
	6 marinated mushrooms	2	6 marinated mushrooms	2	6 marinated mushrooms	2
	¼ cup roasted red peppers	2	¼ cup roasted red pepper	2	¼ cup roasted red pepper	2
			¼ cup marinated artichokes	4	¼ cup marinated artichokes	4

			2 cups romaine with vinaigrette	2	¼ cup garbanzo beans	9
					2 cups romaine with vinaigrette	2
SUBTOTAL		7		13		22
DINNER	Pork Tenderloin with Sweet and Sour Red Cabbage	7.5	Pork Tenderloin with Sweet and Sour Red Cabbage and Apples	12	Pork Tenderloin with Sweet and Sour Red Cabbage and Apples	12
	Small spinach salad with low-carb poppyseed dressing	2	Large spinach salad with low-carb poppyseed dressing	4	½ cup baked butternut squash	9.5
					Large spinach salad with low-carb poppyseed dressing	4
SUBTOTAL		9.5		16		25.5
SNACK	6 black olives	1	6 black olives	1	6 black olives	1
TOTAL		22		38		61.5

MEAL PLAN—DAY 7

	20 GRAMS OF NET CARBS		40 GRAMS OF NET CARBS		60 GRAMS OF NET CARBS	
BREAKFAST	Atkins Morning Start breakfast bar	2	⅔ cup low-carb cereal	4	⅔ cup bran flakes	15
	2 poached eggs	1	½ cup unsweetened soy milk	2	½ cup unsweetened soy milk	2
			⅓ cup raspberries	2	⅓ cup raspberries	2
			1 oz. almonds	2	1 oz. almonds	2
SUBTOTAL		3		10		21
LUNCH	Cream of Broccoli, Ham, and Cheddar Soup	3	Cream of Broccoli, Ham, and Cheddar Soup	3	Cream of Broccoli, Ham, and Cheddar Soup	3
	Small mixed green salad with ½ cup yellow beans and vinaigrette	4	Large mixed green salad with ½ cup yellow beans and vinaigrette	6	Large mixed green salad with ¾ cup yellow beans and vinaigrette	7
			1 large plum	8	1 large plum	8
SUBTOTAL		7		17		18

	Food	Carbs	Food	Carbs	Food	Carbs
DINNER	Broiled chicken breast topped with 2 tbsp. marinara sauce and 1 slice mozzarella cheese	5	Broiled chicken breast topped with 2 tbsp. marinara sauce and 1 slice mozzarella cheese	5	Broiled chicken breast topped with 2 tbsp. marinara sauce and 1 slice mozzarella cheese	5
	Large romaine salad with low-carb Caesar dressing	3	Large romaine salad with low-carb Caesar dressing	3	Large romaine salad with low-carb Caesar dressing	3
			1 slice garlic toast made with low-carb bread	3	¾ cup low-carb pasta with olive oil and Parmesan	12
SUBTOTAL		8		11		20
SNACK	½ cup cucumber slices	1	½ cup cucumber slices	1	½ cup cucumber slices	1
	1 oz. smoked salmon	0	1 oz. smoked salmon	0	1 oz. smoked salmon	0
	1 tbsp. cream cheese	0.5	1 tbsp. cream cheese	0.5	1 tbsp. cream cheese	0.5
TOTAL		19.5		39.5		60.5

MEAL PLAN—DAY 8

	20 GRAMS OF NET CARBS		40 GRAMS OF NET CARBS		60 GRAMS OF NET CARBS	
BREAKFAST	2 scrambled eggs	1	2 scrambled eggs	1	2 scrambled eggs with 1 oz. Cheddar cheese	2
	Atkins Iced Coffee	5.5	Atkins Iced Coffee	5.5	Atkins Iced Coffee	5.5
			1 apricot	3	15 seedless grapes	12.5
SUBTOTAL		6.5		9.5		20
LUNCH	2 roast beef wraps: roast beef and 2 tbsp. bean sprouts wrapped in lettuce leaf with horseradish mayonnaise	2	2 roast beef wraps: roast beef and 2 tbsp. bean sprouts wrapped in lettuce leaf with horseradish mayonnaise	2	1 roast beef wrap: roast beef and 2 tbsp. bean sprouts wrapped in low-carb tortilla with horseradish mayonnaise	5
	¾ cup cucumber slices with vinaigrette	2	½ cup each cucumber slices and baby carrots with vinaigrette	5	½ cup each sugar snap peas and baby carrots with vinaigrette	10
			1 slice low-carb bread	3		
SUBTOTAL		4		10		15

DINNER	Polish sausage	0	Polish sausage	0	Polish sausage	0
	½ cup sauerkraut	0.5	1 cup sauerkraut	1	1 cup sauerkraut	1
	½ cup steamed yellow squash	2.5	1 cup steamed yellow squash	5	1 cup steamed yellow squash	5
	Large iceberg lettuce salad with ranch dressing	4	Large iceberg lettuce salad with ranch dressing	4	Large iceberg lettuce salad with ranch dressing	4
SUBTOTAL		7		10		10
SNACK	Sugar-free gelatin	0	8 seedless grapes	7	½ apple	10
	2 tbsp. heavy cream	1	1 oz. Brie	0	1 oz. Brie	0
			1 oz. pecans	2	1 oz. pecans	2
TOTAL		18.5		38.5		57

MEAL PLAN—DAY 9

	20 GRAMS OF NET CARBS		40 GRAMS OF NET CARBS		60 GRAMS OF NET CARBS	
BREAKFAST	Broccoli and cheese omelet made with ¼ cup cooked broccoli and 2 oz. cheese	3	½ cup plain whole-milk yogurt	5.5	1 cup plain whole-milk yogurt	11
	1 slice low-carb toast	3	½ cup sliced strawberries	4	½ cup sliced strawberries	4
			2 tbsp. slivered almonds	1	2 tbsp. slivered almonds	1
			1 hard-boiled egg	0.5		
SUBTOTAL		6		11		16
LUNCH	Greek Salad with Grilled Chicken Breast	7	Greek Salad with Grilled Chicken Breast	7	Greek Salad with Grilled Chicken Breast	7
			Key Lime Mousse	7.5	½ whole-wheat pita	15
SUBTOTAL		7		14.5		22

DINNER	Baked halibut with dill butter — 0	Baked halibut with dill butter — 0	Baked halibut with dill butter — 0
	½ cup sautéed snow peas and mushrooms — 4	1 cup sautéed snow peas and mushrooms — 8	1 cup sautéed snow peas and mushrooms — 8
	Small butter lettuce salad with vinaigrette — 2	Large butter lettuce salad with vinaigrette — 4	Large butter lettuce salad with vinaigrette — 4
			Key Lime Mousse — 8.5
SUBTOTAL	6	12	20.5
SNACK	1 deviled egg — 1	1 oz. low-carb soy chips — 4	1 oz. low-carb soy chips — 4
TOTAL	20	41.5	62.5

MEAL PLAN—DAY 10

	20 GRAMS OF NET CARBS		40 GRAMS OF NET CARBS		60 GRAMS OF NET CARBS	
BREAKFAST	2 scrambled eggs	1	2 scrambled eggs	1	2 scrambled eggs	1
	¼ Haas avocado, sliced	1	¼ Haas avocado, sliced	1	¼ Haas avocado, sliced	1
	1 oz. grated cheese	0.5	1 oz. grated cheese	0.5	1 oz. grated cheese	0.5
	1 low-carb tortilla	3	1 low-carb tortilla	3	1 low-carb tortilla	3
	2 tbsp. salsa	1	2 tbsp. salsa	1	2 tbsp. salsa	1
			½ cup pineapple	9	½ cup pineapple	9
SUBTOTAL		6.5		15.5		15.5
LUNCH	Sirloin patty with sautéed mushrooms (½ cup raw)	2	Sirloin patty with sautéed mushrooms (½ cup raw)	2	Sirloin patty with sautéed mushrooms (½ cup raw)	2
	Large mixed green salad with vinaigrette	4	Large mixed green salad with ¼ cup red kidney beans and vinaigrette	12	Large mixed green salad with ⅓ cup red kidney beans and vinaigrette	15
SUBTOTAL		6		14		17

		Column 1	Column 2	Column 3
DINNER	Sliced turkey breast	0	0	0
	Cauliflower Purée	3	3	3
	¾ cup sautéed green beans	4		
	1 cup sautéed green beans		5	5
	½ small sweet potato			12
SUBTOTAL		7	8	20
SNACK	1 oz. string cheese	0.5	0.5	0.5
	6 olives	1	1	
	1 medium plum			6
TOTAL		21	39	59

MEAL PLAN—DAY 11

	20 GRAMS OF NET CARBS		40 GRAMS OF NET CARBS		60 GRAMS OF NET CARBS	
BREAKFAST	Spinach Parmesan Egg Puff	4	Spinach Parmesan Egg Puff	4	Spinach Parmesan Egg Puff	4
	3 slices nitrate-free Canadian bacon	1	3 slices nitrate-free Canadian bacon	1	3 slices nitrate-free Canadian bacon	1
			½ cup cantaloupe cubes	6	¾ cup cantaloupe cubes	9
SUBTOTAL		5		11		14
LUNCH	1 slice low-carb rye bread	3	1 slice low-carb rye bread	3	2 slices low-carb rye bread	6
	broiled with 1 slice cheese,	1	broiled with 1 slice cheese,	1	broiled with 1 slice cheese,	1
	¼ sliced Haas avocado,	1	¼ sliced Haas avocado,	1	¼ sliced Haas avocado,	1
	and turkey	0	and turkey	0	and turkey	0
	1 cup chicken broth	1	1 medium sliced tomato with vinaigrette	6	1 medium sliced tomato with vinaigrette	6
			1 cup chicken broth	1		
SUBTOTAL		6		12		14

	Day 1		Day 2		Day 3	
DINNER	Roasted pork tenderloin	0	Roasted pork tenderloin	0	Roasted pork tenderloin	0
	1 cup roasted eggplant and zucchini	4.5	1 cup roasted eggplant and zucchini	4.5	1 cup roasted eggplant and zucchini	4.5
	Small radicchio and arugula salad with vinaigrette	3	Large radicchio and arugula salad with vinaigrette	5	⅓ cup brown rice	14
					Large radicchio and arugula salad with vinaigrette	5
SUBTOTAL		7.5		9.5		23.5
SNACK	Atkins Advantage bar	2	2 tbsp. hummus	6	3 tbsp. hummus	8.5
			2 celery stalks	1.5	3 celery stalks	2.5
TOTAL		20.5		40		62.5

MEAL PLAN—DAY 12

	20 GRAMS OF NET CARBS		40 GRAMS OF NET CARBS		60 GRAMS OF NET CARBS	
BREAKFAST	Smoked salmon	0	Smoked salmon	0	Smoked salmon	0
	Cream cheese and capers	1	Cream cheese and capers	1	Cream cheese and capers	1
	Chopped egg and onion	1	Chopped egg and onion	1	Chopped egg and onion	1
	1 slice low-carb toast	3	1 slice low-carb toast	3	1 slice low-carb toast	3
			½ grapefruit	8.5	½ grapefruit	8.5
SUBTOTAL		5		13.5		13.5
LUNCH	Chicken salad with mayonnaise and celery	1	Chicken salad with mayonnaise and celery	1	Chicken salad with mayonnaise and celery	1
	Large mixed green salad with vinaigrette	4	Large mixed green salad with vinaigrette	4	Large mixed green salad with vinaigrette	4
			2 tbsp. chopped walnuts	1	2 tbsp. chopped walnuts	1

Meal	Plan 1 Item	CHO	Plan 2 Item	CHO	Plan 3 Item	CHO
					3 Kavli Krispy Thin crackers	11
			1 small tangerine	6	1 small tangerine	6
SUBTOTAL		5		12		23
DINNER	Classic Beef Stew	6	Classic Beef Stew	8.5	Classic Beef Stew	10
	2 tbsp. crumbled feta	1	2 tbsp. crumbled feta	1	2 tbsp. crumbled feta	1
	Small red leaf salad with vinaigrette	2	Large red leaf salad with vinaigrette	4	Large red leaf salad and ¼ cup red kidney beans with vinaigrette	12
SUBTOTAL		9		13.5		23
SNACK	Atkins Advantage RTD shake	2	Atkins Advantage RTD shake	2	Atkins Advantage RTD shake	2
NET CHO		21		41		61.5

MEAL PLAN—DAY 13

	20 GRAMS OF NET CARBS		40 GRAMS OF NET CARBS		60 GRAMS OF NET CARBS	
BREAKFAST	Ham and 1 slice cheese on 1 slice low-carb bread	1	**Cinnamon Pancakes**	11	**Cinnamon Pancakes**	11
		3	2 breakfast sausage links	0	2 breakfast sausage links	0
	1 small tomato	3	⅓ cup raspberries	2	½ cup unsweetened applesauce	12
SUBTOTAL		7		13		23
LUNCH	2 hard-boiled eggs and 6 black olives on large spinach and iceberg salad with real bacon bits and vinaigrette	4	2 hard-boiled eggs and 6 black olives on large spinach and iceberg salad with real bacon bits and vinaigrette	4	2 hard-boiled eggs and 6 black olives on large spinach and iceberg salad with real bacon bits and vinaigrette	4
			¼ cup chickpeas	6.5	½ cup chickpeas	13
SUBTOTAL		4		10.5		17

	Barbecued Chicken	4	Barbecued Chicken	4	Barbecued Chicken	4
DINNER	1 cup pattypan squash	2	1 cup pattypan squash	2	1½ cups pattypan squash	3
	½ cup shredded cabbage with	1	1 cup shredded cabbage with	2	1 cup shredded cabbage with	2
	1 tbsp. low-carb poppyseed dressing	0.5	2 tbsp. low-carb poppyseed dressing	1	2 tbsp. low-carb poppyseed dressing	1
SUBTOTAL		7.5		9		10
SNACK	½ cup cucumber slices	1	1 fresh fig	8	1 fresh fig	8
	1 oz. Camembert cheese	0	1 oz. Camembert cheese	0	1 oz. Camembert cheese	0
TOTAL		19.5		40.5		58

MEAL PLAN—DAY 14

	20 GRAMS OF NET CARBS		40 GRAMS OF NET CARBS		60 GRAMS OF NET CARBS	
BREAKFAST	2 scrambled eggs with ¼ cup each green pepper, green onion, and mushrooms	4	2 scrambled eggs with ¼ cup each green pepper, green onion, and mushrooms	4	2 scrambled eggs with ¼ cup each green pepper, green onion, and mushrooms	4
	3 slices nitrate-free Canadian bacon	1	3 slices nitrate-free Canadian bacon	1	3 slices nitrate-free Canadian bacon	1
			1 slice low-carb toast	3	1 slice low-carb toast	3
					8 oz. V-8 juice	10
TOTAL		5		8		18
LUNCH	Grilled chicken breast strips	0	Grilled chicken breast strips	0	Grilled chicken breast strips	0
	1 cup grilled vegetables: eggplant, zucchini, red pepper	5	1½ cups grilled vegetables: eggplant, zucchini, red pepper	7.5	1½ cup grilled vegetables: eggplant, zucchini, red pepper	7.5
	2 oz. goat cheese	1	2 oz. goat cheese	1	⅓ cup corn kernels	9

	Plan 1	CHO	Plan 2	CHO	Plan 3	CHO
			½ medium baked apple with cinnamon	9	2 oz. goat cheese	1
SUBTOTAL		6		17.5		17.5
DINNER	Grilled rib-eye steak	0	Grilled rib-eye steak	0	Grilled rib-eye steak	0
	1 medium steamed artichoke with melted butter or mayonnaise	6.5	1 medium steamed artichoke with melted butter or mayonnaise	6.5	½ cup sautéed mushrooms	2
	Small romaine salad with low-carb Caesar dressing	2	Large romaine salad with low-carb Caesar dressing	4	1 medium boiled artichoke with melted butter or mayonnaise	6.5
					Large romaine salad with low-carb Caesar dressing	4
					½ medium baked apple with cinnamon	9
SUBTOTAL		8.5		10.5		21.5
SNACK	½ Haas avocado	2	Ragin' Nuts	4	Ragin' Nuts	4
NET CHO		21.5		40		61

MEAL PLAN—DAY 15

	20 GRAMS OF NET CARBS		40 GRAMS OF NET CARBS		60 GRAMS OF NET CARBS	
BREAKFAST	1 slice low-carb toast	3	½ cup (cooked) old-fashioned oatmeal	11	½ cup (cooked) old-fashioned oatmeal	11
	2 tbsp. cream cheese	1	1 tbsp. chopped pecans	1	2 tbsp. chopped pecans	2
	2 deviled eggs	2	½ cup dairy beverage	1.5	½ cup dairy beverage	1.5
					½ cup boysenberries	5.5
SUBTOTAL		6		13.5		20
LUNCH	South-of-the-Border Burger with Avocado Salsa	8	South-of-the-Border Burger with Avocado Salsa	8	South-of-the-Border Burger with Avocado Salsa	8
	⅓ cup each jicama and cucumber slices	2	½ cup each jicama and cucumber slices	3	½ cup each jicama and cucumber slices	3
			⅓ cup boysenberries	3.5	¾ cup honeydew melon	11
SUBTOTAL		10		14.5		22

	Plan 1		Plan 2		Plan 3	
DINNER	Veal chop	0	Veal chop	0	Veal chop	0
	½ cup steamed spinach	2	1 cup steamed spinach	4	1 cup roasted Brussels	7.5
	Small endive and watercress salad with low-carb ranch dressing	2	Small endive and watercress salad with low-carb ranch dressing	2	Large endive and watercress salad with low-carb ranch dressing	4
			Chocolate Almond Torte	6.5	**Chocolate Almond Torte**	6.5
					2 tbsp. whipped cream	1
SUBTOTAL		4		12.5		19
SNACK	2 turkey and cheese roll-ups	2	Sliced turkey	0	Sliced turkey	0
			2 slices tomato	1.5	2 slices tomato	1.5
TOTAL		22		42		62.5

MEAL PLAN—DAY 16

	20 GRAMS OF NET CARBS		40 GRAMS OF NET CARBS		60 GRAMS OF NET CARBS	
BREAKFAST	Italian Frittata	5	Italian Frittata	5	Italian Frittata	5
	2 slices tomato	1.5	2 slices tomato	1.5	2 slices tomato	1.5
			½ medium orange	6	½ grapefruit	8.5
SUBTOTAL		6.5		12.5		15
LUNCH	½ Haas avocado stuffed with crabmeat	2	½ Haas avocado stuffed with crabmeat	2	½ Haas avocado stuffed with crabmeat	2
	Small butter lettuce salad with vinaigrette	2	Large butter lettuce salad with vinaigrette	4	Large butter lettuce salad with vinaigrette	4
			8 oz. tomato juice	8	½ cup raw sugar snap peas	5
					8 oz. tomato juice	8
SUBTOTAL		4		14		19

	Day 1	Day 2	Day 3
DINNER	Meatballs (made without bread crumbs) — 0	Meatballs (made without bread crumbs) — 0	Meatballs (made without bread crumbs) — 0
	Spaghetti Squash with Spinach Pesto — 4.5	**Spaghetti Squash with Spinach Pesto** — 9	**Spaghetti Squash with Spinach Pesto** — 9
	Medium romaine salad with 6 black olives and low-carb Caesar dressing — 3	Large romaine salad with 6 black olives and low-carb Caesar dressing — 4	Large romaine salad with 6 black olives and low-carb Caesar dressing — 4
SUBTOTAL	7.5	13	13
SNACK	Atkins Advantage RTD shake — 2	Atkins Advantage RTD shake — 2	Atkins Advantage RTD shake — 2
			1 kiwifruit — 10
TOTAL	20	41.5	59

MEAL PLAN—DAY 17

	20 GRAMS OF NET CARBS		40 GRAMS OF NET CARBS		60 GRAMS OF NET CARBS	
BREAKFAST	2 poached eggs	1	Breakfast Cheesecake	5	Breakfast Cheesecake	5
	2 breakfast sausages	0	1 tbsp. slivered almonds	0.5	2 tbsp. slivered almonds	1
	1 slice low-carb toast	3	½ cup raspberries	3	1 cup raspberries	6
SUBTOTAL		4		8.5		12
LUNCH	1 large grilled portobello mushroom	2	1 large grilled portobello mushroom	2	1 large grilled portobello mushroom	2
	1 small tomato, 3 oz. mozzarella and 1 tbsp. fresh chopped basil with olive oil and red wine vinegar	6	1 small tomato, 3 oz. mozzarella and 1 tbsp. fresh chopped basil with olive oil and red wine vinegar	6	1 small tomato, 3 oz. mozzarella and 1 tbsp. fresh chopped basil with olive oil and red wine vinegar	6
					¼ cup chickpeas	6.5
			½ medium apple	8.5	½ medium apple	8.5
SUBTOTAL		8		16.5		23

DINNER		Day 1		Day 2		Day 3
Grilled chicken breast with butter and 1 tbsp. each capers and lemon juice		1	Grilled chicken breast with butter and 1 tbsp. each capers and lemon juice	1	Grilled chicken breast with butter and 1 tbsp. each capers and lemon juice	1
8 asparagus spears		3	8 asparagus spears	3	8 asparagus spears	3
Small spinach salad with vinaigrette		2	1/3 cup cooked low-carb pasta	6	1/3 cup cooked low-carb pasta	6
			Large spinach salad with vinaigrette	4	Large spinach salad with vinaigrette	4
					1/2 medium apple	8.5
SUBTOTAL		6		14		22.5
SNACK	Atkins Advantage bar	2	Atkins Advantage bar	2	Atkins Advantage bar	2
TOTAL		20		41		59.5

MEAL PLAN—DAY 18

	20 GRAMS OF NET CARBS		40 GRAMS OF NET CARBS		60 GRAMS OF NET CARBS	
BREAKFAST	Fried egg, ham, and 1 slice cheese on low-carb toast	4.5	Lemon Poppyseed Muffin	4	Lemon Poppyseed Muffin	4
			½ cup cottage cheese	4	1 cup cottage cheese	8
			½ cup strawberries	4	¾ cup strawberries	6
SUBTOTAL		4.5		12		18
LUNCH	Beef tacos in lettuce wraps filled with	1	Beef tacos in 2 low-carb tortillas filled with	8	Beef tacos in 2 low-carb tortillas filled with	8
	¼ cup chopped tomato	1.5	¼ cup chopped tomato	1.5	¼ cup chopped tomato	1.5
	1 cup shredded iceberg lettuce	0.5	1 cup shredded iceberg lettuce	0.5	1 cup shredded iceberg lettuce	0.5
	¼ cup shredded cheese	0.5	¼ cup shredded cheese	0.5	¼ cup shredded cheese	0.5

	½ Haas avocado, sliced	2	½ Haas avocado, sliced	2	½ Haas avocado, sliced	2
	Sour cream dressing	1	Sour cream dressing	1	Sour cream dressing	1
					½ medium orange	6
SUBTOTAL		6.5		13.5		19.5
DINNER	Bouillabaisse	6.5	Bouillabaisse	7	Bouillabaisse	7
	Small green leaf salad with vinaigrette	2	⅓ cup steamed peas	6	½ cup steamed peas	8
			Large green leaf salad with vinaigrette	4	Large green leaf salad with vinaigrette	4
					1 slice low-carb toast	3
SUBTOTAL		8.5		17		22
SNACK	½ cup sugar-free gelatin	0	½ cup sugar-free gelatin	0	½ cup sugar-free gelatin	0
	2 tbsp. heavy cream	1	2 tbsp. heavy cream	1	2 tbsp. heavy cream	1
TOTAL		20.5		43.5		60.5

MEAL PLAN—DAY 19

	20 GRAMS OF NET CARBS		40 GRAMS OF NET CARBS		60 GRAMS OF NET CARBS	
BREAKFAST	Omelet made with ¼ cup chopped artichoke hearts and 1 slice Swiss cheese	4	Omelet made with ¼ cup chopped artichoke hearts and 1 slice Swiss cheese	4	Omelet made with ¼ cup chopped artichoke hearts and 1 slice Swiss cheese	4
	1 slice low-carb rye bread	3	1 slice low-carb rye bread	3	2 slices low-carb rye bread	6
			½ cup cantaloupe	6	¾ cup cantaloupe	9
SUBTOTAL		7		13		19
LUNCH	Bacon, Lettuce, and Tomato Salad	5	Bacon, Lettuce, and Tomato Salad	5	Bacon, Lettuce, and Tomato Salad	5
	1 cup chicken consommé with 1 tbsp. green onion	2	Croutons made from 1 slice low-carb bread, toasted	3	Croutons made from 1 slice low-carb bread, toasted	3
			1 cup chicken consommé with 1 tbsp. green onion	2	¾ cup lentil soup	12
SUBTOTAL		7		10		20

	Plan 1		Plan 2		Plan 3	
DINNER	Beef tenderloin kabobs	0	Beef tenderloin kabobs	0	Beef tenderloin kabobs	0
	½ cup yellow squash, on skewers with kabobs	2.5	¾ cup yellow squash, on skewers with kabobs	4	¾ cup yellow squash, on skewers with kabobs	4
	1 cup Bibb lettuce with ¼ cup each sliced radish and cucumbers with vinaigrette	3.5	2 cups Bibb lettuce with ¼ cup each sliced radish and cucumbers with vinaigrette	4	2 cups Bibb lettuce with ¼ cup each sliced radish and cucumbers with vinaigrette	4
					½ cup steamed carrots	5
SUBTOTAL		6		8		13
SNACK	2 oz. cubed provolone	1	4 dried apricot halves	7.5	4 dried apricot halves	7.5
			2 oz. cubed provolone	1	2 oz. cubed provolone	1
TOTAL		21		39.5		60.5

MEAL PLAN—DAY 20

	20 GRAMS OF NET CARBS		40 GRAMS OF NET CARBS		60 GRAMS OF NET CARBS	
BREAKFAST	2 scrambled eggs with chives	1	Egg sandwich: 1 fried egg, 1 slice cheese, ham, and 2 slices low-carb rye bread	7	Egg sandwich: 1 fried egg, 1 slice cheese, ham, and 2 slices low-carb rye bread	7
	3 slices nitrate-free Canadian bacon	1	½ cup tomato juice	4	¾ cup tomato juice	6.5
	1 slice low-carb toast	3				
SUBTOTAL		5		11		13.5
LUNCH	Chicken (or shrimp) Caesar salad: 2 cups romaine lettuce, grilled chicken strips (or shrimp), and 3 tbsp. each low-carb Caesar dressing and Parmesan cheese	3	Chicken (or shrimp) Caesar salad: 2 cups romaine lettuce, grilled chicken strips (or shrimp), and 3 tbsp. each low-carb Caesar dressing and Parmesan cheese	3	Chicken (or shrimp) Caesar salad: 2 cups romaine lettuce, grilled chicken strips (or shrimp), and 3 tbsp. each low-carb Caesar dressing and Parmesan cheese	3

	(Plan A)		(Plan B)		(Plan C)	
			Lemon Ice Cream with Raspberry Sauce	9	2 tbsp. toasted pine nuts	2
					½ cup seedless grapes	13.5
SUBTOTAL		3		12		18.5
DINNER	Leg of lamb	0	Leg of lamb	0	Leg of lamb	0
	Greek Side Salad	5	Greek Side Salad	5	Greek Side Salad	5
	½ cup sautéed green beans	3	1 cup sautéed green beans topped with 2 tbsp. slivered almonds	7	1 cup sautéed green beans topped with 2 tbsp. slivered almonds	7
					Lemon Ice Cream with Raspberry Sauce	9
SUBTOTAL		8		12		21
SNACK	¾ cup raw broccoli florets	2	¾ cup raw broccoli florets	2	1 cup raw broccoli florets	3
	2 tbsp. sour cream dip	2	2 tbsp. sour cream dip	2	2 tbsp. sour cream dip	2
TOTAL		20		39		58

MEAL PLAN—DAY 21

	20 GRAMS OF NET CARBS	40 GRAMS OF NET CARBS	60 GRAMS OF NET CARBS
BREAKFAST	Atkins Iced Coffee 5.5	Soy Fruit Frappe (Raspberry) 7	Soy Fruit Frappe (Strawberry) 12
	2 hard-boiled eggs 1	1 slice low-carb toast 3	1 slice low-carb toast 3
		1 slice Muenster cheese 0.5	1 slice Muenster cheese 0.5
SUBTOTAL	6.5	10.5	15.5
LUNCH	Tuna salad 0	Tuna salad 0	Tuna salad 0
	1 slice low-carb toast 3	2 slices low-carb toast 6	1 slice whole-grain toast 12
	1 large lettuce leaf 0	1 large lettuce leaf 0	1 large lettuce leaf 0
	¼ cup each cucumber slices and snow peas 2.5	¼ cup each cucumber slices and snow peas 2.5	2 slices tomato 1.5
	½ large dill pickle 0.5	½ large dill pickle 0.5	½ cup steamed carrots 5.5
			½ cup snow peas 3.5
			½ large dill pickle 0.5
SUBTOTAL	6	9	23

DINNER	Day 1		Day 2		Day 3	
	Pork loin	0	Pork loin	0	Pork loin	0
	Cauliflower Purée	3	**Cauliflower Purée**	3	**Cauliflower Purée**	3
	Large spinach salad with 1 tbsp. nitrate-free crumbled bacon and vinaigrette	4	Large spinach salad with 1 tbsp. nitrate-free crumbled bacon and vinaigrette	4	Large spinach salad with 1 tbsp. nitrate-free crumbled bacon and vinaigrette	4
			½ pear	10	½ pear	10
					2 oz. blue cheese	2
SUBTOTAL		7		17		19
SNACK	1 slice Muenster cheese	0.5	¼ cup walnut halves	3.5	¼ cup walnut halves	3.5
TOTAL		20		40		61

MEAL PLAN—DAY 22

	20 GRAMS OF NET CARBS		40 GRAMS OF NET CARBS		60 GRAMS OF NET CARBS	
BREAKFAST	Steak and 2 eggs	1	Steak and 2 eggs	1	Steak and 2 eggs	1
	2 slices tomato	1.5	2 slices tomato	1.5	2 slices tomato	1.5
			1 small peach	7	1 cup Ocean Spray Light-Style cranberry juice	10
SUBTOTAL		2.5		9.5		12.5
LUNCH	Corned beef sandwich made with:		Corned beef sandwich made with:		Corned beef sandwich made with:	
	1 slice Swiss cheese	1	1 slice Swiss cheese	1	1 slice Swiss cheese	1
	1 slice low-carb rye bread	3	2 slices low-carb rye bread	6	1 slice rye bread	12
	½ cup sauerkraut	1	½ cup sauerkraut	1	½ cup sauerkraut	1
	Small chopped green salad with vinaigrette	2	Large chopped green salad with vinaigrette	4	Large chopped green salad with vinaigrette	4
SUBTOTAL		7		12		18

	Butterflied Roast Chicken		Butterflied Roast Chicken		Butterflied Roast Chicken	
		0		0		0
DINNER	¾ cup sautéed spinach with olive oil and garlic	3	1 cup sautéed spinach with olive oil and garlic	4	1 cup sautéed spinach with olive oil and garlic	4
	6 mushrooms marinated in vinaigrette	4	¼ cup cannellini beans with	6.5	½ cup cannellini beans with	13
	6 black olives	1	6 mushrooms marinated in vinaigrette	4	6 mushrooms marinated in vinaigrette	4
			1 fresh apricot	3		
SUBTOTAL		8		17.5		21
SNACK	Large celery stalk stuffed with 1 tbsp. herbed cream cheese	2	Large celery stalk stuffed with 1 tbsp. herbed cream cheese	2	2 fresh apricots	6
					1 oz. Brie	0
					¼ cup almonds	2
TOTAL		19.5		41		59.5

MEAL PLAN—DAY 23

	20 GRAMS OF NET CARBS		40 GRAMS OF NET CARBS		60 GRAMS OF NET CARBS	
BREAKFAST	Mexican Frittata	4.5	Mexican Frittata	4.5	Mexican Frittata	4.5
	2 tbsp. salsa	1	2 tbsp. salsa	1	2 tbsp. salsa	1
			2 tbsp. sour cream	1	2 tbsp. sour cream	1
			½ medium orange	6	1 medium orange	12
SUBTOTAL		5.5		12.5		18.5
LUNCH	Turkey sandwich:		Turkey sandwich:		Turkey sandwich:	
	1 slice low-carb bread	3	1 slice low-carb bread	3	2 slices low-carb bread	6
	2 slices tomato and 1 leaf red leaf lettuce	1.5	2 slices tomato and 1 leaf red leaf lettuce	1.5	2 slices tomato and 1 leaf red leaf lettuce	1.5
	Turkey breast	0	Turkey breast	0	Turkey breast	0
	1 slice Colby cheese	0.5	1 slice Colby cheese	0.5	2 slices Colby cheese	1

	Plan 1 (item)	g	Plan 2 (item)	g	Plan 3 (item)	g
	Small mixed lettuce salad with ½ cup hearts of palm and vinaigrette	4	Small mixed lettuce salad with ½ cup hearts of palm and vinaigrette	4	Large mixed lettuce salad with ½ cup hearts of palm and vinaigrette	6
			1 Coconut Pecan Macaroon	3	2 Coconut Pecan Macaroons	6
SUBTOTAL		9		12		20.5
DINNER	Sirloin steak	0	Sirloin steak	0	Sirloin steak	0
			¼ cup sautéed onions	3	⅓ cup sautéed onions	4
	1 cup sautéed kale	4	1 cup sautéed kale	4	1 cup sautéed kale	4
	Small romaine salad with low-carb blue cheese dressing	2	Large romaine salad with low-carb blue cheese dressing	4	Large romaine salad with low-carb blue cheese dressing	4
SUBTOTAL		6		11		12
SNACK	10 green olives	0.5	½ cup raspberries	3	½ cup raspberries	3
			½ cup ricotta cheese	3	½ cup ricotta cheese	3
					2 tbsp. chopped almonds	1.5
TOTAL		21		41.5		58.5

MEAL PLAN—DAY 24

	20 GRAMS OF NET CARBS		40 GRAMS OF NET CARBS		60 GRAMS OF NET CARBS	
BREAKFAST	2 fried eggs	1	1 fried egg	0.5	1 fried egg	0.5
	1 smoked pork chop	0	1 slice French toast made with low-carb bread; with sugar-free syrup	3.5	2 slices French toast made with low-carb bread; with sugar-free syrup	7
	½ cup sautéed spinach	1	⅓ cup blueberries	5.5	½ cup blueberries	8
	1 slice low-carb toast	3				
SUBTOTAL		5		9.5		15.5
LUNCH	Thin-sliced roast beef	0	Thin-sliced roast beef	0	Thin-sliced roast beef	0
	2 oz. Cheddar cheese	1	2 oz. Cheddar cheese	1	2 oz. Cheddar cheese	1
	4 leaves lettuce	0.5	4 leaves lettuce	0.5	4 leaves lettuce	0.5
	2 slices tomato	1.5	4 slices tomato	3	4 slices tomato	3
	6 black olives	1	6 black olives	1	6 black olives	1

Sour cream and horseradish dressing 1	Sour cream and horseradish dressing 1	Sour cream and horseradish dressing 1
	8 baby carrots 6	12 baby carrots 9
SUBTOTAL 5	12.5	15.5
DINNER **Spicy Orange Stir-Fry** 7	**Spicy Orange Stir-Fry** 9.5	**Spicy Orange Stir-Fry** 11.5
Small shredded Napa cabbage salad with natural rice vinegar and oil 1	Large shredded Napa cabbage salad with natural rice vinegar and oil 2	Large shredded Napa cabbage salad with natural rice vinegar and oil 2
		¼ cup steamed brown rice 10.5
SUBTOTAL 8	11.5	24
SNACK ½ cup sugar-free gelatin 0	1 oz. hazelnuts 2	2 oz. hazelnuts 4
2 tbsp. heavy cream, whipped 1	3 dried apricot halves 5	
TOTAL 19	40.5	59

MEAL PLAN—DAY 25

	20 GRAMS OF NET CARBS		40 GRAMS OF NET CARBS		60 GRAMS OF NET CARBS	
BREAKFAST	Omelet made with 2 oz. cheese	2	Omelet made with 2 oz. cheese and 6 asparagus spears	4	Omelet made with 2 oz. cheese and 6 asparagus spears	4
	4 slices tomato	3	1 slice low-carb rye toast	3	2 slices low-carb rye toast	6
			⅓ cup seedless grapes	9	⅓ cup seedless grapes	9
SUBTOTAL		5		16		19
LUNCH	Turkey burger	0	Turkey burger	0	Turkey burger	0
	Sautéed Swiss Chard	4.5	Sautéed Swiss Chard	4.5	Sautéed Swiss Chard	4.5
	Small lettuce salad with ½ cup shredded red cabbage and vinaigrette	3	Small lettuce salad with ½ cup shredded red cabbage, ¼ cup shredded carrot, and vinaigrette	5	1 small tomato, sliced	4

	Column 1	Column 2	Column 3
			Small lettuce salad with ½ cup shredded red cabbage, ¼ cup shredded carrot, and vinaigrette — 5
SUBTOTAL	7.5	9.5	13.5
DINNER	Herb-roasted chicken — 0	Herb-roasted chicken — 0	Herb-roasted chicken — 0
	⅔ cup braised leeks — 4.5	⅔ cup braised leeks — 4.5	⅔ cup braised leeks — 4.5
	Small endive and radicchio salad with low-carb ranch dressing — 2	¾ cup steamed cubed rutabaga — 9	¾ cup steamed cubed rutabaga — 9
		Small endive and radicchio salad with low-carb ranch dressing — 2	Large endive and radicchio salad with low-carb ranch dressing — 4
SUBTOTAL	6.5	15.5	17.5
SNACK	Nitrate- and sugar-free beef jerky — 0	Nitrate- and sugar-free beef jerky — 0	½ pear — 10
	1 oz. Cheddar cheese — 0.5		1 oz. blue cheese — 0.5
TOTAL	19.5	41	60.5

MEAL PLAN—DAY 26

	20 GRAMS OF NET CARBS		40 GRAMS OF NET CARBS		60 GRAMS OF NET CARBS	
BREAKFAST	Atkins Advantage RTD shake	3	Lemon Poppyseed Muffin	4	Lemon Poppyseed Muffin	4
	1 deviled egg	1	½ cup creamed cottage cheese	3	1 cup plain whole-milk yogurt	11
			½ cup boysenberries	5.5	½ cup boysenberries	5.5
SUBTOTAL		4		12.5		20.5
LUNCH	Grilled tuna	0	Grilled tuna	0	Grilled tuna	0
	Small mixed green salad with ¼ cup snow peas and ½ cup cucumber slices dressed with:	4.5	Medium mixed green salad dressed with:	3	Large mixed green salad dressed with:	4
	2 tbsp. sugar-free rice wine vinegar, 2 tbsp. sesame oil, 1 tsp. soy sauce, and ¼ tsp. grated fresh ginger	1	1 tbsp. red wine vinegar, 2 tbsp. olive oil, 1 tsp. Dijon mustard, and pinch of salt	1	1 tbsp. red wine vinegar, 2 tbsp. olive oil, 1 tsp. Dijon mustard, and pinch of salt	1
			½ cup green beans	3	½ cup green beans	3
			¼ cup water chestnuts	6	¼ cup water chestnuts	6

	Item	g carb	Item	g carb	Item	g carb
	6 green olives and capers	0.5	6 green olives and capers	0.5		
	½ cup papaya chunks	5.5				5.5
SUBTOTAL		20		13.5		5.5
DINNER	Sliced beef fajita style	0	Sliced beef fajita style	0	Sliced beef fajita style	0
	⅔ cup sautéed onions and green peppers	5	⅔ cup sautéed onions and green peppers	5	½ cup sautéed onions and green peppers	3.5
	1 cup shredded lettuce	0.5	1 cup shredded lettuce	0.5	1 cup shredded lettuce	0.5
	½ Haas avocado	2	½ Haas avocado	2	½ Haas avocado	2
	2 tbsp. each sour cream and salsa	2	2 tbsp. each sour cream and salsa	2	2 tbsp. each sour cream and salsa	2
	2 large low-carb tortillas	10	½ cup papaya chunks	5.5	1 small low-carb tortilla	3
SUBTOTAL		19.5		15		11
SNACK	2 tbsp. almonds	2	1 deviled egg	1	6 black olives	1
TOTAL		62		42		21.5

MEAL PLAN—DAY 27

	20 GRAMS OF NET CARBS		40 GRAMS OF NET CARBS		60 GRAMS OF NET CARBS	
BREAKFAST	Smoked salmon and	0	Cinnamon Pancakes	11	Cinnamon Pancakes	11
	4 tbsp. cream cheese rolled up in	2	Breakfast sausage links	0	Breakfast sausage links	0
	2 lettuce leaves	0	Sugar-free syrup	0	Sugar-free syrup	0
			½ cup sliced strawberries	4	¾ cup sliced strawberries	6
SUBTOTAL		2		15		17
LUNCH	Cobb salad:		Cobb salad:		Cobb salad:	
	2 cups Bibb lettuce	1.5	2 cups Bibb lettuce	1.5	2 cups Bibb lettuce	1.5
	½ cup watercress	0	½ cup watercress	0	½ cup watercress	0
	Diced turkey breast	0	Diced turkey breast	0	Diced turkey breast	0
	2 slices nitrate-free bacon	0	2 slices nitrate-free bacon	0	2 slices nitrate-free bacon	0
	¼ Haas avocado, sliced	1	½ Haas avocado, sliced	2	½ Haas avocado, sliced	2
	1 boiled egg, chopped	0.5	1 boiled egg, chopped	0.5	1 boiled egg, chopped	0.5

	Menu 1	(g)	Menu 2	(g)	Menu 3	(g)
	3 tbsp. chunky blue cheese dressing	3	3 tbsp. chunky blue cheese dressing	3	3 tbsp. chunky blue cheese dressing	3
	½ cup melon balls	8				
SUBTOTAL		15		7		6
DINNER	Roasted Cornish game hen	0	Roasted Cornish game hen	0	Roasted Cornish game hen	0
	Zucchini Gratin	4	**Zucchini Gratin**	4	**Zucchini Gratin**	4
	Large red leaf lettuce salad with ½ cup sliced cucumber and vinaigrette	4	Large red leaf lettuce salad with ½ cup sliced cucumber and vinaigrette	4	Large red leaf lettuce salad with ½ cup sliced cucumber and vinaigrette	4
	¼ cup baby lima beans	7	¼ cup lima beans	7		
	½ cup low-carb pasta	8				
SUBTOTAL		23		15		8
SNACK	Atkins Advantage shake mix with water and 6 tbsp. heavy cream	5.5	Atkins Advantage shake mix with water and 4 tbsp. heavy cream	4.5	Atkins Advantage shake mix with water and 4 tbsp. heavy cream	4.5
TOTAL		60.5		41.5		20.5

MEAL PLAN—DAY 28

	20 GRAMS OF NET CARBS		40 GRAMS OF NET CARBS		60 GRAMS OF NET CARBS	
BREAKFAST	2 pancakes made from low-carb pancake mix	3	½ cup Wheatena cereal	11	½ cup Wheatena cereal	11
			½ cup dairy beverage	1.5	½ cup dairy beverage	1.5
	Sugar-free pancake syrup	0	Sugar-free pancake syrup	0	Sugar-free pancake syrup	0
	2 slices nitrate-free bacon	0			1 small peach	7
SUBTOTAL		3		12.5		19.5
LUNCH	Italian sausage	0	Italian sausage	0	Italian sausage	0
	½ cup spaghetti squash	4	1 cup spaghetti squash	8	1 cup spaghetti squash	8
	1 tbsp. Parmesan	0.5	1 tbsp. Parmesan	0.5	1 tbsp. Parmesan	0.5
	Small romaine salad with low-carb Caesar dressing	2	Large romaine salad with low-carb Caesar dressing	4	Large romaine salad with low-carb Caesar dressing	4
					¼ cup cannellini beans	6
SUBTOTAL		6.5		12.5		18.5

DINNER			
New York strip steak	0		
Medium grilled tomato	4		
2 oz. grilled portobello mushroom slices	2		
Small iceberg salad with low-carb blue cheese dressing	3		
SUBTOTAL	**9**		
SNACK			
Sliced turkey	0		
2 oz. string cheese	1		
TOTAL	**19.5**		

DINNER			
New York strip steak	0		
Medium grilled tomato	4		
2 oz. grilled portobello mushroom slices	2		
Small iceberg salad with low-carb blue cheese dressing	3		
Key Lime Mousse	**8.5**		
SUBTOTAL	**17.5**		
SNACK			
Sliced turkey	0		
1 oz. string cheese	0.5		
TOTAL	**43**		

DINNER			
New York strip steak	0		
Large grilled tomato	6		
2 oz. grilled portobello mushroom slices	2		
Large spinach salad with 4 tbsp. sunflower seeds and vinaigrette	4.5		
Key Lime Mousse	**8.5**		
SUBTOTAL	**21**		
SNACK			
Sliced turkey	0		
2 oz. string cheese	1		
TOTAL	**60**		

MEAL PLAN—DAY 29

	20 GRAMS OF NET CARBS		40 GRAMS OF NET CARBS		60 GRAMS OF NET CARBS	
BREAKFAST	Vegetable Frittata	4	Vegetable Frittata	4	Vegetable Frittata	4
	1 slice low-carb toast	3	1 slice low-carb toast	3	1 slice whole-wheat toast	12
			½ cup tomato juice	4	¾ cup V-8 juice	7
SUBTOTAL		7		11		23
LUNCH	1 cup low-carb soup	2	1 cup low-carb soup	2	1 cup low-carb soup	2
	Sliced ham and 2 slices Swiss cheese rolled up in 2 lettuce leaves with mustard	2	Sliced ham and 2 slices Swiss cheese melted on 1 slice low-carb rye toast	5	Sliced ham and 2 slices Swiss cheese melted on 1 slice low-carb toast	5
			Small green lettuce salad with 6 black olives and low-carb ranch dressing	3	Small green lettuce salad with 6 black olives and low-carb ranch dressing	3
					2 fresh apricots	6
SUBTOTAL		4		10		16

DINNER	Barbecued Ribs	4	Barbecued Ribs	4	Barbecued Ribs	4
	½ cup green beans	3	1 cup green beans	6	½ cup mashed turnips	3.5
	Small cabbage salad with vinaigrette	2	Large cabbage salad with vinaigrette	4	1 cup green beans	6
					Large cabbage salad with vinaigrette	4
SUBTOTAL		9		14		17.5
SNACK	½ cup sugar-free gelatin	0	½ cup raspberries	3	2 tbsp. shelled pistachios	3
	2 tbsp. heavy cream, whipped	1	2 tbsp. heavy cream, whipped	1		
TOTAL		21		39		59.5

MEAL PLAN—DAY 30

	20 GRAMS OF NET CARBS		40 GRAMS OF NET CARBS		60 GRAMS OF NET CARBS	
BREAKFAST	Open-face burrito:		Egg burrito:		Egg burrito:	
	2 scrambled eggs	1	2 scrambled eggs	1	2 scrambled eggs	1
	2 tbsp. chopped green onion	0.5	2 tbsp. chopped green onion	0.5	2 tbsp. chopped green onion	0.5
	⅓ cup shredded cheese	0.5	⅓ cup shredded cheese	0.5	⅓ cup shredded cheese	0.5
	2 tbsp. salsa	1	2 tbsp. salsa	1	2 tbsp. salsa	1
	1 small low-carb tortilla	3	1 large low-carb tortilla	5	1 large low-carb tortilla	5
					½ orange	6
SUBTOTAL		6		8		14
LUNCH	Chicken salad with mayonnaise in ½ Haas avocado	2	Chicken salad with mayonnaise and 2 tbsp. pecans in ½ Haas avocado	4	Chicken Salad with mayonnaise and 2 tbsp. pecans in ½ Haas avocado	4

	Plan 1		Plan 2		Plan 3	
	Large mixed green salad with vinaigrette	4	Small mixed green salad with vinaigrette	2	Small mixed green salad with vinaigrette	2
			1 slice low-carb bread	3	½ cup seedless grapes	14
SUBTOTAL		6		9		20
DINNER	Shrimp scampi	0	Shrimp scampi	0	Shrimp scampi	0
	½ cup sautéed snow peas	3.5	1 cup sautéed snow peas	7	½ cup sautéed snow peas	3.5
	Small spinach salad with ¼ cup red peppers and vinaigrette	4	Large spinach salad with ½ cup red peppers and vinaigrette	8	Small spinach salad with vinaigrette	2
					⅓ cup brown rice	14
SUBTOTAL		7.5		15		19.5
SNACK	½ cup cucumber slices	1	Chocolate Almond Torte	6.5	Chocolate Almond Torte	6.5
	1 oz. Brie	0	2 oz. mascarpone cheese	1		
TOTAL		20.5		39.5		60

Chapter 27

RECIPES FOR SUCCESS

SALMON EN PAPILLOTE WITH TOMATO-BASIL RELISH

Sealing the salmon "en papillote," or in a packet, keeps it moist. When the packet is opened, the fresh basil and garlic lend a wonderfully intoxicating aroma. Using foil makes this quick and easy, but parchment gives an elegant presentation for special occasions.

Prep Time: 15 minutes
Cook Time: 20 to 30 minutes
Makes 2 Servings

2 large Roma tomatoes, seeded and diced (1 cup)
2 tablespoons fresh basil, julienned
2 tablespoons shallots, finely chopped
2 teaspoons garlic, minced
2 teaspoons extra virgin olive oil
1 teaspoon lemon juice
Dash of cayenne pepper
¼ teaspoon salt
1 cup loosely packed spinach leaves
2 (6-ounce) wild salmon fillets, skinned

2 (10 x 15-inch) pieces of aluminum foil

1. Preheat the oven to 375°F. Mix the first 8 ingredients in a small bowl. Set aside.

2. Place half of the spinach leaves in the center of foil. Lay one piece of salmon on top of the spinach. Spoon half of the tomato mixture over the fish. Fold foil over and seal edges securely. Repeat. Cook packets for 20 to 30 minutes, or until the fish is opaque in the center.

NOTE: You can prepare the packets ahead of time and keep them in the refrigerator. Allow 10 to 15 minutes more cooking time.

To cook the salmon in parchment, cut two pieces of parchment paper, each 12 x 16 inches. Fold in half to form 12 x 8-inch rectangles. Cut a half-shaped heart away from the fold on each piece, then unfold, to create 2 full hearts. Lay the open heart on the pan and spray lightly with cooking spray. Layer the spinach, fish, and topping on half of the heart as directed. Fold the remaining flap of the heart over the fish to create a package. Seal by turning the edges under one small portion at a time, starting at the top and working to the point, creasing and overlapping at each turn as you work your way down the "package." Bake as directed. Place the packets onto plates and allow your guests to open them.

Per serving:
Carbohydrate: 6 grams; Net Carbs: 4 grams; Fiber: 2 grams; Protein: 42 grams; Fat: 20 grams; Calories: 380

GRILLED CHICKEN AND AVOCADO SALAD WITH SWEET MUSTARD VINAIGRETTE AND OLIVES

This entrée salad has it all—protein, healthy fats, nutritious carbs, and fiber. You may substitute spinach, chopped romaine, or any other of your favorite greens for all or part of the lettuce and roasted or leftover shredded chicken for the grilled chicken breasts. The red peppers and almonds suitable for people able to have higher carb counts add vitamins and healthy monounsaturated fat, respectively.

Prep Time: 15 minutes
Cook Time: 12 minutes
Makes 2 Servings

Mustard Vinaigrette
2 tablespoons extra virgin olive oil
2 tablespoons sugar-free natural rice wine vinegar
1 to 2 packets sugar substitute
1 teaspoon prepared yellow mustard
1 tablespoon water
¼ teaspoon salt
Black pepper to taste

4 cups mixed lettuce
½ cup red pepper strips (for 40- and 60-gram meal plans only)
1 Haas avocado, peeled, pitted, and sliced
2 (5-ounce) chicken breasts, grilled (see Note)
¼ cup chopped green onions, green ends only
10 pitted black olives, halved
¼ cup slivered almonds (for 40- and 60-gram meal plans only)

1. In a small bowl, whisk together the vinaigrette ingredients. Set aside.

2. Place 2 cups of lettuce on each of two large plates. Mix in the red pepper strips (if permitted). Top with sliced avocado. Slice the chicken breasts thinly on the diagonal, and lay on top of the lettuce.

3. Sprinkle on the green onions and garnish with the black olives. Drizzle half of the dressing over each salad. Sprinkle with almonds (if permitted).

Note: Grill the chicken on a stovetop grill pan set over medium heat for 12 minutes, turning halfway during the cooking.

Per serving (basic recipe):
Carbohydrate: 12 grams; Net Carbs: 4 grams: Fiber: 8 grams; Protein: 33 grams; Fat: 33 grams; Calories: 485

With additions:
Per serving, add 2 grams of Net Carbs for the red peppers and 1 gram of Net Carbs for the almonds.

CONFETTI SLAW

This colorful and nutritious salad uses both green and red cabbage. The trick to making this beautiful slaw is to use a knife, not a grater or food processor, to shred the cabbage. Cut the cabbage head in half and then core it. Cut the halves lengthwise once more to make quarters, and then use a sharp knife to cut long julienne shreds of cabbage. Use a large-hole grater for shredding the carrot. The finishing touch: a tangy dressing that coats the slaw without weighing it down.

Prep Time: 20 minutes
Makes 6 servings

4 cups shredded green cabbage
2 cups shredded red cabbage
½ to 1 cup shredded carrot (for 40- and 60-gram meal plans only)
¼ medium red onion, peeled and cored
¼ cup fresh chopped parsley (or cilantro)
3 tablespoons cider vinegar
2 tablespoons extra virgin olive oil
2 tablespoons mayonnaise
2 to 3 packets sugar substitute
1 teaspoon Dijon mustard
1 teaspoon celery seed
½ teaspoon salt
¼ teaspoon black pepper

1. Place the cabbages and carrot in a large bowl. Cut the onion into thin slices. Add to the bowl. Toss in the parsley.

2. In a small bowl, whisk together the remaining ingredients. Pour over the slaw and toss. Chill before serving.

Per serving (basic recipe):
Carbohydrate: 5 grams; Net Carbs: 3 grams; Fiber: 2 grams; Protein: 1 gram; Fat: 8 grams; Calories: 100

With additions:
For 40-gram meal plan, use ½ cup grated carrot, which adds 1 gram of Net Carbs per serving.
For 60-gram meal plan, add 1 cup grated carrot, which adds 2 grams of Net Carbs per serving.

FABULOUS FRITTATAS

Frittatas are excellent low-carb fare. In these "flat omelets," eggs are used simply to bind together vegetables, seasonings, and meats, making them not only easy to make, but incredibly versatile, as shown by these six different options. You may also mix and match or substitute other low-carb ingredients to create your own fabulous frittata.

Prep Time: 20 minutes
Cook Time: 20 minutes
Makes 4 servings

BASIC RECIPE
1 tablespoon olive oil
1 tablespoon butter
2 garlic cloves, minced
½ cup chopped onion
Vegetables, herbs, and/or meat (see chart on page 407)
8 large eggs
2 tablespoons water
¼ teaspoon salt
Freshly ground pepper to taste
Cheese (see chart on page 407)

1. Heat the olive oil and butter in a large, preferably nonstick skillet over medium heat. Add the garlic and onion and sauté for 2 to 3 minutes, or until softened. Add the vegetables and herbs and cook for 5 to 6 minutes, stirring occasionally, until soft but not limp. Add the meat and cook for 2 to 3 minutes, stirring occasionally.

2. Heat the broiler. In a large bowl, whisk together the eggs, water, salt, and pepper. Pour the eggs into the hot pan over the meat and/or vegetable mixture. Let cook for a few seconds, undisturbed, then use a spatula to move the eggs toward the center while tilting the pan to let the uncooked eggs to run to the sides.

3. Continue cooking and moving the egg mixture for 4 to 5 minutes, or until the eggs are almost set (they will still be moist on the top). Sprinkle with the cheese and place under the broiler until the

eggs are cooked on top and the cheese is melted and bubbly, about 2 to 3 minutes. Cut into quarters and serve.

	VEGETABLE	**ITALIAN**	**MEXICAN**
Vegetables	2 cups sliced mushrooms and 1 cup artichoke hearts (8 oz.), chopped	1 large zucchini, sliced	1¾ cups thinly sliced red and green bell peppers
Herbs	1 tsp. dried thyme leaves	1 tsp. dried basil	½ tsp. dried oregano
Meat		8 oz. Italian sausage, uncooked, crumbled	8 oz. diced chorizo, cooked, drained
Cheese	1 cup Swiss cheese, shredded	⅓ cup Parmesan cheese, grated	¾ cup Monterey Jack cheese, shredded

	VEGETABLE	**ITALIAN**	**MEXICAN**
Per serving:			
Calories	340	460	430
Carbohydrates	9.5 g	6 g	5 g
Net Carbs	6.5 g	5 g	4.5 g
Fiber	3 g	1 g	0.5 g
Fat	24 g	37 g	34 g
Saturated Fat	10 g	13 g	13 g
Protein	22 g	25 g	25 g

MEXICAN CHICKEN SOUP

Traditional chicken soup is left out in the cold when compared to this zesty Mexican version. The bold flavor of the nutrient-rich broth replaces the need for noodles and the broth is a good source of phosphorus, potassium, and vitamins A, B₃, and C. The turmeric adds color, but is optional. Garnish if you like with additional fresh cilantro, shredded cheese, or avocado slices, but be sure to add the carbs to your daily tally. Olé.

Prep Time: 15 minutes
Cook Time: 18 minutes
Makes 4 servings

1 tablespoon olive oil
¾ cup chopped onion
¾ teaspoon cumin
⅛ teaspoon turmeric (optional)
4 cups reduced-sodium chicken broth
2 cups shredded cooked chicken
¾ teaspoon jalapeño pepper, seeded and minced (or jarred
    jalapeño slices, finely chopped)
½ cup canned corn niblets, drained (40- and 60-gram meal
    plans only)
1 small tomato, seeded and chopped
3 tablespoons fresh cilantro, chopped

1. Heat the oil in a medium saucepan over medium-low heat. Add the onion and sauté for 2 to 3 minutes to soften. Add the cumin and turmeric and stir for 30 seconds to heat.

2. Add the broth, chicken, jalapeño, and corn (if using). Simmer, uncovered, for 10 minutes. Stir in the tomato and cilantro; simmer for 5 minutes longer.

Per serving (basic recipe):
Carbohydrate: 3 grams; Net Carbs: 3 grams; Fiber: 0 gram; Protein: 22 grams; Fat: 9 grams;
Calories: 380

With addition of corn:
Add 3 grams of Net Carbs per serving.

RICOTTA CREAM, BERRIES, AND ALMONDS

Sweetened, puréed ricotta cheese makes an elegant topping for fresh berries in this easy-to-make dessert.

Prep Time: 10 minutes
Makes 4 servings

¾ cup ricotta cheese
6 tablespoons sour cream
⅓ cup granular sugar substitute
½ teaspoon vanilla extract
¼ teaspoon almond extract
1 teaspoon lemon zest and 2 cups raspberries (40-gram meal plan only), or 1 teaspoon orange zest and 2 cups boysenberries (60-gram meal plan only)
½ cup sliced almonds, toasted

1. Place the ricotta, sour cream, sugar substitute, and vanilla and almond extracts in a food processor. Purée until smooth.

2. Place ½ cup of the berries into four glass bowls or glasses. Spoon the ricotta cream over the berries (about ¼ cup each). Sprinkle with toasted almonds. (The ricotta cream may be made up to 2 days ahead. Cover and refrigerate until ready to use.)

Per serving:
Carbohydrate: 13.5 grams; Net Carbs: 8.5 grams; Fiber: 5 grams; Protein: 9 grams; Fat: 17 grams; Calories: 235

With substitution:
Add 2.5 grams Net Carbs if you substitute boysenberries for raspberries.

PORK TENDERLOIN WITH SWEET AND SOUR RED CABBAGE

Tender pork pairs beautifully with bright red cabbage in this hearty en-trée that's pretty enough to serve to company. Horseradish cream makes a tangy accompaniment. Simply mix sour cream and a small amount of mayonnaise with enough horseradish to suit your taste and place a dollop on top of the sliced pork just before serving.

Prep Time: 25 minutes
Cook Time: 15 to 20 minutes
Makes 4 servings

2 pounds pork tenderloin, trimmed (two 1-pound tenderloins)
2 tablespoons olive oil
Salt to taste
Pepper to taste
¼ cup diced red onion
1 small red cabbage (1 pound), cored, quartered, and thinly sliced
1 medium apple, peeled and sliced (40- and 60-gram meal plans only)
½ cup water
¼ cup red wine vinegar
1 tablespoon balsamic vinegar
3 to 4 packets sugar substitute

1. Preheat the oven to 425°F. Rub the pork tenderloins with 1 tablespoon of the olive oil and season with salt and pepper. Place the pork in a hot 12-inch skillet over medium heat and cook for 5 to 6 minutes, turning the pork to brown well on all sides. Remove the pork and place onto a baking sheet. Place the pork in the oven.

2. While the pork cooks, add the remaining tablespoon of oil to the sauté pan. Add the onion and cook for 2 minutes, stirring occasionally, or until the onion softens. Add the cabbage and apple (if using) to the pan. Stir in the water, vinegars, sugar substitute, and ½ teaspoon salt. Cover and cook for 10 minutes. Uncover and cook for an additional 10 minutes, stirring occasionally. Check the pork after 15 or 20 minutes and remove from the oven when an instant-read

meat thermometer reads 145° to 150°F. Let the meat rest for 10 minutes. Slice the pork on the diagonal and serve with the red cabbage.

Per serving (basic recipe):
Carbohydrate: 9.5 grams; Net Carbs: 7.5 grams; Fiber: 2 grams; Protein: 48 grams; Fat: 13 grams;
Calories; 390

With addition of apple:
Add 4.5 grams of Net Carbs per serving.

CREAM OF BROCCOLI, HAM, AND CHEDDAR SOUP

*This warm and hearty entrée delivers a healthy dose of antioxidant vita-
mins A and C along with bone-building calcium. To serve as a side dish
or as a first course, omit the ham and use only ½ cup of cheese.*

Prep Time: 15 minutes
Cook Time: 18 minutes
Makes 4 Servings

    1 tablespoon olive oil
    ¾ cup chopped green onion
    2 garlic cloves, minced
    ¾ teaspoon dried, crushed thyme leaves
    2 (14-ounce) cans reduced-sodium chicken broth plus
        ¼ cup water
    3½ cups fresh broccoli florets
    6 tablespoons heavy cream
    Salt to taste
    Pinch of cayenne pepper
    1½ cups diced ham (cut into ¼-inch dice)
    ¾ cup shredded Cheddar cheese

    1. Heat the oil in a medium saucepan over medium-low heat. Add
the green onion and garlic. Cook for 1 to 2 minutes until the onion is
soft. Stir in the thyme.
    2. Add the chicken broth and broccoli. Simmer for 8 to 10 minutes
until the broccoli is tender but not mushy. In a blender or food proces-

sor, purée the soup until smooth. Add the cream, salt, and cayenne. Pour the soup back into the pot, add the ham, and gently heat for 5 to 10 minutes until the soup thickens slightly. Remove from the heat and stir the cheese into the soup until blended.

Per serving:
Carbohydrate: 5 grams; Net Carbs: 3 grams; Fiber: 2 grams; Protein: 24 grams; Fat 24: grams; Calories: 330

ATKINS ICED COFFEE

So simple—so good! This cool and creamy coffee is a terrific low-carb alternative to the offerings at popular coffee shops. Using Atkins Advantage Shake Mix adds extra protein as well as fiber and plenty of vitamins and minerals. It also contributes to the creamy texture and flavor.

Makes 1 serving

½ cup warm water
2 teaspoons instant decaf coffee powder
2½ tablespoons light cream
1 scoop Atkins Advantage shake mix (cappuccino, chocolate, or
    vanilla)
½ cup crushed ice (about 5 medium ice cubes)

Pour the water and coffee powder into a blender. When the coffee powder dissolves, add the cream, sugar substitute, and shake mix. Blend. Add the crushed ice and blend until cold and creamy.

Per serving:
Carbohydrate: 8 grams; Net Carbs: 5.5 grams; Fiber: 2.5 grams; Protein: 8.5 grams; Fat: 14 grams; Calories: 190

GREEK SALAD WITH GRILLED CHICKEN BREAST

Nothing beats a classic Greek salad for a touch of the Mediterranean. Here we have paired it with grilled chicken for a filling entrée. For a side salad, omit the chicken, but be sure to include the briny Kalamata olives for their authentic Greek flavor.

Prep Time: 20 minutes
Cook Time: 12 minutes
Makes 4 servings as an entrée; 6 servings as a side salad

DRESSING
¼ cup extra virgin olive oil
3 tablespoons red wine vinegar
1 tablespoon water
2 teaspoons dried oregano
1 garlic clove, finely minced
¼ teaspoon salt
Freshly ground black pepper to taste
Pinch of sugar substitute (optional)

Four 5-ounce chicken breasts, pounded flat
6 cups torn romaine leaves
2 medium tomatoes, cored and cut into wedges or chunks
1 medium cucumber, peeled, seeded, and cut into chunks
½ cup thinly sliced red onion
1 cup feta cheese, crumbled (4 ounces)
12 Kalamata olives, pitted and quartered

1. In a small bowl, whisk together the oil, vinegar, water, oregano, garlic, salt, pepper, and sugar substitute, if using. Adjust to taste.

2. Season the chicken with salt and pepper. Preheat a stovetop grill pan over medium heat. Brush the pan with oil and add the chicken. Cook for 12 minutes, turning halfway during the cooking, until the chicken is no longer pink in the center. Set aside, covered, for 10 minutes.

3. In a large salad bowl, combine the romaine, tomatoes, cucum-

ber, and red onion. Gently toss with half of the dressing. Divide the salad among four serving plates. Top with feta and the chicken breasts. Drizzle with the remaining dressing and garnish with olives.

Per serving as an entrée (with chicken):
Carbohydrate: 10 grams; Net Carbs: 7 grams; Fiber: 3 grams; Protein: 38 grams; Fat: 31 grams; Calories: 460

Per serving as a side salad:
5 grams of Net Carbs.

KEY LIME MOUSSE

With the classic flavor of key lime pie but no high-carb crust, this sumptuous mousse is sure to please. If you can't find fresh key limes, don't worry, simply use unsweetened bottled key lime juice found in the juice section of most markets.

Prep Time: 20 minutes
Cook Time: 8 minutes
Chilling Time: 4½ hours
Makes 6 servings

⅔ cup key lime juice
1 envelope unflavored gelatin
1 cup whole milk
1 large egg
2 large eggs, separated
⅔ cup granular sugar substitute
Zest of 2 key limes or 1 regular lime
8 ounces cream cheese, softened

1. Place the lime juice in a medium saucepan. Sprinkle the gelatin over the juice. Let set for 3 minutes. Thoroughly whisk in the milk, whole egg, 2 egg yolks, and sugar substitute.
2. Place the pan over low heat and warm the mixture while stirring. Increase the temperature to medium, add the zest, and continue

cooking for 6 to 8 minutes, stirring, until the mixture thickens. Remove from the heat and cool until the mixture is lukewarm, about 1½ hours.

3. In a medium bowl, beat the cream cheese with an electric mixer until very smooth. Beat in the lime mixture. Refrigerate until cool, about 1 hour, stirring occasionally.

4. In a small bowl, beat the 2 egg whites until soft peaks form. Fold the egg whites into the lime mixture. Pour into six individual dishes or custard cups, if desired, and refrigerate until set, about 1 hour. Garnish with additional lime zest.

Per serving:
Carbohydrate: 8.5 grams; Net Carbs: 8.5 grams; Fiber: 0 gram; Protein: 9 grams; Fat: 15 grams; Calories: 205

CAULIFLOWER PURÉE

When properly puréed, cauliflower tastes like mashed potatoes. The trick is to get the right texture and the right taste. For the perfect texture, be sure to press down on the cooked cauliflower when draining to remove excess moisture. The perfect flavor comes from a winning combination of butter, garlic, and Parmesan cheese.

Prep Time: 10 minutes
Cook Time: 15 minutes
Makes 4 servings

1 (1-pound head) fresh cauliflower, trimmed into florets
2 large fresh garlic cloves, peeled
1 tablespoon light cream
2 tablespoons sour cream
¼ cup Parmesan cheese
½ teaspoon salt
⅛ teaspoon ground black pepper

1. Set a steamer basket in a large saucepan filled with 1 inch of water and bring to a simmer. Add the cauliflower and garlic, cover, and

steam for 12 to 15 minutes, or until tender. Pour the cauliflower and garlic into a colander to drain. Using a small plate or a pot lid, press down on the cauliflower to remove as much water as possible. Transfer the cauliflower and garlic to a food processor.

2. Add the light cream, sour cream, Parmesan, salt, and pepper; process until smooth. (Add more salt and pepper to taste.)

Per serving:
Carbohydrate: 6 grams; Net Carbs: 3 grams; Fiber: 3 grams; Protein: 5 grams; Fat: 9 grams; Calories: 120

SPINACH PARMESAN EGG PUFF

Egg puffs are fancier than omelets yet sturdier than soufflés. Protein powder not only adds extra protein, but helps to keep the puff from rapidly deflating. Wonderful for entertaining, a puff makes a great breakfast centerpiece when placed on the table right out of the oven.

Prep Time: 20 minutes
Bake Time: 35 minutes
Makes 4 servings

1 (10-ounce) package frozen chopped spinach, thawed
2 tablespoons butter
½ cup chopped green onions
6 large eggs, at room temperature
¾ cup cottage cheese
½ cup grated Parmesan cheese
2 tablespoons unflavored soy isolate protein powder
1 teaspoon dried dill
½ teaspoon salt
¼ teaspoon pepper

1. Preheat the oven to 350°F. Coat a 2-quart soufflé dish with non-stick cooking spray. Squeeze the spinach dry and chop; set aside.

2. Heat the butter in a small saucepan over medium-low heat. Add

the green onions and cook for 2 minutes, stirring occasionally. Add the spinach and cook for 3 minutes, stirring occasionally. Set aside on a plate to cool.

3. In the large bowl of an electric mixer set on high speed, beat the eggs for 8 minutes, or until frothy, lemon colored, and doubled in volume. Stir in the cottage cheese, ⅓ cup of the Parmesan, the protein powder, dill, salt, pepper, and spinach mixture. Pour into the prepared soufflé dish.

4. Sprinkle the remaining Parmesan cheese on top and bake for 30 to 35 minutes, or until browned and puffed. Serve immediately.

Per serving:
Carbohydrate: 6 grams; Net Carbs: 4 grams; Fiber: 2 grams; Protein: 24 grams; Fat: 19 grams; Calories: 285

CLASSIC BEEF STEW

Fork-tender beef takes center stage in this traditional entrée. Add turnips for the 40-carbohydrate-gram meal plan and carrots for the 60-gram meal plan.

Prep Time: 35 minutes
Cook Time: 2½ hours
Makes 6 servings

2¼ pounds beef stew meat, cut into 1½-inch pieces
1 teaspoon each dried oregano and thyme
½ teaspoon salt
⅛ teaspoon pepper
2 tablespoons olive oil
½ cup chopped onions
1 cup chopped celery
1 (14-ounce) can reduced-sodium beef broth
1 cup canned chopped tomatoes, drained
½ cup red wine (40- and 60-gram meal plans only)
2 bay leaves

2 cups fresh green beans, trimmed and cut in half

8 ounces fresh mushrooms, quartered

2 cups peeled turnip cubes, cut into ½-inch cubes
    (40-gram meal plan only)

4 medium carrots, cut diagonally (60-gram meal plan only)

1 teaspoon salt

¼ teaspoon ground black pepper

3 to 5 teaspoons ThickenThin Not/Starch thickener (see Note)

¼ cup chopped fresh parsley

1. Season the beef with ½ teaspoon oregano, ½ teaspoon thyme, and the salt and pepper. Heat 1 tablespoon oil in a large pot over medium-high heat. Add half of the meat and cook for 6 to 8 minutes, turning to brown on all sides. Transfer to a bowl and repeat with the remaining tablespoon oil and meat. Add the onions and celery to the pot and sauté for 3 to 4 minutes to soften.

2. Return the beef to the pan. Add the broth, tomatoes, wine (if using), bay leaves, and remaining oregano and thyme. Bring to a bare simmer, cover, and cook for 1½ to 2 hours, or until the beef is just tender. Discard the bay leaves. Add the green beans and mushrooms (and either the turnip cubes or cut carrots as indicated). Cook for an additional 20 to 30 minutes until the vegetables are tender.

3. Season with salt and pepper. Stir in ThickenThin to the desired consistency. Bring to a low boil. Sprinkle with chopped parsley before serving.

NOTE: This thickener is available at www.atkins.com.

Per serving (basic recipe):
Carbohydrate: 9 grams; Net Carbs: 6 grams; Fiber: 3 grams; Protein: 30 grams; Fat: 19 grams;
Calories: 377

With additions:
The turnips add 2.5 grams Net Carbs per serving; the carrots add 4 grams per serving.

CINNAMON PANCAKES

These cinnamon-scented pancakes cook up light and fluffy just like the old-fashioned kind, but they are filled with high-quality protein rather than refined carbohydrates. They taste just great by themselves, but can be topped with butter and sugar-free syrup if you like.

Prep Time: 10 minutes
Cook Time: 12 minutes
Makes eight 4-inch pancakes; serves 4

½ cup whole wheat pastry flour
¼ cup soy flour
¼ cup unflavored soy-isolate protein powder
2 to 3 tablespoons granulated sugar substitute
1 teaspoon baking powder
1 teaspoon cinnamon
¼ teaspoon salt (optional)
½ cup light cream mixed with ⅔ cup water
2 eggs, lightly beaten
Canola oil

1. In a medium bowl, whisk together all the dry ingredients. Make a well in the center and pour in the cream mixture and eggs. Combine the dry and liquid ingredients, stirring just until blended. (Whisk just until smooth.)

2. Place a griddle or skillet over medium heat. Brush with oil. For each pancake, pour a scant ¼ cup of batter onto the griddle and lightly spread to a 4-inch circle. Cook the pancake for 2 to 3 minutes on the first side until the underside browns. Flip and cook the other side for 1 to 2 minutes more, or until the pancake puffs up and springs back when lightly touched in the center.

Per serving:
Carbohydrate: 13 grams; Net Carbs: 11 grams; Fiber: 2 grams; Protein: 12 grams; Fat: 8 grams; Calories: 160

BARBECUED CHICKEN OR RIBS

East meets West in this tangy sugar-free barbecue sauce, where soy sauce and ginger add depth and punch to traditional barbecue sauce. Be sure to use sugar-free hoisin sauce.

Prep Time: 20 minutes
Cook Time: 50 minutes (chicken); 3 hours (ribs)
Makes 4 servings (sauce only without hoisin)

BARBECUE SAUCE
1 tablespoon canola oil
1 teaspoon minced garlic
1 ½ cups water
1 (6-ounce) can tomato paste
2 tablespoons each vinegar and
    Worcestershire sauce
¼ cup soy sauce
¼ teaspoon powdered ginger
¼ cup granular sugar substitute
¾ teaspoon chili powder
½ teaspoon dry mustard
1 tablespoon Steel's sugar-free hoisin sauce

1 whole cut-up chicken (about 4 pounds), or 3 pounds pork or
    beef ribs

1. For the barbecue sauce: In a medium saucepan, heat the oil and garlic over medium heat for 1 minute. Add the water and tomato paste. Whisk until smooth. Add the remaining ingredients as specified, stir well, and simmer for 15 to 20 minutes.

2. If using chicken, preheat the oven to 350°F. Coat a shallow roasting pan with nonstick cooking spray. Place the chicken skin side down into the pan. Bake for 25 minutes. Turn the chicken with tongs and coat with 1 cup barbecue sauce. Bake for 20 to 25 minutes longer until the juices from all the pieces run clear when pricked deeply with a fork.

3. If using ribs, preheat the oven to 300°F. Arrange the ribs in a single layer in a 9 x 13-inch pan. Brush with 1 cup barbecue sauce and seal the pan with foil. Bake for 3 hours. Uncover, increase the temperature to 350°F, and bake for 1 additional hour until the ribs are tender and the meat easily separates from the bone. (Keep the remaining cup of sauce in the refrigerator for up to two weeks.)

Note: Total protein, fat, and calories will differ if pork is used but will not affect the carbohydrate content of the recipe.

Chicken per serving:
Carbohydrate: 5 grams; Net Carbs: 4 grams; Fiber: 1 gram; Protein: 31 grams; Fat: 25 grams; Calories: 374

RAGIN' NUTS

Hot and spicy or sweet and salty, these snack nuts fill the bill. Simple to make and delicious to eat, the only problem with them is the temptation to eat the whole batch in one sitting!

Prep Time: 15 minutes
Bake Time: 15 minutes
Makes eight ¼-cup servings: 2 cups

>   1 large egg white
>   6 tablespoons granular sugar substitute
>   2 teaspoons Cajun spice blend
>   ¼ teaspoon dried thyme leaves, crushed
>   ⅛ teaspoon cayenne pepper
>   1 tablespoon melted butter
>   2 cups pecans (or almonds or walnuts)
>   ¼ teaspoon salt (optional)

1. Preheat the oven to 350°F. Line a baking sheet with foil and coat with nonstick cooking spray. Set the whole egg (in the shell) in a small bowl of very warm tap water (130°F); let stand 5 minutes to warm.

2. Meanwhile, combine the sugar substitute, spice blend, thyme, and cayenne in a medium bowl. Separate the egg white into a small dish and reserve the yolk for another use. Add the egg white and melted butter to the bowl and stir until well blended. Toss in the nuts, stirring until well coated. Spread the nuts in a single layer on a baking sheet. Sprinkle with salt, if using. Bake for 12 to 15 minutes, or until fragrant and crisped. Loosen the nuts from the foil with a spatula and set aside to cool completely. Store in an airtight container.

Per serving:
Carbohydrate: 6 grams; Net Carbs: 4 grams; Fiber: 2 grams; Protein: 3 grams; Fat: 18 grams; Calories: 190

SOUTH-OF-THE-BORDER BURGERS WITH AVOCADO SALSA

These salsa-filled burgers make a great "fork and knife" sandwich. Cheese lovers can melt Jack cheese on the burgers before topping with salsa. Be sure to count the added carbs.

Prep Time: 20 minutes
Cook Time: 8 minutes
Makes 4 servings

1 medium tomato, seeded and diced
3 tablespoons diced red onion
3 tablespoons finely chopped cilantro
1 small jalapeño, seeded and minced
Salt
1 tablespoon fresh lime juice
1 large Haas avocado, peeled, seeded, and diced
1½ pounds lean ground beef
⅛ teaspoon ground black pepper
¼ cup drained prepared medium-hot tomato salsa
4 large lettuce leaves

1. Place the tomato in a medium bowl. Stir in the red onion, cilantro, jalapeño, and a pinch of salt. Gently stir in the lime juice and then the avocado. Do not overmix. Set aside.

2. Season the ground beef with ½ teaspoon salt and the pepper. Divide the mixture into fourths. To make one patty, divide one-fourth of the meat in half; shape each into a thin 3½-inch patty with an in-dent in the center. Spoon 1 tablespoon of the salsa in the center and top with the other patty, indented side down. Press the edges to seal well and shape into a 4-inch patty, flattening slightly. Repeat with the remaining meat and salsa to make 4 burgers.

3. Preheat a stovetop grill pan over medium heat. Grill the burgers for 6 to 8 minutes, turning halfway during the cooking, or until medium-well. Place each burger on a lettuce leaf and top with ½ cup of the avocado salsa.

Per serving:
Carbohydrate: 14 grams; Net Carbs: 8 grams; Fiber: 6 grams; Protein: 72 grams; Fat: 68 grams; Calories: 860

CHOCOLATE ALMOND TORTE

In Europe you will find that many delicious cakes or tortes are made with little to no flour. Nut meals or flours (made by grinding the nuts into powder) are used instead. This sweet, moist, chocolaty cake uses almonds, but hazelnuts and walnuts can easily be substituted.

Prep Time: 20 minutes
Bake Time: 60 minutes
Makes 8 servings

1½ cups natural raw almonds (or 1½ cups almond flour or meal)
3 Endulge Chocolate Candy Bars, chopped
½ cup softened butter (1 stick)
6 large eggs, separated
1 (3.5-ounce) jar prune and apple baby food
½ cup granular sugar substitute
¾ teaspoon almond extract
Sugar-free sweetened whipped cream (optional)

1. Preheat the oven to 300°F. Grease and line the bottom of an 8-inch round cake pan with parchment or wax paper. Set aside.

2. Place the nuts in a food processor and pulse into a coarse meal. Add the chocolate and process until the mixture is a coarse powder.

3. In a medium bowl, cream the butter and egg yolks until light and lemon colored. Blend in the baby food, sugar substitute, and almond extract. Stir in the ground almond mixture.

4. In a separate bowl, beat the egg whites until soft peaks form. Fold a small amount of egg whites into the batter to loosen and then carefully fold in the remaining whites. Pour the mixture into the prepared pan. Bake for 60 minutes until the cake springs back when lightly touched and a toothpick inserted in the center comes out clean. Cool on a wire rack. Serve with a dollop of whipped cream if desired. (The cake can be frozen.)

Per serving (without cream topping):
Carbohydrate: 10.5 grams; Net Carbs: 6.5 grams; Fiber: 4 grams; Protein: 11 grams; Fat: 33 grams; Calories: 390

SPAGHETTI SQUASH WITH SPINACH PESTO

The long thin strands and subtle taste of spaghetti squash make this a wonderful alternative to high-carb pasta. With only 1 gram of carbohydrate per tablespoon and high in vitamin A, calcium, and iron, this pesto is a terrific topping to spread on chicken or fish, to use in soups, or to spread on low-carb sandwiches.

Prep Time: 15 minutes
Cook Time: 10 minutes
Makes eight ½-cup servings or four 1-cup servings

½ cup fresh spinach leaves, packed
½ cup fresh basil leaves
¼ cup pine nuts
¼ cup grated Parmesan cheese
⅛ teaspoon salt
2 garlic cloves, peeled
⅓ cup extra virgin olive oil
2 tablespoons chicken broth
1 medium spaghetti squash (about 2 pounds)

1. Place the spinach, basil, pine nuts, Parmesan, salt, and garlic in a food processor. Pulse for 1 minute until finely chopped. Add the oil and pulse until smooth. Add the chicken broth to thin the pesto.

2. Wash the whole squash and pierce in several places with a fork. Microwave on high heat for 10 minutes. Remove from the microwave and cut lengthwise in half. Scoop out the seeds. Using a fork, lift and tease out "spaghetti" strands of squash. Pile the squash onto a serving dish or individual plates (½ cup each for 20-gram meal plan and 1 cup each for 40- and 60-gram meal plans). Top with either ½ cup of squash with 1 tablespoon pesto or 1 cup of squash with 2 tablespoons pesto. Garnish with additional Parmesan if desired.

Per serving (8 servings, each ½ cup squash and sauce):
Carbohydrate: 7.5 grams; Net Carbs: 4.5 grams; Fiber: 3 grams; Protein: 3 grams; Fat: 7.5 grams; Calories: 115

Per serving (4 servings, each 1 cup squash and sauce):
Carbohydrate: 15 grams; Net Carbs: 9 grams; Fiber: 6 grams; Protein: 6 grams; Fat: 15 grams; Calories: 230

BREAKFAST CHEESECAKES

These creamy and filling cups of cheesecake are fun for breakfast and great for snacks or even dessert. Scented with fresh orange zest and not overly sweet, they pack the protein of 2 eggs and are a good source of calcium. You can also use lemon or lime zest if you prefer.

Prep Time: 15 minutes
Cook Time: 35 minutes
Chill Time: 4 hours
Makes 6 servings

2 cups creamed cottage cheese
8 ounces tub-style cream cheese at room temperature
½ cup granular sugar substitute
½ teaspoon almond extract
¾ teaspoon orange zest
2 large eggs
2 large egg whites

1. Preheat the oven to 325°F. Set six 6-ounce custard cups in a large baking pan (with at least 2-inch sides).
2. In a food processor, purée the cottage cheese until *completely* smooth. Add the cream cheese, sugar substitute, almond extract, and orange zest; process until smooth. Add the eggs and egg whites, one at a time, pulsing briefly just to incorporate.
3. Pour the batter into the custard cups. Add hot water to the pan until halfway up the sides of the custard cups. Bake for 30 to 35 minutes until the sides are firm and the center is barely set. Chill for at least 4 hours.

Per serving:
Carbohydrate: 5 grams; Net Carbs: 5 grams; Fiber: 0 gram; Protein: 15 grams; Fat: 18 grams; Calories: 240

LEMON POPPYSEED MUFFINS

If these muffins were made the usual way, with sugar and refined flour, they would contain 34 grams of carbs per muffin! Here, our moist and light muffins clock in at a mere 4 grams of carbohydrates each.

Prep Time: 15 minutes
Cook Time: 20 minutes
Makes 12 servings

    1 cup almonds (or 1 cup almond meal or flour)
    1 cup vanilla-flavored protein powder
    1 teaspoon baking soda
    2 teaspoons baking powder
    ½ cup butter (1 stick), softened
    3 large eggs
    ½ cup sour cream
    1 cup granular sugar substitute
    1 tablespoon poppyseeds
    1½ teaspoons lemon extract
    ½ teaspoon almond extract
    Zest of 1 lemon

1. Preheat the oven to 375°F. Lightly spray 12 muffin cups with nonstick cooking spray.

2. Process the nuts in a food processor to a fine meal. Place in a medium bowl; stir in the protein powder, baking soda, and baking powder. Set aside.

3. In another medium bowl, cream the butter with an electric mixer. Beat in the eggs one at a time. Blend in the sour cream and sugar substitute. Stir in the poppyseeds, lemon and almond extracts, and lemon zest. Gently stir in the almond mixture just until all dry ingredients are wet. Divide the batter among the muffin tins (¼ cup each). Bake for 20 minutes, or until a toothpick inserted in the center comes out clean. Do not overbake. Cool on a wire rack.

Per serving:
Carbohydrate: 6 grams; Net Carbs: 4 grams; Fiber: 2 grams; Protein: 11 grams; Fat: 17 grams; Calories: 220

BOUILLABAISSE

Fresh fish and shellfish combine beautifully in this classic French fisherman's stew. Mussels can be added or substituted for the clams, and any firm-fleshed white fish can be used. A hallmark of bouillabaisse is the distinctive flavor and color added by saffron threads. Just a touch of this exotic (and expensive) spice goes a long way. Don't be intimidated by the number of ingredients or the time to prepare; this one-pot stew makes up the time with an easy clean-up and fantastic flavor.

Prep Time: 30 minutes
Cook Time: 35 minutes
Makes 4 servings

2 tablespoons olive oil
1 tablespoon butter
2 garlic cloves, minced
½ cup chopped leeks
½ cup chopped fennel
    (40- and 60-gram meal plans only)
1 cup chopped celery
½ teaspoon dried thyme leaves
¼ teaspoon saffron threads (or ⅛ teaspoon ground saffron or
    turmeric)
1 tablespoon tomato paste
One (8-ounce) bottle clam juice
1 cup chicken broth
½ cup clam juice or reduced-sodium chicken broth
    (20-gram meal plans only)
¾ cup white wine (40- and 60-gram meal plans only)
One (14-ounce) can chopped or plum tomatoes, with juice
½ teaspoon salt
¼ to ½ teaspoon cayenne pepper
12 clams, rinsed and scrubbed
1 pound halibut, red snapper, orange roughy, or cod, or a
    combination, cut into 2-inch pieces

½ pound each shelled, deveined shrimp and scallops
2 tablespoons chopped fresh flat-leaf parsley

1. Heat the olive oil and butter in a large saucepan. Add the garlic, leeks, fennel, celery, thyme, and saffron. Sauté over medium heat for 4 to 5 minutes, or until vegetables are softened.

2. Add the tomato paste, clam juice, chicken broth, and wine. Stir. Add the tomatoes and juice, and season with the salt and cayenne. Bring to a boil, reduce the heat, and simmer for 15 minutes. (The broth may be made a day in advance.)

3. Add the clams and cook for 3 minutes. Add the fish, then the shrimp and scallops. Tuck the seafood into the broth, cover, and cook for 5 minutes until the fish is opaque and the clams have opened. Sprinkle with the parsley and ladle into four large serving bowls.

Per serving:
Carbohydrates: 8 grams; Net Carbs: 6.5 grams; Fiber: 1.5 grams; Protein: 40 grams; Fat: 12 grams; Calories: 305

With additions:
Wine and fennel add .5 gram Net Carbs and 35 calories per serving.

BACON, LETTUCE, AND TOMATO SALAD

Here's a new twist on a great American tradition. Butter lettuce is now the base for bacon, tomato, and luscious avocado slices, all topped with a creamy mayonnaise dressing. There is no need for bread with this rendition; however, croutons made with low-carb bread add a nice touch.

Prep Time: 10 minutes
Makes 4 servings

8 cups Bibb lettuce
2 medium tomatoes, cut into wedges
8 ounces nitrate-free bacon, cooked and drained
1½ Haas avocados, ripe but firm, sliced
½ cup mayonnaise
3 tablespoons each light cream and water
1 tablespoon finely chopped green onion
1 teaspoon cider vinegar
¼ teaspoon horseradish
⅛ teaspoon salt
Pinch of sugar substitute (optional)
Freshly ground black pepper

1. Wash, drain, and pat the lettuce dry. Place 2 cups of lettuce on each of four plates. Top with tomato wedges. Crumble the bacon in large pieces and divide among the salads. Arrange the avocado on top of the salads.

2. In a blender or food processor, combine the remaining ingredients (except the black pepper). Process until smooth. Ladle 3 tablespoons of dressing over each salad. Top with ground pepper.

Per serving:
Carbohydrate: 13 grams; Net Carbs: 5 grams; Fiber: 8 grams; Protein: 10 grams; Fat: 40 grams;
Calories: 440

LEMON ICE CREAM WITH RASPBERRY SAUCE

Very easy, very quick, and very elegant, this dessert complements almost any meal. The recipe can be doubled or tripled for entertaining.

Prep Time: 15 minutes, plus chilling time
Makes 2 servings

1¼ cups Atkins Endulge Super Premium vanilla ice cream
⅓ cup frozen unsweetened raspberries
2 packets sugar substitute
Juice of ½ lemon (or 3 tablespoons)
Grated lemon zest of ½ lemon
Fresh mint garnish (optional)

1. Microwave ice cream on high for 15 seconds to soften it.
2. Purée the raspberries with one packet of sugar substitute. Press the berry purée through a strainer.
3. In a small bowl, whisk the lemon juice and the second packet of sugar substitute and zest into the ice cream until creamy but not melted. Place the ice cream back in the freezer until firm, 15 minutes.
4. To serve, place ½ cup ice cream in a bowl or parfait glass. Spoon one-half of the raspberry sauce over the ice cream. Garnish with mint, if desired.

Per serving:
Carbohydrate: 10 grams; Net Carbs: 9 grams; Fiber: 1 gram; Protein: 3 grams; Fat: 4 grams; Calories: 180

SOY FRUIT FRAPPE

Soy can be a great addition to your diet. Research has shown that isoflavones found in soy may reduce the risk for heart disease. The problem is, many soy milks are full of hidden sugars. Fortunately, low-carb versions are increasingly available.

Prep Time: 5 minutes
Makes 1 serving

1 cup vanilla soy milk (like Westsoy Soy Slender with sucralose)
½ cup frozen unsweetened raspberries, blackberries, or
   strawberries
¼ teaspoon orange or almond extract
2 packets sugar substitute
½ cup crushed ice or 3 ice cubes

1. In a blender, purée all ingredients except the ice, on high until smooth.
2. Add the ice and blend until smooth.

	RASPBERRY	BLACKBERRY	STRAWBERRY
Per serving:			
Carbohydrate	16 g	18 g	16 g
Net Carbs	7 g	11 g	12 g
Fiber	9 g	7 g	5 g
Protein	7 g	7 g	6 g
Fat	3.5 g	3.5 g	3 g
Calories	120	130	120

BUTTERFLIED ROAST CHICKEN

Nothing beats a good home-cooked roast chicken—especially one that cooks in only 45 minutes! The trick is to butterfly the chicken open (or to save more time, ask the butcher to do it for you), lay it directly into a roasting pan, and put it into a very hot oven. The result is a chicken with beautiful crispy skin and juicy tender meat. This one is simply seasoned with salt, garlic, and fresh rosemary, but any of your favorite herbs will work.

Prep Time: 25 minutes
Cook Time: 45 minutes
Makes 4 servings

1 roasting chicken (about 4 pounds)
1 tablespoon olive oil
¾ teaspoon seasoned salt
½ teaspoon garlic powder
½ teaspoon finely minced fresh rosemary
Freshly ground black pepper

1. Set the cooking rack in the middle of the oven. Preheat the oven to 450°F. Coat the bottom of a large roasting pan with olive oil or cooking spray.

2. Remove the giblets from the chicken and rinse the cavity. Pat dry. With poultry shears or a sharp knife, cut down the center of the chicken's backbone (not the breast side). Open the chicken and flatten by pressing down on the breast. Cut away the backbone by making a vertical cut ½ inch on either side of the original cut. Rub the chicken with the oil and dust with the seasoned salt. Sprinkle on the garlic powder and rosemary. Grind fresh pepper over the chicken to taste.

3. Place the chicken in a roasting pan, breast side up. Roast for 30 minutes. Cover the breast skin if necessary with foil. Cook for an additional 10 to 15 minutes, or until the juices run clear when pierced and the thigh meat registers 175° to 180°F on a meat thermometer.

Per serving:
Carbohydrate: 0 gram; Net Carbs: 0 gram; Fiber: 0 gram; Protein: 56 grams; Fat: 35 grams; Calories: 560

COCONUT PECAN MACAROONS

Traditional coconut is paired with tasty pecans in these chewy low-carb macaroons. To get the maximum volume out of the beaten egg whites, be sure to allow them to warm to room temperature before whipping them in a clean, grease-free bowl.

Prep Time: 15 minutes
Bake Time: 20 minutes
Makes 16 servings (1 cookie each)

> 2 large egg whites
> Pinch of cream of tartar
> 1 cup granular sugar substitute
> 1 cup unsweetened shredded coconut
> 1 cup finely chopped pecans
> ½ teaspoon vanilla extract
> ¼ teaspoon orange extract (optional)

1. Preheat the oven to 300°F. Line a cookie sheet with ungreased parchment paper, a silicon mat, or aluminum foil.

2. In a medium bowl, beat the egg whites and cream of tartar with an electric mixer until very soft peaks begin to form. Gradually add the sugar substitute at medium speed until all the substitute is added and stiff peaks form. With a spoon or spatula, fold in the coconut, pecans, vanilla, and orange extract, if using.

3. Spoon the batter by tablespoons onto the prepared pan. Using the back of a spoon, flatten each cookie into a 2-inch round. Bake for 20 minutes, or until the bottoms are lightly browned. (Tops will not brown.) Remove and cool on a wire rack. Store in a covered container or wrap tight and freeze.

Per serving (1 cookie):
Carbohydrate: 4 grams; Net Carbs: 3 grams; Fiber: 1 gram; Protein: 1 gram; Fat: 8 grams;
Calories: 90

SPICY ORANGE STIR-FRY

Delicious orange-tinged stir-fries are some of the most popular Asian dishes. Unfortunately, they are also typically laden with sugar. We've kicked the sugar and added some heat to create an equally delicious sauce for this simple stir-fry. Chicken is specified, but you may use thin-sliced beef, shrimp, or for a vegetarian option, firm tofu (which will add just 1 additional gram of Net Carbs per serving). Most important, have all your ingredients measured out and ready to go before you fire up your wok.

Prep Time: 25 minutes
Marinate Time: 15 minutes
Cook Time: 12 minutes
Makes 4 servings

¼ cup lite soy sauce
2 tablespoons dry sherry
2 teaspoons each sesame oil and orange zest
½ teaspoon chili flakes (or more to taste)
1 pound chicken breast, skinned and cut into 1- to 1½-inch cubes
3 tablespoons canola oil
1 teaspoon minced garlic
¼ pound fresh snow peas, cleaned and trimmed
½ pound mushrooms, washed and thickly sliced
½ pound broccoli florets
1 cup carrots, peeled and diagonally sliced (40- and 60-gram meal plans only)
¼ cup chicken broth
½ cup sliced water chestnuts (60-gram meal plan only)
1 teaspoon ThickenThin Not/Starch thickener for sauce (optional)
4 green onions, trimmed and sliced diagonally

1. In a small bowl, mix together the soy sauce, sherry, sesame oil, orange zest, and chili flakes. Place the chicken in a separate small bowl; toss with 3 tablespoons sauce mix. Marinate for 15 minutes.
2. Heat a wok or large skillet over high heat until hot. Add 1

tablespoon of the oil and the garlic. Add the chicken, quickly stirring and separating for 3 to 4 minutes, or until browned. Remove from the pan. Add the snow peas and cook for 30 seconds. Remove from the pan.

3. Add the remaining 2 tablespoons oil and the mushrooms to the pan. Stir briefly. Add the broccoli and carrots. Stir to coat with oil; add the broth; cover and steam the vegetables for 2 minutes. Remove the lid; stir in the chicken, snow peas, water chestnuts, and the remaining sauce mix. Stir briefly to coat. If desired, to thicken the sauce, push the meat and vegetables to the side, and whisk ThickenThin into the simmering sauce. Sprinkle chopped green onions over the stir-fry and serve.

Per serving:
Carbohydrate: 10.5 grams; Net Carbs: 7 grams; Fiber: 3.5 grams; Protein: 28 grams; Fat: 6 grams; Calories: 300

With additions:
Per serving, add 2.5 grams of Net Carbs for the carrots and 2 grams of Net Carbs for the water chestnuts.

SAUTÉED SWISS CHARD

Full of vitamins and antioxidants, Swiss chard is a great addition to any diet. This often overlooked vegetable actually gives you two different tastes and textures. The dark green leaves resemble spinach and the stems have the crunch and taste of celery. Separating the leaves from the stems before cooking ensures that each is cooked just right.

Prep Time: 10 minutes
Cook Time: 8 minutes
Makes 2 servings

  1 bunch fresh Swiss chard (about ¾ pound)
  2 tablespoons olive oil
  2 garlic cloves, minced
  ¼ cup chicken broth
  ½ teaspoon seasoned salt
  Ground black pepper

1. Rinse the Swiss chard and pat dry. Separate the leaves from the stems and cut the stems into 1-inch pieces. Set aside.

2. Heat the oil and garlic in a medium sauté pan. Add the stems and sauté for 4 minutes. Stir in the leaves and pour in the broth; cover the pan and cook for 3 additional minutes. Uncover; stir in seasoned salt and add ground pepper to taste.

Per serving:
Carbohydrate: 7.5 grams; Net Carbs: 4.5 grams; Fiber: 3 grams; Protein: 3 grams; Fat: 14 grams;
Calories: 160

ZUCCHINI GRATIN

Gratins are characterized by their attractive browned tops of cheese and/or bread crumbs. You will find that versatile zucchini reaches new heights when prepared this way.

Prep Time: 10 minutes
Cook Time: 30 minutes
Makes 4 servings

> 2 pounds fresh zucchini
> Salt to taste
> 1 teaspoon garlic powder
> 2 tablespoons butter, melted
> ⅓ cup grated Parmesan cheese

1. Preheat the oven to 400°F. Bring a large pot of water to a boil.

2. Trim the ends of the zucchini and slice on the diagonal ¼-inch-thick. Place in the boiling water for 4 minutes. Drain and rinse the zucchini under cold water to stop the cooking process.

3. Arrange the zucchini into the bottom of a pie plate by overlapping them in circles, starting with the outside edge and working toward the center. Sprinkle with salt and ½ teaspoon of the garlic powder. Drizzle 1 tablespoon of the melted butter over the bottom layer. Add the second layer of zucchini and sprinkle with salt and the remaining garlic powder and butter. Sprinkle the cheese evenly over the top.

4. Place in the oven and bake for 20 minutes. Turn the oven up to 450°F and bake for an additional 10 minutes, or until the cheese is lightly browned.

Per serving:
Carbohydrate: 7 grams; Net Carbs: 4 grams; Fiber: 3 grams; Protein: 6 grams; Fat: 9 grams; Calories: 120

Glossary

A1C: *See* Glycated hemoglobin test.

Acanthosis nigricans: Dark skin patches often found in children and adults who have prediabetes or diabetes; they are caused by insulin resistance.

ACE: *See* Atkins Carbohydrate Equilibrium.

ACE inhibitor drugs: Angiotensin-converting enzyme drugs used to treat hypertension, such as benazepril (Lotensin), captopril (Capoten), and lisinopril (Prinivil, Zestril).

Advanced glycated end products (AGEs): The result of glucose in the body binding with proteins; a major cause of blood vessel damage and other complications of diabetes.

Aerobic exercise: Exercise that increases your heart rate and the consumption of oxygen.

AGEs: *See* Advanced glycated end products.

AGR: *See* Atkins Glycemic Ranking.

Amino acids: The building blocks of protein; necessary for maintaining normal metabolism.

Anaerobic exercise: Also called resistance exercise. Any exercise that builds muscle strength.

Antioxidants: Substances that neutralize free radicals in the body.

ARB drugs: Angiotensin receptor blocker drugs used to treat hypertension, such as irbesartan (Avapro), losartan (Cozaar), and valsartan (Diovan).

Atherosclerosis: Blood vessels clogged, narrowed, and hardened by deposits known as plaques.

Atkins Carbohydrate Equilibrium (ACE): The amount of Net Carbs in grams an individual can eat on a daily basis without gaining or losing weight.

Atkins Glycemic Ranking (AGR): A comparative ranking of carbohydrate-containing foods based on their glycemic index and glycemic load.

Beta-blocker drugs: Drugs such as metoprolol (Lopressor, Toprol), nadolol (Corgard), and propranolol (Inderal); most commonly used to treat hypertension.

Beta cells: Specialized cells in the pancreas that produce insulin.

Biguanide drugs: Oral medications used to treat diabetes by reducing the amount of glucose produced by the liver and increasing insulin sensitivity. *See also* Metformin.

Blood lipids: Refers to total cholesterol, triglycerides, and HDL and LDL cholesterol circulating in the blood; the blood test that measures these factors.

Blood pressure: A measure of the force your bloodstream exerts against the walls of your arteries as your heart beats and rests.

Blood sugar: The amount of glucose in the bloodstream.

BMI: *See* Body mass index.

Body mass index (BMI): A measure of your body weight relative to your height, used to indicate weight ranges for underweight, normal weight, overweight, and obesity.

Calcium channel blockers: Drugs used to treat hypertension, such as amlopidine (Norvasc), diltiazam (Cardizem), felodipine (Plendil), nifedipine (Procardia), and verapamil (Covera).

Carbohydrate: A macronutrient found in plant foods that is broken down into glucose during the digestive process.

Cholesterol: A waxy substance necessary for many body functions, including making cell walls and hormones.

Coenzyme Q_{10} (CoQ_{10}): An enzyme needed for normal production of energy in the mitochondria within the body's cells.

CoQ_{10}: *See* Coenzyme Q_{10}.

C-peptide: A small protein normally produced as a by-product of insulin. The level of c-peptide in the blood is an indirect way of measuring insulin production.

C-reactive protein (CRP): A natural chemical in the blood used as a marker of inflammation.

CRP: *See* C-reactive protein.

Diabetes mellitus: Hyperglycemia due to an inability to use blood sugar for energy. *See also* Gestational diabetes; Type 1 diabetes; Type 2 diabetes.

Diastolic blood pressure: The pressure in your blood vessels when the heart rests between beats; the second, lower number in a blood pressure reading.

Dietary reference intakes (DRI): Reference values for nutrient and energy intake for use in dietary plans and assessments.

Digestible fiber: Dietary fiber in the form of pectin and other substances. Also called soluble fiber.

Diuretics: Drugs that remove fluid from the body by causing increased urination.

DNA: The molecule that encodes genetic information in the nucleus of a cell and determines its structure, function, and behavior.

Endothelial dysfunction: Inflammation of the lining of the blood vessels, or endothelium.

Endothelium: The thin layer of cells lining all blood vessels.

Essential fatty acids: Dietary fats necessary for your body, which must be obtained from food or supplements.

Fasting blood sugar (FBS): The amount of sugar (blood glucose) in the blood after a fast of 8 to 12 hours.

Fasting plasma glucose: *See* Fasting blood sugar.

Fat: Oily, organic compounds that don't dissolve in water but do dissolve in other oils; also known as lipids. Fat is one of the three macronutrients in foods.

FBS: *See* Fasting blood sugar.

Fiber: The nondigestible parts of plant foods, such as cell walls.

Fibrinogen: A protein in the blood that is important for blood clotting. High levels can cause dangerous blood clots within blood vessels.

Free radicals: Harmful molecules created as part of normal metabolism. Excess free radicals can cause damage to cells and cause oxidation.

Fructose: A simple sugar found in fruit and fruit juices.

Gestational diabetes: A form of diabetes that sometimes occurs during pregnancy.

GI: *See* Glycemic index.

GL: *See* Glycemic load.

Glitazone drugs: *See* Thiazolidinedione drugs.

Glucophage: *See* Metformin.

Glucose: A simple form of sugar burned as fuel by your body.

Glucose tolerance test (GTT): A test used to diagnose blood sugar abnormalities. Blood glucose is measured before and several times after drinking a high-glucose solution. The results show how the body uses blood sugar over a specific period of time.

Glycated hemoglobin test: A blood test that reflects blood sugar control over the past two to three months; also known as A1C.

Glycation: The process causing damage to protein in the body as a result of high levels of blood sugar.

Glycemic index (GI): A ranking of carbohydrate-containing foods based on the food's impact on blood sugar relative to the same amount of glucose or white bread.

Glycemic load (GL): A ranking of carbohydrate-containing foods based on the food's fiber content, glycemic index, and portion size.

Glycogen: Glucose stored in the liver and muscle tissues.

GTT: *See* Glucose tolerance test.

HDL cholesterol: High-density lipoprotein cholesterol. Also known as "good" cholesterol, a type of lipoprotein used to carry cholesterol back to the liver.

High blood pressure: *See* Hypertension.

Homocysteine: A by-product of metabolizing the amino acid methionine. High levels of homocysteine are associated with an increased risk of heart disease.

Hormone: A chemical such as insulin produced in a gland or organ and carried in the blood to another part of the body to stimulate a particular function.

Hydrogenated vegetable oil: *See* Trans fat.

Hyperglycemia: Excessive sugar in the blood.

Hyperinsulinism: Excessive insulin in the blood.

Hypertension: A condition in which blood flows through blood vessels with more force than normal; also known as high blood pressure.

Hypoglycemia: Lower than normal blood sugar.

Hypothyroidism: A decrease in thyroid activity resulting in slowed metabolism. *See also* Thyroid gland.

Impaired fasting glucose: A fasting blood sugar level between 100 mg/dL and 125 mg/dL; also known as prediabetes.

Impaired glucose tolerance: Blood sugar that rises to between 140 mg/dL and 199 mg/dL two hours after the start of an oral glucose tolerance test or after a high-carb meal; also known as prediabetes.

Inflammation: Redness, swelling, heat, and dysfunction of a body part for a variety of reasons, including infection or injury.

Insulin: A hormone produced by the pancreas and used to carry glucose into the cells for energy.

Insulin resistance: The inability of cells to respond properly to insulin, the first stage of the metabolic syndrome.

Ketoacidosis: An emergency condition usually caused by extremely high blood sugar levels combined with a severe lack of insulin. This dangerous metabolic imbalance results in an abnormal acid state. If not immediately treated, this condition can lead to coma. Not to be confused with the perfectly safe production of ketones, resulting solely from following a low-carb dietary program.

Ketones: A by-product of fat that the body uses for energy.

Ketosis: Having ketones in the blood and urine, often as a result of following a low-carbohydrate eating plan; also known as benign dietary ketosis.

Lactose: A simple sugar found in milk and other dairy products.

LADA: *See* Latent autoimmune diabetes in adults.

Latent autoimmune diabetes in adults (LADA): A condition in which adults develop Type 1 diabetes.

LDL cholesterol: Low-density lipoprotein cholesterol. Also known as "bad" cholesterol; a lipoprotein found in the blood and used to carry cholesterol to the cells.

Lipid profile: *See* Blood lipids.

Lipids: A general term for fats in the body.

Lipoic acid. An antioxidant related to the B vitamins; used to treat peripheral neuropathy. Also known as alpha lipoic acid, or ALA.

Lipoprotein(a). A form of LDL cholesterol that has been shown to be an independent risk factor for heart disease.

Lp(a). *See* Lipoprotein(a).

Macronutrient. The dietary sources of calories and nutrients; specifically protein, fat, and carbohydrate.

Meglitinide drugs. Short-acting oral drugs for Type 2 diabetes, such as repaglinide (Prandin), that help the pancreas produce insulin immediately after meals.

Metabolic syndrome. A group of several signs or conditions, which include central obesity, hypertension, low HDL, high triglycerides, and high blood sugar. A major risk factor for heart disease, prediabetes, and diabetes. Also known as syndrome X.

Metformin. An oral drug (brand name Glucophage) used primarily for treating Type 2 diabetes; it reduces the amount of glucose produced by the liver and improves insulin sensitivity.

Microalbuminuria. Small amounts of protein in the urine.

Mitochondria. The portion of each cell that is responsible for energy production for that cell.

Mmol/L: Millimoles per liter, a unit of measure used outside the United States for indicating blood glucose levels and measurements of other specific substances in the blood.

Monounsaturated fat: Dietary fat with one missing hydrogen atom; found in foods such as olive oil, nuts, seeds, and avocados.

Morbid obesity: A BMI of 40 or more.

Nateglinide: An oral drug (brand name Starlix) for treating Type 2 diabetes; it helps the pancreas produce more insulin immediately after a meal.

Nephropathy: Kidney disease caused by hyperglycemia and/or hypertension.

Net Carbs: The carbohydrates in a whole food that have an impact on your blood sugar, represented by subtracting the fiber grams in the food from the total carbohydrate grams. In a low-carb product, sugar alcohols and glycerine are also deducted.

Neuropathy: Damage to the nerves, often caused by hyperglycemia. *See also* Peripheral neuropathy.

Neurotransmitters: Chemicals that transmit nerve impulses across synapses, or gaps, in the brain.

Nondigestible fiber: Dietary fiber consisting mostly of cellulose from plant walls; also called insoluble fiber.

Omega-3 fatty acids: A form of polyunsaturated dietary fat found in fish oil, flaxseed oil, and some other vegetable oils.

Omega-6 fatty acids: A form of polyunsaturated dietary fat found in many vegetable oils.

Oral glucose tolerance test: *See* Glucose tolerance test.

Oxidation: A chemical reaction that involves combining a substance with oxygen, similar to the process of metal rusting.

Pancreas: An organ found in the abdomen behind the stomach; the pancreas secretes the hormone insulin and other chemicals.

Partially hydrogenated vegetable oil: *See* Trans fat.

PCOS: *See* Polycystic ovary syndrome.

Peripheral neuropathy: Nerve damage affecting the feet, legs, and hands; causes pain, tingling, and numbness.

Polycystic ovary syndrome (PCOS): A hormonal imbalance in women; associated with enlarged or cystic ovaries, it causes irregular menstruation, infertility, weight gain, high blood sugar, and excessive hair growth.

Polyunsaturated fat: Dietary fat that is missing more than one hydrogen atom, such as corn and soybean oil.

Postprandial blood sugar: The amount of sugar (glucose) in the blood after a meal.

Prediabetes: Blood sugar levels that are higher than normal but not yet high enough to qualify as Type 2 diabetes.

Prehypertension: Elevated blood pressure that is between 120/80 and 139/89. The stage before hypertension.

Protein: Complex, intricately folded and coiled chains of amino acids. One of the three macronutrients found in foods.

Proteinuria: The presence of protein in the urine; an indication of possible kidney disease.

Prothrombotic state: Having blood that is more likely to form a dangerous clot within a blood vessel.

Reactive hypoglycemia: Also known as unstable blood sugar. A sharp drop in blood sugar following a sharp rise.

Retinopathy: Damage to the tiny blood vessels that nourish the retina, the light-sensitive area at the back of the eye.

Saturated fat: Dietary fat that contains as many hydrogen atoms as possible, such as palm and coconut oil. Usually solid at room temperature.

Statin drugs: Drugs such as atorvastatin (Lipitor), lovastatin (Mevacor), pravastatin (Pravachol), and simvastatin (Zocor) that block the action of HMG Co-A reductase and used to lower total and LDL cholesterol.

Sucrose: Table sugar; a two-part sugar consisting of glucose and fructose.

Sugar alcohols: Sweeteners such as manitol and sorbitol that have negligible impact on blood sugar in most people.

Sulfonylureas: A group of oral medications used to treat diabetes by helping the pancreas secrete more insulin; they include glimepiride (Amaryl), glipizide (Glucotrol), glyburide (Micronase), tolazamide (Tolinase), and tolbutamide (Orinase).

Syndrome X: *See* Metabolic syndrome.

Systolic pressure: Blood pressure when the heart contracts and pumps the blood; the first, higher number in a blood pressure reading.

Thiazolidinedione drugs: Oral drugs for treating Type 2 diabetes, including pioglitazone (Actos) and rosiglitazone (Avandia). These drugs improve insulin sensitivity.

Thyroid gland: A butterfly-shaped gland in the neck that secretes hormones crucial for regulating metabolism.

Trans fat: Partially hydrogenated or hydrogenated vegetable oil; a manufactured form of fat widely used in baked goods, fried foods, and snack foods.

Triglycerides: Fats that circulate in the bloodstream and are stored as body fat. Elevated levels are an independent risk factor for heart disease.

Type 1 diabetes: High blood sugar levels caused by a lack of insulin resulting from destruction of the beta cells in the pancreas.

Type 2 diabetes: High blood sugar caused by an inability to use insulin properly, and in later stages of the disease, an insufficiency of insulin.

TZD drugs: *See* Thiazolidinedione drugs.

Unsaturated fat: Dietary fat that has some unfilled hydrogen bonds; polyunsaturated and monounsaturated fats.

Unstable blood sugar: Blood sugar levels that rise and fall too much, too quickly, or both, as reflected in a more than 50-point drop in one hour on the GTT or a 100-point drop overall. Symptoms include headaches, irritability, mood swings, sweating, and heart pounding.

Very low density lipoprotein (VLDL): A form of LDL cholesterol associated with an increased risk of heart disease.

VLDL: *See* Very low density lipoprotein.

Waist-to-hip ratio: The size of your waist compared with the size of your hips. A high waist-to-hip ratio indicates abdominal obesity.

Scientific Studies That Validate the Atkins Nutritional Approach

Until recently, only a handful of serious research studies had looked at low-carbohydrate nutritional programs. Most conventional medical theories, such as the belief that low-carb diets increase the risk for heart disease by raising cholesterol, were based on the simple and unsupported opinion that "you are what you eat." Now all that's changing.

In the past few years, 27 studies and two review papers investigating low-carb approaches have been published in peer-reviewed journals, or were presented at medical conferences. (Several longer-term studies are under way.) Some focused mainly on weight loss and others looked at the effect on blood lipid levels such as total cholesterol, HDL ("good"), LDL ("bad"), and triglycerides. Still others looked at inflammation indicators, which are now considered a risk factor for heart disease. And a few looked at the effect of low-carb programs on medication dosages, particularly in Type 2 diabetics.

Some of the studies used only men or only women, and others were mixed. Some included only obese subjects, others included normal-weight subjects, and still others included primarily diabetics. Yet the picture that is beginning to emerge is increasingly clear. There is now an arsenal of hard facts validating the efficacy and safety of controlling carbohydrate intake.

These 27 studies are listed on the following pages.

Bailes, J. R. J., Strow, M. T., Werthammer, J., et al., "Effect of Low-Carbohydrate, Unlimited Calorie Diet on the Treatment of Childhood Obesity: A Prospective Controlled Study," *Metabolic Syndrome and Related Disorders*, 1(3), 2003, pages 221–225.

Brehm, B. J., Seeley, R. J., Daniels, S. R., et al., "A Randomized Trial Comparing a Very Low Carbohydrate Diet and a Calorie-Restricted Low Fat Diet on Body Weight and Cardiovascular Risk Factors in Healthy Women," *Journal of Clinical Endocrinology and Metabolism*, 88(4), 2003, pages 1617–1623.

Dansinger, M. L., Gleason, J. L., Griffith, J. L., et al., "One Year Effectiveness of the Atkins, Ornish, Weight Watchers, and Zone Diets in Decreasing Body Weight and Heart Disease Risk," presented at the American Heart Association Scientific Sessions November 12, 2003 in Orlando, Florida.

Foster, G. D., Wyatt, H. R., Hill, J. O., et al., "A Randomized Trial of a Low-Carbohydrate Diet for Obesity," *New England Journal of Medicine*, 348(21), 2003, pages 2082–2090.

Greene, P., Willett, W., Devecis, J., et al., "Pilot 12-Week Feeding Weight-Loss Comparison: Low-Fat Vs Low-Carbohydrate (Ketogenic) Diets," abstract presented at The North American Association for the Study of Obesity Annual Meeting 2003, *Obesity Research*, 11S, 2003, page 95OR.

Gutierrez, M., Akhavan, M., Jovanovic, L., et al., "Utility of a Short-Term 25% Carbohydrate Diet on Improving Glycemic Control in Type 2 Diabetes Mellitus," *Journal of the American College of Nutrition*, 17(6), 1998, pages 595–600.

Hays, J. H., Gorman, R. T., Shakir, K. M., "Results of Use of Metformin and Replacement of Starch with Saturated Fat in Diets of Patients with Type 2 Diabetes," *Endocrine Practice*, 8(3), 2002, pages 177–183.

Hays, J. H., DiSabatino, A., Gorman, R. T., et al., "Effect of a High Saturated Fat and No-Starch Diet on Serum Lipid Subfractions in Patients with Documented Atherosclerotic Cardiovascular Disease," *Mayo Clinic Proceedings*, 78(11), 2003, pages 1331–1336.

Hickey, J. T., Hickey, L., Yancy, W .S. J., et al., "Clinical Use of a Carbohydrate-Restricted Diet to Treat the Dyslipidemia of the Metabolic

Syndrome," *Metabolic Syndrome and Related Disorders,* 1(3), 2003, pages 227–232.

Kossoff, E. H., Krauss, G. L., McGrogan, J. R., et al., "Efficacy of the Atkins Diet as Therapy for Intractable Epilepsy," *Neurology,* 61(12), 2003, pages 1789–1791.

O'Brien, K. D., Brehm, B. J., Seeley, R. J., "Greater Reduction in Inflammatory Markers with a Low Carbohydrate Diet Than with a Calorically Matched Low Fat Diet," presented at American Heart Association's Scientific Sessions 2002 on Tuesday, November 19, 2002, Abstract ID: 2081.

Samaha, F. F., Iqbal, N., Seshadri, P., et al., "A Low-Carbohydrate as Compared with a Low-Fat Diet in Severe Obesity," *New England Journal of Medicine,* 348(21), 2003, pages 2074–2081.

Sharman, M. J., Gomez, A. L., Kraemer, W. J., et al., "Very Low-Carbohydrate and Low-Fat Diets Affect Fasting Lipids and Postprandial Lipemia Differently in Overweight Men," *Journal of Nutrition,* 134(4), 2004, pages 880–885.

Sharman, M. J., Kraemer, W. J., Love, D. M., et al., "A Ketogenic Diet Favorably Affects Serum Biomarkers for Cardiovascular Disease in Normal-Weight Men," *Journal of Nutrition,* 132(7), 2002, pages 1879–1885.

Sondike, S. B., Copperman, N., Jacobson, M. S., "Effects of a Low Carbohydrate Diet on Weight Loss and Cardiovascular Risk Factor in Overweight Adolescents," *Journal of Pediatrics,* 142(3), 2003, pages 253–258.

Stadler, D. D., Burden, V., Connor, W., et al., "Impact of 42-Day Atkins Diet and Energy-Matched Low-Fat Diet on Weight and Anthropometric Indices," *FASEB Journal,* 17(4–5), abstract of the 12th Annual FASEB Meeting on Experimental Biology: Translating the Genome; Abstract ID: 453.3, San Diego, California, April 11–15, 2003.

Stern, L., Iqbal N., Seshadri, P., et al., "The Effects of Low-Carbohydrate Versus Conventional Weight-Loss Diets in Severely Obese Adults: One-Year Follow-up of a Randomized Trial," *Annals of Internal Medicine,* 140(10), 2004, pages 778–785.

Vernon, M. C., Mavropoulos, J., Transue, M., et al., "Clinical Experience of a Carbohydrate-Restricted Diet: Effect on Diabetes Mellitus," *Metabolic Syndrome and Related Disorders,* 1(3), 2003, pages 233–237.

Volek, J. S., Gomez, A. L., Kraemer, W. J., "Fasting Lipoprotein and Postprandial Triacylglycerol Responses to a Low-Carbohydrate Diet Supplemented with N-3 Fatty Acids," *Journal of the American College of Nutrition,* 19(3), 2000, pages 383–391.

Volek, J. S., Sharman, M. J., Gomez, A. L., et al., "An Isoenergetic Very Low Carbohydrate Diet Improves Serum HDL Cholesterol and Triacylglycerol Concentrations, the Total Cholesterol to HDL Cholesterol Ratio and Postprandial Pipemic Responses Compared with a Low-Fat Diet in Normal Weight, Normolipidemic Women," *Journal of Nutrition,* 133(9), 2003, pages 2756–2761.

Volek, J. S., Sharman, M. J., Gomez, A. L., et al., "Comparison of a Very Low Carbohydrate and Low-Fat Diet on Fasting Lipids, LDL Subclasses, Insulin Resistance, and Postprandial Lipemic Responses in Overweight Women," *Journal of the American College of Nutrition,* 23(2), 2004, pages 177–184.

Volek, J. S., Westman, E. C., "Very Low Carbohydrate Weight-Loss Diets Revisited," *Cleveland Clinic Journal of Medicine,* 69(11), 2002, pages 849–862.

Westman, E. C., Mavropoulos, J., Yancy, W. S., et al., "A Review of Low-Carbohydrate Ketogenic Diets," *Current Atherosclerosis Reports,* 5(6), 2003, pages 476–483.

Westman, E. C., Yancy, W. S., Edman, J. S., et al., "Effect of 6-Month Adherence to a Very Low Carbohydrate Diet Program," *American Journal of Medicine,* 113(1), 2002, pages 30–36.

Yancy, W. S., Jr., Olsen, M. K., Guyton, J. R., et al., "A Low-Carbohydrate, Ketogenic Diet Versus a Low-Fat Diet to Treat Obesity and Hyperlipidemia: A Randomized, Controlled Trial," *Annals of Internal Medicine,* 140(10), 2004, pages 769–777.

Yancy, W. S., Jr., Provenzale, D., Westman, E. C., "Improvement of Gastroesophageal Reflux Disease after Initiation of a Low-Carbohydrate Diet: Five Brief Case Reports," *Alternative Therapies in Health and Medicine,* 7(6), 2001, pages 116–129.

Yancy, W. S., Vernon, M. C., Westman, E. C., "A Pilot Trial of a Low-Carbohydrate, Ketogenic Diet in Patients with Type 2 Diabetes," *Metabolic Syndrome and Related Disorders,* 1(3), 2003, pages 239–243.

Appendixes

As we discussed in the body of the text, there are differences between the standard Atkins Nutritional Approach (ANA) and the Atkins Blood Sugar Control Program (ABSCP). The main distinctions are related to how rapidly you will advance from Induction to Lifetime Maintenance and the flexibility of your Atkins Carbohydrate Equilibrium (ACE), which is determined by the degree of metabolic correction you are able to achieve. In the ANA, finding your ACE is primarily related to your ability to manage your weight. In the ABSCP, your ACE depends upon weight management but, more important, it takes into account your ability to control cardiovascular risk factors, blood pressure, and blood sugar. Chapters 10 and 11 provide far more detailed information on personalizing your program and should be reviewed regularly as you proceed.

To further refine your knowledge, *Dr. Atkins' New Diet Revolution* and *Atkins for Life* are required reading. In addition to these books, *Dr. Atkins' New Carbohydrate Gram Counter* can assist you in calculating Net Carbs, and several Atkins cookbooks will assist you in adding variety to your meal plans. The Atkins Web site, www.atkins.com, is an up-to-the-minute resource for recipes, food products, breaking news, and the latest research on Atkins.

Before you begin, reviewing the following information can make it easier to prepare your Atkins kitchen and understand the acceptable carbs for the initial phase of the ABSCP and the order in which they should be added to your meals.

Appendix 1

ACCEPTABLE INDUCTION FOODS

FOODS YOU DO NOT NEED TO LIMIT IN INDUCTION:

Eat these foods in portions that make you feel satisfied. Do not stuff yourself.

Poultry
Fish
Shellfish
Meat
Eggs

Exceptions:

1. Oysters, mussels, and clams are higher in carbs than other shellfish, so eat no more than 4 ounces a day.
2. Processed meats, such as ham, bacon, pepperoni, salami, hot dogs, and other luncheon meats—and some fish—may be cured with sugar or contain fillers that contribute carbs.
3. Avoid meat and fish products cured with nitrates, which are known carcinogens.
4. Also beware of products that are not exclusively meat, fish,

or fowl, such as imitation crabmeat, fish sticks, meat loaf, and all breaded foods.

5. Do not consume more than 4 ounces of organ meats a day.

FOODS YOU NEED TO LIMIT IN INDUCTION

Cheese: A Maximum of 4 Ounces per Day

All cheeses contain some carbohydrate. You can consume 3 to 4 ounces daily of full-fat, firm, soft, and semisoft aged cheeses (for example, Cheddar, Swiss, Gouda, goat cheese, mozzarella, blue cheese). Count 1 ounce of cheese as 1 gram of Net Carbs. Full-fat cream cheese is also permitted, as are cheeses made from soy or rice, but check the carbohydrate content so that you consume no more than 4 grams of Net Carbs from cheese.

NOT ALLOWED

Cottage cheese
Farmer cheese
Ricotta cheese
Other fresh cheeses
Reduced-fat or low-calorie cheeses
Processed cheeses such as cheese spreads

Other Dairy

Butter (unlimited)
A maximum of 4 ounces (4 tablespoons to ½ cup) of light or
heavy cream *or* sour cream

Salad Vegetables: 2 to 3 Cups

You can have 2 to 3 loosely packed cups per day of the following raw vegetables:

Alfalfa sprouts
Arugula
Cabbage
Celery
Chicory
Chives
Cucumber
Daikon
Endive
Escarole
Fennel
Jicama
Lettuce (all types)
Mache
Mushrooms
Parsley
Peppers
Radicchio
Radishes
Romaine
Scallions
Sorrel
Spinach
Tomato
Watercress
Any other leafy green vegetables

Cooked Vegetables: 1 Cup per Day

You can have 1 cup (measured cooked) per day of these vegetables, if salad does not exceed 2 cups. A few vegetables, such as spinach or tomatoes, that cook down significantly, should be measured raw. Some of the following vegetables are slightly higher in carbohydrate content than the salad vegetables:

Artichoke hearts
Artichokes

Asparagus
Bamboo shoots
Bean sprouts
Beet greens
Bok choy
Broccoli
Broccoli rabe
Brussels sprouts
Cabbage
Cauliflower
Celery root
Chard
Collard greens
Dandelion greens
Eggplant
Hearts of palm
Kale
Kohlrabi
Leeks
Okra
Onion
Pumpkin
Rhubarb
Sauerkraut
Snow peas
Spaghetti squash
String or wax beans
Summer squash
Tomato
Turnips
Water chestnuts
Zucchini or summer squash

Note that certain vegetables appear on both this list and the preceding salad list.

Garnishes

Crumbled crisp bacon (look for nitrate-free products)
Grated cheese (figure into your cheese count)
Minced hard-boiled egg
Sautéed mushrooms (figure into your vegetable count)
Spices and herbs (as long as they contain no added sugar)

Salad Dressings

Oil and vinegar
Prepared salad dressings without added sugars, such as sugar, corn syrup, or honey (no more than 2 grams Net Carbs per serving)

NOT ALLOWED

Balsamic vinegar (contains added sugar)
Rice vinegar with added sugar
Prepared salad dressings with added sugar

Condiments

Caponata (eggplant relish)
Mayonnaise (regular, not low-fat)
Mustard (not honey mustard)
Horseradish
Pesto (after first two weeks of Induction)
Pickles (but not "bread and butter" or other sweet pickles); be sure to calculate the grams of Net Carbs
Soy sauce (tamari, others made without wheat)
Tabasco sauce
Tapenade (black olive purée)
Worcestershire sauce

Also, low-carb ketchup, hoisin, and sweet-and-sour and other sauces, made without added sugar, are acceptable. Always check carb counts. A serving should contain no more than 2 grams of Net Carbs.

Not Allowed

Barbecue sauce
Ketchup
Pickle relish
Russian dressing
Cranberry sauce
Any sauce with added sugar, corn syrup, or bleached flour, such as
    steak sauce, jarred gravies, etc.

Oils

You may use any type of oil, preferably cold-pressed or expeller-pressed. Olive oil or butter is preferred, but you may use margarine spreads made of vegetable oils as long as they do not contain added trans fats (hydrogenated oils).

Artificial Sweeteners

The words *sugarless, sugar-free,* or *no added sugar* are not sufficient. You must also look at carbohydrate counts. We recommend the following sweeteners:

Sucralose (marketed as Splenda)
Saccharin (marketed as Sweet'n Low)
Acesulfame-K (Sweet One)

Note: Most chewing gum, breath mints, cough syrups, and cough drops are filled with sugar or other caloric sweeteners and must be avoided. However, there are many sugar-free products available.

Beverages:

Be sure to drink a minimum of eight 8-ounce glasses of water each day, including:

Filtered water
Mineral water

Spring water
Tap water

The following beverages are acceptable but should be consumed only in addition to the recommended 64 ounces of water:

Decaffeinated coffee or tea
Diet soda made with one of the acceptable artificial sweeteners (no more than three cans a day; be sure to add in the Net Carbs)
Essence-flavored seltzer (must say "no calories")
Herb tea (without barley or any fruit sugar, or fructose, added)
Clear broth/bouillon (not all brands; read the label)
Club soda

NOT ALLOWED

Coffee substitutes made from grains
Alcoholic beverages
Caffeinated cola drinks
Fruit or vegetable juices

Special Category Foods

Each day you can also eat the following, but add to your carb count:

10 green olives or 6 black olives
Half a Haas avocado
2 to 3 tablespoons of lemon juice or lime juice

If you stay on Induction past the second week, you can add 1 ounce of nuts and/or seeds to your daily intake. The best choices are macadamias, almonds, walnuts, pecans, Brazil nuts, pumpkin or sunflower seeds.

Note: These foods occasionally slow down weight loss in some people, and may need to be avoided at first. If you seem to be losing slowly, moderate your intake of these foods or avoid them altogether.

ATKINS CONTROLLED-CARB INGREDIENTS SUITABLE FOR INDUCTION

These ingredients can come in handy when planning meals:

Atkins Quick Quisine Sugar Free Flavored Syrups
Atkins Quick Quisine Salad Dressings
Atkins Quick Quisine Ketch-A-Tomato Sauce
Atkins Quick Quisine Barbecue Sauce
Atkins Quick Quisine Steak Sauce
Atkins Quick Quisine Teriyaki Sauce
Atkins Quick Quisine Bake Mix
Atkins Quick Quisine Pancake & Waffle Mix (not all flavors)
Atkins Quick Quisine Muffin & Bread Mixes (not all flavors)
Atkins Kitchen Quick & Easy Bread Mix

As new products are developed, be sure to check the phase coding on the packaging.

ATKINS CONTROLLED-CARB CONVENIENCE FOODS SUITABLE FOR INDUCTION

It is important that you eat primarily unprocessed foods, but some controlled-carb food products can come in handy when you are unable to find appropriate foods, can't take time for a meal, or need a quick snack. Atkins products suitable for Induction include:

Atkins Advantage Bars
Atkins Advantage Shakes (as mixes or in ready-to-drink cans)
Atkins Morning Start Breakfast Bars
Atkins Bakery Ready-to-Eat Sliced Bread (1 slice only)

Note: Do not consume more than two servings of low-carb alternative foods a day during Induction and remember that you still must count your Net Carbs. If you have trouble losing weight, you may want to replace these products with whole foods during Induction.

Appendix 2

MOVING BEYOND INDUCTION

When they're ready to move on from Induction, most people find it best to add back foods in a certain order. In "Atkins language," this is known as the Carbohydrate Ladder (see below). When you are following the Atkins Nutritional Approach, weight loss is the primary indicator of when to advance through the four phases, adding additional grams of carbs and broadening your choices among foods that contain carbohydrates. When you follow the ABSCP, correction of metabolic markers such as improved blood pressure control, loss of inches especially around the waist, and improvement in blood sugar and lipid levels, as well as pounds lost, will determine your ability to advance through the phases. (For more detail, refer to Chapters 10 and 11.) Following this order tends to minimize blood sugar surges that could reactivate cravings:

CARBOHYDRATE LADDER

1. More salad and other vegetables on the acceptable foods list
2. Fresh cheeses (as well as more aged cheese)
3. Seeds and nuts

4. Berries
5. Legumes
6. Fruits other than berries
7. Starchy vegetables
8. Whole grains

Appendix 3

THE POWER OF FIVE AND TEN

What constitutes approximately 5 grams of Net Carbs when it comes to the foods on the Carbohydrate Ladder? This list will help you get a handle on a 5-gram portion of those items.

VEGETABLES

¾ cup cooked spinach
½ cup red peppers
1 medium tomato
⅔ cup cooked broccoli
8 medium asparagus
1 cup cauliflower
⅓ cup chopped onions
½ Haas avocado
⅔ cup summer squash

DAIRY

5 ounces farmer cheese or pot cheese
½ cup cottage cheese

⅔ cup ricotta cheese
½ cup heavy cream

NUTS AND SEEDS

1 ounce of:
Macadamias (approximately 10–12 nuts)
Walnuts (approximately 14 halves)
Almonds (approximately 24 nuts)
Pecans (approximately 31 nuts)
Hulled sunflower seeds (3 tablespoons)

½ ounce cashews (approximately 9 nuts)

FRUITS

¼ cup blueberries, raspberries
½ cup strawberries
¼ cup cantaloupe, honeydew

JUICES

¼ cup lemon juice
½ cup tomato juice

What constitutes roughly 10 grams of Net Carbs?

LEGUMES (COOKED)

⅓ cup lentils
⅓ cup kidney beans
⅓ cup chickpeas
⅓ cup baby lima beans

FRUITS

½ large apple
1 medium kiwifruit

¼ small cantaloupe
1 medium tangerine
3 small plums

Starchy Vegetables (Cooked)

¼ cup carrots
1 cup pumpkin
¾ cup mashed turnip
¾ cup chestnuts

Whole Grains (Cooked)

¼ cup brown rice
½ cup plain old-fashioned oatmeal
⅓ cup corn kernels

Appendix 4

THE ATKINS GLYCEMIC RANKING

ATKINS FOREVER: LIFETIME MAINTENANCE

After you've achieved your goals and you're in the Lifetime Maintenance phase of the ABSCP, you may be able to enjoy the foods that were deemed unacceptable in the earlier phases.

That said, you must always consume the highest-quality carbohydrates. To make it simpler to discern which foods fill that bill, the Atkins Glycemic Ranking (AGR) was created. In brief, this ranking system compares foods based on their impact on blood sugar. Here is a series of charts that can help you understand which foods most of you can eat regularly (low AGR). Depending on your degree of metabolic improvement, some of you will be able to choose from the medium AGR foods and occasionally from the high AGR foods.

VEGETABLES

1. EAT REGULARLY	2. EAT IN MODERATION	3. EAT SPARINGLY
Artichokes	Beets	Corn, sweet
Asparagus	Carrots	Parsnips
Bamboo shoots	Peas, green	Pea soup
Beans, string or other green varieties	Squash, acorn	Potatoes
Bok choy	Squash, butternut	
Broccoli	Taro	
Broccoli rabe	Tomato juice	
Brussels sprouts	Tomato soup	
Butter beans	Sweet potato	
Cabbage, all varieties	Yucca	
Cauliflower		
Celeriac		
Celery		
Chard		
Chayote		
Collards		
Cucumber		
Dandelion greens		
Eggplant		
Endive		
Fennel		
Jicama		
Kale		
Kohlrabi		
Lettuce, all varieties		
Lima beans, baby		
Mushrooms, all varieties		
Mustard greens		
Okra		
Onion		
Pea pods/snow peas		
Peppers, all varieties		

VEGETABLES

1. EAT REGULARLY	2. EAT IN MODERATION	3. EAT SPARINGLY

Pumpkin
Radishes
Rutabaga
Sauerkraut
Spinach
Sprouts, all varieties
Squash, zucchini
Tomato
Turnip greens
Water chestnuts

DAIRY PRODUCTS

1. EAT REGULARLY	2. EAT IN MODERATION	3. EAT SPARINGLY
Butter	Buttermilk	Other milk (skim,
Cheese, all nonprocessed	Milk, whole	2 percent)
hard varieties*	Low-carb ice cream	Yogurt, low-fat,
Cottage cheese	Yogurt, full-fat, plain	plain
Cream, heavy and light*		
Farmer cheese		
Half-and-half*		
Low-carb dairy beverages		
Low-carb yogurt		
Pot cheese		
Ricotta cheese		
Sour cream*		

* Keep portions small.

NUTS AND SEEDS

1. Eat regularly	2. Eat in moderation	3. Eat sparingly
Almonds	Cashews	Chestnuts
Brazil nuts	Peanuts	
Coconut	Soybeans, roasted	
Hazelnuts/filberts		
Macadamias		
Pecans		
Pine nuts/pignolis		
Pistachios		
Pumpkin seeds		
Sesame seeds		
Sunflower seeds		
Walnuts		

LEGUMES

1. Eat regularly	2. Eat in moderation	3. Eat sparingly
Chickpeas	Kidney beans	Black-eyed peas
Hummus	Peas, dried	Lima beans (dried)
Lentils		Navy beans
Lentil soup		Pinto beans
Minestrone soup		
Soybeans		
Soymilk, no added sugar		
Tofu/bean curd		

GRAINS

1. Eat regularly	2. Eat in moderation	3. Eat sparingly
Barley, cooked	Amaranth	Bagel, 100%
Low-carb bagels	Bran flakes	whole grain
Low-carb bread	Bread, 100% whole grain	Cornflakes, no
Low-carb cereal	Bread, 100% whole wheat	added sugar
Low-carb muffins	Bread, dark rye, 100%	Cream of Wheat
Low-carb rolls	whole grain	Crackers, 100%
Low-carb snack chips	Bread, multigrain,	whole wheat
Low-carb pasta	unrefined	Grapenuts
Low-carb tortillas	Bread, pumpernickel,	Grits
Low-carb wraps	100% whole grain,	Millet
Oat bran	no molasses	Pasta, whole
Oatmeal, old-fashioned	Bread, rye, 100%	wheat
Wheat bran	whole grain	Pasta, brown
Wheat germ, no added	Bread, sourdough,	rice
sugar	100% whole grain	Pita, 100%
	Buckwheat (kasha)	whole wheat
	Bulgur	Pizza, cheese,
	Cornmeal	100% whole
	Couscous, whole wheat	wheat crust
	Crispbread, 100%	Pretzels, whole
	whole grain	wheat

GRAINS

1. EAT REGULARLY	2. EAT IN MODERATION	3. EAT SPARINGLY
	Flatbread, 100% whole grain	Puffed brown rice cereal, no added sugar
	Melba toast, 100% rye or whole wheat	Rice cake, 100% brown rice
	Müesli, without added sugar	Rice, basmati, unprocessed brown
	Pizza, low-carb	Rice, brown
	Popcorn, without hydrogenated oils	Shredded wheat
	Tortilla, corn or 100% whole wheat	Wild rice
	Wrap, 100% whole wheat	

FRUITS

1. EAT REGULARLY	2. EAT IN MODERATION	3. EAT SPARINGLY
Apple	Apricots, canned in juice	Banana
Blackberries	Apricots, dried	Cranberry cocktail, no added sugar
Blueberries	Apricots, fresh	Cranberry juice, no added sugar
Cherries	Grapes, green and red	Fruit cocktail, canned in juice
Cranberries	Grapefruit juice, no added sugar	Grape juice
Grapefruit	Kiwifruit	Orange juice
Orange	Mango	Prunes
Peach	Melon, cantaloupe	Raisins
Pear	Melon, Crenshaw	
Plum	Melon, honeydew	
Pomegranate	Nectarine	
Raspberries	Papaya	
Strawberries	Pineapple, fresh	
Tangerine	Watermelon	

Appendix 5

THE ATKINS LIFESTYLE FOOD GUIDE PYRAMID

ATKINS CAN HELP

Atkins Nutritional, Inc., is constantly working toward improving the health and nutrition of people around the world. One step toward accomplishing this monumental task has been the development of the Atkins Lifestyle Food Guide Pyramid, a nutritional strategy based on a controlled-carbohydrate lifestyle and a way to help the more than 100 million Americans who are currently fighting the battles against obesity and diabetes to lose weight and keep it off. Members of the Atkins Physicians Council recently presented the Pyramid (shown on the following page) to the White House domestic-policy staff on health and nutrition, as well as to representatives of both the United States Department of Agriculture (USDA) Dietary Guidelines Committee and the Department of Health and Human Services, including representatives of the Food and Drug Administration.

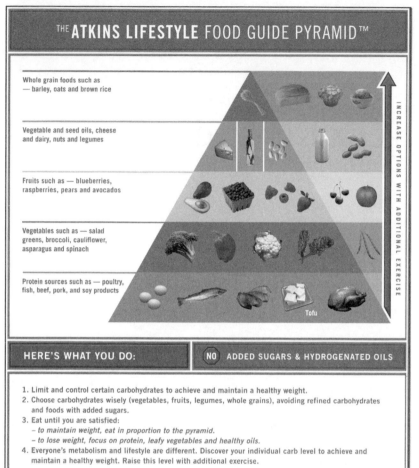

THE ATKINS LIFESTYLE FOOD GUIDE PYRAMID™

Whole grain foods such as
— barley, oats and brown rice

Vegetable and seed oils, cheese
and dairy, nuts and legumes

Fruits such as — blueberries,
raspberries, pears and avocados

Vegetables such as — salad
greens, broccoli, cauliflower,
asparagus and spinach

Protein sources such as — poultry,
fish, beef, pork, and soy products

Tofu

INCREASE OPTIONS WITH ADDITIONAL EXERCISE

HERE'S WHAT YOU DO:

NO ADDED SUGARS & HYDROGENATED OILS

1. Limit and control certain carbohydrates to achieve and maintain a healthy weight.
2. Choose carbohydrates wisely (vegetables, fruits, legumes, whole grains), avoiding refined carbohydrates
   and foods with added sugars.
3. Eat until you are satisfied:
   – to maintain weight, eat in proportion to the pyramid.
   – to lose weight, focus on protein, leafy vegetables and healthy oils.
4. Everyone's metabolism and lifestyle are different. Discover your individual carb level to achieve and
   maintain a healthy weight. Raise this level with additional exercise.

Appendix 6

DRUGS FOR HYPERTENSION

This list is provided simply to help you understand the classification of a drug you may be presently taking or your doctor is advising you to take. It is not an endorsement of any drug.

DIURETICS

Thiazides

Generic ingredient: bendroflumethiazide
Brand name: Naturetin

Generic ingredient: benzthiazide
Brand name: Exna

Generic ingredient: chlorothiazide
Brand names: Diurigen, Diuril

Generic ingredient: chlorthalidone
Brand names: Hygroton, Thalitone

Generic ingredient: hydrochlorothiazide
Brand names: Esidrex, Ezide, Hydrodiuril, Hydro-Par,
  Microzide, Oretic

Generic ingredient: hydroflumethiazide
Brand names: Diucardin, Saluron

Generic ingredient: indapamide
Brand name: Lozol

Generic ingredient: methylclothiazide
Brand names: Aquatensen, Enduron

Generic ingredient: metolazone
Brand names: Mykrox, Zaroxolyn

Generic ingredient: polythiazide
Brand name: Renese

Generic ingredient: quinethazone
Brand name: Hydromox

Generic ingredient: trichlormethiazide
Brand names: Diurese, Metahydrin, Naqua

Loop Diuretics

Generic ingredient: bumetanide
Brand name: Bumex

Generic ingredient: ethacrynic acid
Brand name: Edecrin

Generic ingredient: Furosemide
Brand name: Lasix

Generic ingredient: torsemide
Brand name: Demadex

Diuretic/Loop Diuretic

Generic ingredient: hydrochlorthiazide and triamterene
Brand names: Maxzide, Maxzide-25

Diuretic/aldosterone antagonists

Generic ingredient: spironolactone
Brand name: Aldactone

Generic ingredient: spironolactone and hydrochlorothiazide
Brand name: Aldactazide

ACE Inhibitors

Generic ingredient: benazepril
Brand name: Lotensin

Generic ingredient: captopril
Brand name: Capoten

Generic ingredient: enalapril
Brand name: Vasotec

Generic ingredient: fosinopril
Brand name: Monopril

Generic ingredient: lisinopril
Brand names: Prinivil, Zestril

Generic ingredient: quinapril
Brand name: Accupril

Generic ingredient: ramipril
Brand name: Altace

Generic ingredient: trandolapril
Brand name: Mavik

Calcium Channel Blockers

Generic ingredient: amlopidine
Brand name: Norvasc

Generic ingredient: diltiazam
Brand names: Cardizem, Cartia, Dilacor, Diltia, Tiamate, Tiazac

Generic ingredient: felodipine
Brand name: Plendil

Generic ingredient: isradipine
Brand name: DynaCirc

Generic ingredient: nicardipine
Brand name: Cardene

Generic ingredient: nifedipine
Brand names: Adalat, Procardia

Generic ingredient: verapamil
Brand names: Calan, Covera, Isoptin, Verelan

Beta-Blockers

Generic ingredient: atenolol
Brand name: Tenormin

Generic ingredient: labetalol
Brand names: Nomodyne, Trandate

Generic ingredient: metoprolol
Brand names: Lopressor, Toprol

Generic ingredient: nadolol
Brand name: Corgard

Generic ingredient: penbutolol
Brand name: Levatol

Generic ingredient: propranolol
Brand name: Inderal

Generic ingredient: sotalol
Brand names: Betapace, Sorine

Generic ingredient: timolol
Brand name: Blocadren

ARBs

Generic ingredient: irbesartan
Brand name: Avapro

Generic ingredient: losartan
Brand name: Cozaar

Generic ingredient: valsartan
Brand name: Diovan

Reference Notes

Introduction

1. Centers for Disease Control and Prevention, "At a Glance: Diabetes: Disabling, Deadly, and on the Rise 2004," available at: http://www.cdc.gov/nccdphp/aag/aag_ddt.htm, accessed on April 7, 2004.
2. American Diabetes Association, "Diabetes and Cardiovascular (Heart) Disease," available at: http://www.diabetes.org/diabetes-statistics/heart-disease.jsp, accessed on April 7, 2004.
3. Garnt, P. J., Davies, J. A., "Cardiovascular Diseases and Diabetes," 2002, In: Textbook of Diabetes, Pickup, J. C. et al. (Eds.), Blackwell Publishing, 3rd Edition.
4. American Diabetes Association, "Diabetes and Cardiovascular (Heart) Disease," available at: http://www.diabetes.org/diabetes-statistics/heart-disease.jsp, accessed on April 7, 2004.
5. Piette, J. D., Heisler, M., Wagner, T. H., "Problems Paying out-of-Pocket Medication Costs Among Older Adults with Diabetes," *Diabetes Care,* 27(2), 2004, pages 384–391.
6. Centers for Disease Control and Prevention, "At a Glance: Diabetes: Disabling, Deadly, and on the Rise 2004," available at: http://www.cdc.gov/nccdphp/aag/aag_ddt.htm, accessed on April 7, 2004.

7. Centers for Disease Control and Prevention, "National Diabetes Fact Sheet: United States, November 2003," available at: http://www.cdc.gov/diabetes/pubs/factsheet.htm, accessed on April 7, 2004.

Chapter 1: The Diabetes Crossroads

1. National Institute of Diabetes and Digestive and Kidney Diseases. National Diabetes Statistics Fact Sheet: General Information and National Estimates on Diabetes in the United States, 2003. Bethesda, MD: U. S. Department of Health and Human Services, National Institutes of Health, 2003.
2. National Institute of Diabetes and Digestive and Kidney Diseases. National Diabetes Statistics Fact Sheet: General Information and National Estimates on Diabetes in the United States, 2003. Bethesda, MD: U. S. Department of Health and Human Services, National Institutes of Health, 2003.
3. Expert Committee on the Diagnosis and Classification of Diabetes Mellitus, "Report of the Expert Committee on the Diagnosis and Classification of Diabetes Mellitus," *Diabetes Care*, 26(1S), 2003, pages S5–S20.
4. Genuth, S., Alberti, K. G., Bennett, P., et al., "Follow-up Report on the Diagnosis of Diabetes Mellitus," *Diabetes Care*, 26(11), 2003, pages 3160–3167.
5. King, H., Aubert, R. E., Herman, W. H., "Global Burden of Diabetes, 1995–2025: Prevalence, Numerical Estimates, and Projections," *Diabetes Care*, 21(9), 1998, pages 1414–1431.
6. World Health Organization. "Diabetes Estimates and Projections," available at: http://www.who.int/ncd/dia/databases4.htm, accessed on February 24, 2004.
7. Expert Committee on the Diagnosis and Classification of Diabetes Mellitus, "Report of the Expert Committee on the Diagnosis and Classification of Diabetes Mellitus," *Diabetes Care*, 26(1S), 2003, pages S5–S20.
8. Expert Committee on the Diagnosis and Classification of Diabetes Mellitus, "Report of the Expert Committee on the Diagnosis and

Classification of Diabetes Mellitus," *Diabetes Care,* 26(1S), 2003, pages S5–20.

9. National Institute of Diabetes and Digestive and Kidney Diseases. National Diabetes Statistics Fact Sheet: General Information and National Estimates on Diabetes in the United States, 2003. Bethesda, MD: U. S. Department of Health and Human Services, National Institutes of Health, 2003.

10. "Diagnosis and Classification of Diabetes Mellitus," *Diabetes Care,* 27(1S), 2004, pages S5-S10.

11. Ovalle, F., Azziz, R., "Insulin Resistance, Polycystic Ovary Syndrome, and Type 2 Diabetes Mellitus," *Fertility and Sterility,* 77(6), 2002, pages 1095–1105.

12. Knochenhauer, E. S., Key, T. J., Kahsar-Miller, M., et al., "Prevalence of the Polycystic Ovary Syndrome in Unselected Black and White Women of the Southeastern United States: A Prospective Study," *Journal of Clinical Endocrinology and Metabolism,* 83(9), 1998, pages 3078–3082.

13. Knochenhauer, E. S., Key, T. J., Kahsar-Miller, M., et al., "Prevalence of the Polycystic Ovary Syndrome in Unselected Black and White Women of the Southeastern United States: A Prospective Study," *Journal of Clinical Endocrinology and Metabolism,* 83(9), 1998, pages 3078–3082.

14. "Diagnosis and Classification of Diabetes Mellitus," *Diabetes Care,* 27(1S), 2004, pages S5-S10.

15. Fagot-Campagna, A., Pettitt, D. J., Engelgau, M. M., et al., "Type 2 Diabetes Among North American Children and Adolescents: An Epidemiologic Review and a Public Health Perspective," *Journal of Pediatrics,* 136(5), 2000, pages 664–672.

16. Michels, K. B., Solomon, C. G., Hu, F. B., et al., "Type 2 Diabetes and Subsequent Incidence of Breast Cancer in the Nurses' Health Study," *Diabetes Care,* 26(6), 2003, pages 1752–1758.

17. National Institute of Diabetes and Digestive and Kidney Diseases. National Diabetes Statistics Fact Sheet: General Information and National Estimates on Diabetes in the United States, 2003. Bethesda, MD: U. S. Department of Health and Human Services, National Institutes of Health, 2003.

18. National Institute of Diabetes and Digestive and Kidney Diseases.

National Diabetes Statistics Fact Sheet: General Information and National Estimates on Diabetes in the United States, 2003. Bethesda, MD: U. S. Department of Health and Human Services, National Institutes of Health, 2003.

Chapter 2: Wrong Turn: The Long Road to Diabetes

1. DeFronzo, R. A., Bonadonna, R. C., Ferrannini, E., "Pathogenesis of NIDDM. A Balanced Overview," *Diabetes Care,* 15(3), 1992, pages 318–368.
2. Barzilay, J. I., Freedland, E. S., "Inflammation and Its Relationship to Insulin Resistance, Type 2 Diabetes Mellitus, and Endothelial Dysfunction," *Metabolic Syndrome and Related Disorders,* 1(1), 2003, pages 55–67.
3. Grundy, S. M., "Inflammation, Hypertension, and the Metabolic Syndrome," *Journal of the American Medical Association,* 290(22), 2003, pages 3000–3002.
4. Caballero, A. E., "Endothelial Dysfunction in Obesity and Insulin Resistance: A Road to Diabetes and Heart Disease," *Obesity Research,* 11(11), 2003, pages 1278–1289.
5. Vernon, M. C., Mavropoulos, J., Transue, M., et al., "Clinical Experience of a Carbohydrate-Restricted Diet: Effect on Diabetes Mellitus," *Metabolic Syndrome and Related Disorders,* 1(3), 2003, pages 233–237.
6. Yancy, W. S., Vernon, M. C., Westman, E. C., "A Pilot Trial of a Low-Carbohydrate, Ketogenic Diet in Patients with Type 2 Diabetes," *Metabolic Syndrome and Related Disorders,* 1(3), 2003, pages 239–243.
7. National Institute of Diabetes and Digestive and Kidney Diseases. National Diabetes Statistics Fact Sheet: General Information and National Estimates on Diabetes in the United States, 2003. Bethesda, MD: U. S. Department of Health and Human Services, National Institutes of Health, 2003.
8. Harris, M. I., "Undiagnosed NIDDM: Clinical and Public Health Issues," *Diabetes Care,* 16(4), 1993, pages 642–652.
9. Expert Committee on the Diagnosis and Classification of Diabetes Mellitus, "Report of the Expert Committee on the Diagnosis and

Classification of Diabetes Mellitus," *Diabetes Care,* 26(1S), 2003, pages S5-S20.

Chapter 3: Weighing In: The Number One Risk Factor

1. Chan, J. M., Rimm, E. B., Colditz, G. A., et al., "Obesity, Fat Distribution, and Weight Gain as Risk Factors for Clinical Diabetes in Men," *Diabetes Care,* 17(9), 1994, pages 961–969.
2. Colditz, G. A., Willett, W. C., Rotnitzky, A., et al., "Weight Gain as a Risk Factor for Clinical Diabetes Mellitus in Women," *Annals of Internal Medicine,* 122(7), 1995, pages 481–486.
3. Pi-Sunyer, F. X., "The Obesity Epidemic: Pathophysiology and Consequences of Obesity," *Obesity Research,* 10(2S), 2002, pages 97S-104S.
4. Burke, J. P., Williams, K., Narayan, K. M., et al., "A Population Perspective on Diabetes Prevention: Whom Should We Target for Preventing Weight Gain?" *Diabetes Care,* 26(7), 2003, pages 1999–2004.
5. National Heart, Lung, and Blood Institute, "Clinical Guidelines on the Identification, Evaluation, and Treatment of Overweight and Obesity in Adults: Executive Summary. Expert Panel on the Identification, Evaluation, and Treatment of Overweight in Adults," 1998.
6. Heiat, A. National Institutes of Health (NIH: the NIH Consensus Conference on Health Implications of Obesity in 1985); United States Department of Agriculture (the 1990 Department of Agriculture's Dietary Guidelines for Americans); National Heart, Lung, and Blood Institute., "Impact of Age on Definition of Standards for Ideal Weight," *Preventive Cardiology,* 6(2), 2003, pages 104–107.
7. Aronne, L. J., Segal, K. R., "Adiposity and Fat Distribution Outcome Measures: Assessment and Clinical Implications," *Obesity Research,* 10(1S), 2002, pages 14S-21S.
8. Chan, J. M., Rimm, E. B., Colditz, G. A., et al., "Obesity, Fat Distribution, and Weight Gain as Risk Factors for Clinical Diabetes in Men," *Diabetes Care,* 17(9), 1994, pages 961–969.
9. Colditz, G. A., Willett, W. C., Rotnitzky, A., et al., "Weight Gain as a

Risk Factor for Clinical Diabetes Mellitus in Women," *Annals of Internal Medicine,* 122(7), 1995, pages 481–486.

10. Colditz, G. A., Willett, W. C., Rotnitzky, A., et al., "Weight Gain as a Risk Factor for Clinical Diabetes Mellitus in Women," *Annals of Internal Medicine,* 122(7), 1995, pages 481–486.

11. Chan, J. M., Rimm, E. B., Colditz, G. A., et al., "Obesity, Fat Distribution, and Weight Gain as Risk Factors for Clinical Diabetes in Men," *Diabetes Care,* 17(9), 1994, pages 961–969.

12. Seidell, J. C., Kahn, H. S., Williamson, D. F., et al., "Report from a Centers for Disease Control and Prevention Workshop on Use of Adult Anthropometry for Public Health and Primary Health Care," *American Journal of Clinical Nutrition,* 73(1), 2001, pages 123–126.

13. Kahn, H. S., Valdez, R., "Metabolic Risks Identified by the Combination of Enlarged Waist and Elevated Triacylglycerol Concentration," *American Journal of Clinical Nutrition,* 78(5), 2003, pages 928–934.

14. Janssen, I., Katzmarzyk, P. T., Ross, R., "Waist Circumference and Not Body Mass Index Explains Obesity-Related Health Risk," *American Journal of Clinical Nutrition,* 79(3), 2004, pages 379–384.

15. Janssen, I., Katzmarzyk, P. T., Ross, R., "Waist Circumference and Not Body Mass Index Explains Obesity-Related Health Risk," *American Journal of Clinical Nutrition,* 79(3), 2004, pages 379–384.

16. Wannamethee, S. G., Shaper, A. G., "Alcohol, Body Weight, and Weight Gain in Middle-Aged Men," *American Journal of Clinical Nutrition,* 77(5), 2003, pages 1312–1317.

17. Bernstein, R. K., "Dr. Bernstein's Diabetes Solution: The Complete Guide to Achieving Normal Blood Sugars Revised & Updated," 2003, Little Brown & Company, Revised Edition, page 480.

Chapter 4: A Deadly Quintet: Meet the Metabolic Syndrome

1. Reaven, G. M., "Banting Lecture 1988. Role of Insulin Resistance in Human Disease," *Diabetes,* 37(12), 1988, pages 1595–1607.

2. Calle, E. E., Thun, M. J., Petrelli, J. M., et al., "Body-Mass Index and

Mortality in a Prospective Cohort of U. S. Adults," *New England Journal of Medicine*, 341(15), 1999, pages 1097–1105.

3. Arcaro, G., Cretti, A., Balzano, S., et al., "Insulin Causes Endothelial Dysfunction in Humans: Sites and Mechanisms," *Circulation*, 105(5), 2002, pages 576–582.

4. Reaven, G. M., "Banting Lecture 1988. Role of Insulin Resistance in Human Disease," *Diabetes*, 37(12), 1988, pages 1595–1607.

5. Expert Panel on Detection, Evaluation, and Treatment of High Blood Cholesterol in Adults, "Executive Summary of the Third Report of the National Cholesterol Education Program (NCEP) Expert Panel on Detection, Evaluation, and Treatment of High Blood Cholesterol in Adults (Adult Treatment Panel III)," *Journal of the American Medical Association*, 285(19), 2001, pages 2486–2497.

6. Ford, E. S., Giles, W. H., "A Comparison of the Prevalence of the Metabolic Syndrome Using Two Proposed Definitions," *Diabetes Care*, 26(3), 2003, pages 575–581.

7. Expert Panel on Detection, Evaluation, and Treatment of High Blood Cholesterol in Adults, "Executive Summary of the Third Report of the National Cholesterol Education Program (NCEP) Expert Panel on Detection, Evaluation, and Treatment of High Blood Cholesterol in Adults (Adult Treatment Panel III)," *Journal of the American Medical Association*, 285(19), 2001, pages 2486–2497.

8. Ford, E. S., Giles, W. H., Dietz, W. H., "Prevalence of the Metabolic Syndrome Among US Adults: Findings from the Third National Health and Nutrition Examination Survey," *Journal of the American Medical Association*, 287(3), 2002, pages 356–359.

9. Alberti, K. G., Zimmet, P. Z., "Definition, Diagnosis and Classification of Diabetes Mellitus and Its Complications. Part 1: Diagnosis and Classification of Diabetes Mellitus Provisional Report of a WHO Consultation," *Diabetic Medicine*, 15(7), 1998, pages 539–553.

10. Alberti, K. G., Zimmet, P. Z., "Definition, Diagnosis and Classification of Diabetes Mellitus and Its Complications. Part 1: Diagnosis and Classification of Diabetes Mellitus Provisional Report of a WHO Consultation," *Diabetic Medicine*, 15(7), 1998, pages 539–553.

11. Ford, E. S., Giles, W. H., "A Comparison of the Prevalence of the

Metabolic Syndrome Using Two Proposed Definitions," *Diabetes Care*, 26(3), 2003, pages 575–581.

12. Alexander, C. M., Landsman, P. B., Teutsch, S. M., et al., "NCEP-Defined Metabolic Syndrome, Diabetes, and Prevalence of Coronary Heart Disease among NHANES III Participants Age 50 Years and Older," *Diabetes*, 52(5), 2003, pages 1210–1214.

13. Seidell, J. C., Kahn, H. S., Williamson, D. F., et al., "Report from a Centers for Disease Control and Prevention Workshop on Use of Adult Anthropometry for Public Health and Primary Health Care," *American Journal of Clinical Nutrition*, 73(1), 2001, pages 123–126.

14. Kahn, H. S., Valdez, R., "Metabolic Risks Identified by the Combination of Enlarged Waist and Elevated Triacylglycerol Concentration," *American Journal of Clinical Nutrition*, 78(5), 2003, pages 928–934.

15. Janssen, I., Katzmarzyk, P. T., Ross, R., "Waist Circumference and Not Body Mass Index Explains Obesity-Related Health Risk," *American Journal of Clinical Nutrition*, 79(3), 2004, pages 379–384.

16. Aronne, L. J., Segal, K. R., "Adiposity and Fat Distribution Outcome Measures: Assessment and Clinical Implications," *Obesity Research*, 10(1S), 2002, pages 14S-21S.

17. Pi-Sunyer, F. X., "The Obesity Epidemic: Pathophysiology and Consequences of Obesity," *Obesity Research*, 10(2S), 2002, pages 97S-104S.

18. Ruderman, N., Chisholm, D., Pi-Sunyer, X., et al., "The Metabolically Obese, Normal-Weight Individual Revisited," *Diabetes*, 47(5), 1998, pages 699–713.

19. Sattar, N., Gaw, A., Scherbakova, O., et al., "Metabolic Syndrome with and Without C-Reactive Protein as a Predictor of Coronary Heart Disease and Diabetes in the West of Scotland Coronary Prevention Study," *Circulation*, 108(4), 2003, pages 414–419.

20. Hudgins, L. C., "Effect of High-Carbohydrate Feeding on Triglyceride and Saturated Fatty Acid Synthesis," *Proceedings of the Society for Experimental Biology and Medicine*, 225(3), 2000, pages 178–183.

21. Hudgins, L. C., Hellerstein, M. K., Seidman, C. E., et al., "Relation-

ship Between Carbohydrate-Induced Hypertriglyceridemia and Fatty Acid Synthesis in Lean and Obese Subjects," *Journal of Lipid Research*, 41(4), 2000, pages 595–604.

22. American Heart Association, "Carbohydrates and Sugars," available at: http://www.americanheart.org, accessed February 27, 2004.

23. Volek, J. S., Sharman, M. J., Love, D. M., et al., "Body Composition and Hormonal Responses to a Carbohydrate-Restricted Diet," *Metabolism: Clinical and Experimental*, 51(7), 2002, pages 864–870.

24. Layman, D. K., "The Role of Leucine in Weight Loss Diets and Glucose Homeostasis," *Journal of Nutrition*, 133(1), 2003, pages 261S–267S.

25. Layman, D. K., Boileau, R. A., Erickson, D. J., et al., "A Reduced Ratio of Dietary Carbohydrate to Protein Improves Body Composition and Blood Lipid Profiles During Weight Loss in Adult Women," *Journal of Nutrition*, 133(2), 2003, pages 411–417.

26. Westerterp-Plantenga, M. S., "The Significance of Protein in Food Intake and Body Weight Regulation," *Current Opinion in Clinical Nutrition and Metabolic Care*, 6(6), 2003, pages 635–638.

27. Asztalos, B., Lefevre, M., Wong, L., et al., "Differential Response to Low-Fat Diet Between Low and Normal HDL-Cholesterol Subjects," *Journal of Lipid Research*, 41(3), 2000, pages 321–328.

28. Aro, A., Pietinen, P., Valsta, L. M., et al., "Effects of Reduced-Fat Diets with Different Fatty Acid Compositions on Serum Lipoprotein Lipids and Apolipoproteins," *Public Health Nutrition*, 1(2), 1998, pages 109–116.

29. Berglund, L., Oliver, E. H., Fontanez, N., et al., "HDL-Subpopulation Patterns in Response to Reductions in Dietary Total and Saturated Fat Intakes in Healthy Subjects," *American Journal of Clinical Nutrition*, 70(6), 1999, pages 992–1000.

30. Brehm, B. J., Seeley, R. J., Daniels, S. R., et al., "A Randomized Trial Comparing a Very Low Carbohydrate Diet and a Calorie-Restricted Low Fat Diet on Body Weight and Cardiovascular Risk Factors in Healthy Women," *Journal of Clinical Endocrinology and Metabolism*, 88(4), 2003, pages 1617–1623.

31. Foster, G. D., Wyatt, H. R., Hill, J. O., et al., "A Randomized Trial of a Low-Carbohydrate Diet for Obesity," *New England Journal of Medicine*, 348(21), 2003, pages 2082–2090.

32. O'Brien, K. D., Brehm, B. J., Seeley, R. J., "Greater Reduction in Inflammatory Markers with Low Carbohydrate Diet Than with a Calorically Matched Low Fat Diet," Presented at American Heart Association's Scientific Sessions 2002 on Tuesday, November 19, 2002, Abstract ID: 117597.

33. Samaha, F. F., Iqbal, N., Seshadri, P., et al., "A Low-Carbohydrate as Compared with a Low-Fat Diet in Severe Obesity," *New England Journal of Medicine*, 348(21), 2003, pages 2074–2081.

34. Sharman, M. J., Kraemer, W. J., Love, D. M., et al., "A Ketogenic Diet Favorably Affects Serum Biomarkers for Cardiovascular Disease in Normal-Weight Men," *Journal of Nutrition*, 132(7), 2002, pages 1879–1885.

35. Sondike, S. B., Copperman, N., Jacobson, M. S., "Effects of a Low-Carbohydrate Diet on Weight Loss and Cardiovascular Risk Factor in Overweight Adolescents," *Journal of Pediatrics*, 142(3), 2003, pages 253–258.

36. Volek, J. S., Sharman, M. J., Gomez, A. L., et al., "An Isoenergetic Very Low Carbohydrate Diet Improves Serum HDL Cholesterol and Triacylglycerol Concentrations, the Total Cholesterol to HDL Cholesterol Ratio and Postprandial Pipemic Responses Compared with a Low Fat Diet in Normal Weight, Normolipidemic Women," *Journal of Nutrition*, 133(9), 2003, pages 2756–2761.

37. Westman, E. C., Yancy, W. S., Edman, J. S., et al., "Effect of 6-Month Adherence to a Very Low Carbohydrate Diet Program," *American Journal of Medicine*, 113(1), 2002, pages 30–36.

38. Westman, E. C., Yancy, W. S., Jr., Guyton, J. S., "Effect of a Low Carbohydrate Ketogenic Diet Program on Fasting Lipid Subfractions," *Circulation*, 106(19(SII)), 2002, page 727.

39. Chobanian, A. V., Bakris, G. L., Black, H. R., et al., "Seventh Report of the Joint National Committee on Prevention, Detection, Evaluation, and Treatment of High Blood Pressure," *Hypertension*, 42(6), 2003, pages 1206–1252.

40. Ford, E. S., Giles, W. H., "A Comparison of the Prevalence of the Metabolic Syndrome Using Two Proposed Definitions," *Diabetes Care*, 26(3), 2003, pages 575–581.

41. Ridker, P. M., Morrow, D. A., "C-Reactive Protein, Inflammation, and Coronary Risk," *Cardiology Clinics*, 21(3), 2003, pages 315–325.

42. Reaven, G., "Syndrome X," *Current Treatment Options in Cardio-vascular Medicine,* 3(4), 2001, pages 323–332.

43. Layman, D. K., Boileau, R. A., Erickson, D. J., et al., "A Reduced Ratio of Dietary Carbohydrate to Protein Improves Body Composition and Blood Lipid Profiles During Weight Loss in Adult Women," *Journal of Nutrition,* 133(2), 2003, pages 411–417.

44. Volek, J. S., Sharman, M. J., Love, D. M., et al., "Body Composition and Hormonal Responses to a Carbohydrate-Restricted Diet," *Metabolism: Clinical and Experimental,* 51(7), 2002, pages 864–870.

Chapter 5: Warning: Prediabetes!

1. Expert Committee on the Diagnosis and Classification of Diabetes Mellitus, "Report of the Expert Committee on the Diagnosis and Classification of Diabetes Mellitus," *Diabetes Care,* 26(1S), 2003, pages S5-S20.

2. Expert Committee on the Diagnosis and Classification of Diabetes Mellitus, "Report of the Expert Committee on the Diagnosis and Classification of Diabetes Mellitus," *Diabetes Care,* 26(1S), 2003, pages S5-S20.

3. National Institute of Diabetes and Digestive and Kidney Diseases, "Insulin Resistance and Pre-Diabetes," November 2003, available at: http://www.diabetes.niddk.nih.gov/dm/pubs/insulinresistance/index. htm, accessed on February 27, 2004.

4. American Diabetes Association, "Standards of Medical Care for Patients with Diabetes Mellitus," *Diabetes Care,* 26(1S), 2003, pages S33-S50.

5. Dallo, F. J., Weller, S. C., "Effectiveness of Diabetes Mellitus Screening Recommendations," *Proceedings of the National Academy of Sciences of the United States of America,* 100(18), 2003, pages 10574–10579.

6. Dallo, F. J., Weller, S. C., "Effectiveness of Diabetes Mellitus Screening Recommendations," *Proceedings of the National Academy of Sciences of the United States of America,* 100(18), 2003, pages 10574–10579.

7. Bjornholt, J. V., Erikssen, G., Aaser, E., et al., "Fasting Blood Glu-

cose: An Underestimated Risk Factor for Cardiovascular Death. Results from a 22-Year Follow-up of Healthy Nondiabetic Men," *Diabetes Care,* 22(1), 1999, pages 45–49.

8. Saydah, S. H., Loria, C. M., Eberhardt, M. S., et al., "Subclinical States of Glucose Intolerance and Risk of Death in the U. S," *Diabetes Care,* 24(3), 2001, pages 447–453.

9. Norhammar, A., Tenerz, A., Nilsson, G., et al., "Glucose Metabolism in Patients with Acute Myocardial Infarction and no Previous Diagnosis of Diabetes Mellitus: A Prospective Study," *Lancet,* 359(9324), 2002, pages 2140–2144.

10. de Vegt, F., Dekker, J. M., Jager, A., et al., "Relation of Impaired Fasting and Postload Glucose with Incident Type 2 Diabetes in a Dutch Population: The Hoorn Study," *Journal of the American Medical Association,* 285(16), 2001, pages 2109–2113.

Chapter 6: Diagnosis: Diabetes

1. Reaven, G., "Syndrome X," *Current Treatment Options in Cardiovascular Medicine,* 3(4), 2001, pages 323–332.

2. Saydah, S. H., Fradkin, J., Cowie, C. C., "Poor Control of Risk Factors for Vascular Disease among Adults with Previously Diagnosed Diabetes," *Journal of the American Medical Association,* 291(3), 2004, pages 335–342.

Chapter 8: Twin Peaks: High Blood Pressure and High Blood Sugar

1. Chobanian, A. V., Bakris, G. L., Black, H. R., et al., "The Seventh Report of the Joint National Committee on Prevention, Detection, Evaluation, and Treatment of High Blood Pressure: The JNC 7 Report," *Journal of the American Medical Association,* 289(19), 2003, pages 2560–2572.

2. Chobanian, A. V., Bakris, G. L., Black, H. R., et al., "The Seventh Report of the Joint National Committee on Prevention, Detection, Evaluation, and Treatment of High Blood Pressure: The JNC 7 Report," *Journal of the American Medical Association,* 289(19), 2003, pages 2560–2572.

3. "Research Notebook, New Guidelines Set Lower Mark for High

Blood Pressure," *FDA Consumer Magazine,* 37(4), available at http://www.fda.gov/fdac/403_toc.html, accessed on April 24, 2004.

4. Nesbitt, S. D., Julius, S., "Prehypertension: A Possible Target for Antihypertensive Medication," *Current Hypertension Reports,* 2(4), 2000, pages 356–361.

5. US Department of Health and Human Services, "JNC 7 Express: The Seventh Report of the Joint National Committee on Prevention, Detection, Evaluation, and Treatment of High Blood Pressure," May 2003, NIH Publication No. 03–4233, available at: http://www.nhbli.nih.gov/guidelines/hypertension/jncintro.htm, accessed on February 27, 2004.

6. US Department of Health and Human Services, "JNC 7 Express: The Seventh Report of the Joint National Committee on Prevention, Detection, Evaluation, and Treatment of High Blood Pressure," May 2003, NIH Publication No. 03–4233, available at: http://www.nhbli.nih.gov/guidelines/hypertension/jncintro.htm, accessed on February 27, 2004.

7. Sowers, J. R., Epstein, M., Frohlich, E. D., "Diabetes, Hypertension, and Cardiovascular Disease: An Update," *Hypertension,* 37(4), 2001, pages 1053–1059.

8. US Department of Health and Human Services, "JNC 7 Express: The Seventh Report of the Joint National Committee on Prevention, Detection, Evaluation, and Treatment of High Blood Pressure," May 2003, NIH Publication No. 03–4233, available at: http://www.nhbli.nih.gov/guidelines/hypertension/jncintro.htm, accessed on February 27, 2004.

9. Gress, T. W., Nieto, F. J., Shahar, E., et al., "Hypertension and Antihypertensive Therapy as Risk Factors for Type 2 Diabetes Mellitus. Atherosclerosis Risk in Communities Study," *New England Journal of Medicine,* 342(13), 2000, pages 905–912.

10. Henry, P., Thomas, F., Benetos, A., et al., "Impaired Fasting Glucose, Blood Pressure and Cardiovascular Disease Mortality," *Hypertension,* 40(4), 2002, pages 458–463.

11. American Diabetes Association, "Treatment of Hypertension in Adults with Diabetes," *Diabetes Care,* 25(1), 2002, pages 199–201.

12. Arauz-Pacheco, C., Parrott, M. A., Raskin, P., "Hypertension Man-

agement in Adults with Diabetes," *Diabetes Care,* 27(1S), 2004, pages S65-S67.

13. Vaskonen, T., "Dietary Minerals and Modification of Cardiovascular Risk Factors," *Journal of Nutritional Biochemistry,* 14(9), 2003, pages 492–506.

14. Quinones-Galvan, A., Ferrannini, E., "Renal Effects of Insulin in Man," *Journal of Nephrology,* 10(4), 1997, pages 188–191.

15. Phinney, S. D., Bistrian, B. R., Evans, W. J., et al., "The Human Metabolic Response to Chronic Ketosis without Caloric Restriction: Preservation of Submaximal Exercise Capability with Reduced Carbohydrate Oxidation," *Metabolism: Clinical and Experimental,* 32(8), 1983, pages 769–776.

16. Whelton, S. P., Chin, A., Xin, X., et al., "Effect of Aerobic Exercise on Blood Pressure: A Meta-Analysis of Randomized, Controlled Trials," *Annals of Internal Medicine,* 136(7), 2002, pages 493–503.

17. Bjorntorp, P., "Do Stress Reactions Cause Abdominal Obesity and Comorbidities?" *Obesity Reviews,* 2(2), 2001, pages 73–86.

18. Brunner, E. J., Hemingway, H., Walker, B. R., et al., "Adrenocortical, Autonomic, and Inflammatory Causes of the Metabolic Syndrome: Nested Case-Control Study," *Circulation,* 106(21), 2002, pages 2659–2665.

19. Bjorntorp, P., "Do Stress Reactions Cause Abdominal Obesity and Comorbidities?" *Obesity Reviews,* 2(2), 2001, pages 73–86.

20. Brunner, E. J., Hemingway, H., Walker, B. R., et al., "Adrenocortical, Autonomic, and Inflammatory Causes of the Metabolic Syndrome: Nested Case-Control Study," *Circulation,* 106(21), 2002, pages 2659–2665.

21. Leproult, R., Van Reeth, O., Byrne, M. M., et al., "Sleepiness, Performance, and Neuroendocrine Function During Sleep Deprivation: Effects of Exposure to Bright Light or Exercise," *Journal of Biological Rhythms,* 12(3), 1997, pages 245–258.

22. Vgontzas, A. N., Tsigos, C., Bixler, E. O., et al., "Chronic Insomnia and Activity of the Stress System: A Preliminary Study," *Journal of Psychosomatic Research,* 45(1S), 1998, pages 21–31.

23. Arauz-Pacheco, C., Parrott, M. A., Raskin, P., "Hypertension Man-

agement in Adults with Diabetes," *Diabetes Care*, 27(1S), 2004, pages S65-S67.

24. Gress, T. W., Nieto, F. J., Shahar, E., et al., "Hypertension and Antihypertensive Therapy as Risk Factors for Type 2 Diabetes Mellitus. Atherosclerosis Risk in Communities Study," *New England Journal of Medicine*, 342(13), 2000, pages 905–912.

25. Pollare, T., Lithell, H., Berne, C., "A Comparison of the Effects of Hydrochlorothiazide and Captopril on Glucose and Lipid Metabolism in Patients with Hypertension," *New England Journal of Medicine*, 321(13), 1989, pages 868–873.

26. Alderman, M. H., Cohen, H., Madhavan, S., "Diabetes and Cardiovascular Events in Hypertensive Patients," *Hypertension*, 33(5), 1999, pages 1130–1134.

27. Dunder, K., Lind, L., Zethelius, B., et al., "Increase in Blood Glucose Concentration During Antihypertensive Treatment as a Predictor of Myocardial Infarction: Population Based Cohort Study," *British Medical Journal*, 326(7391), 2003, page 681–686.

28. Quinones-Galvan, A., Ferrannini, E., "Renal Effects of Insulin in Man," *Journal of Nephrology*, 10(4), 1997, pages 188–191.

29. Mora-Rodriguez, R., Hodgkinson, B. J., Byerley, L. O., et al., "Effects of Beta-Adrenergic Receptor Stimulation and Blockade on Substrate Metabolism During Submaximal Exercise," *American Journal of Physiology. Endocrinology and Metabolism*, 280(5), 2001, pages E752–760.

30. Imazu, M., "Hypertension and Insulin Disorders," *Current Hypertension Reports*, 4(6), 2002, pages 477–482.

31. Mills, G. A., Horn, J. R., "Beta-Blockers and Glucose Control," *Drug Intelligence and Clinical Pharmacy*, 19(4), 1985, pages 246–251.

32. Marcus, A. O., "Safety of Drugs Commonly Used to Treat Hypertension, Dyslipidemia, and Type 2 Diabetes (the Metabolic Syndrome): Part 1," *Diabetes Technology & Therapeutics*, 2(1), 2000, pages 101–110.

33. Devoy, M. A., Tomson, C. R., Edmunds, M. E., et al., "Deterioration in Renal Function Associated with Angiotensin Converting Enzyme Inhibitor Therapy Is Not Always Reversible," *Journal of Internal Medicine*, 232(6), 1992, pages 493–498.

34. Wargo, K. A., Chong, K., Chan, E. C., "Acute Renal Failure Secondary to Angiotensin II Receptor Blockade in a Patient with Bilateral Renal Artery Stenosis," *Pharmacotherapy,* 23(9), 2003, pages 1199–1204.

Chapter 9: The Cardiac Connection

1. Garnt, P. J., Davies, J. A., "Cardiovascular Diseases and Diabetes," In: Textbook of Diabetes, Pickup, J. C. & Williams, G. (Eds.), Blackwell Publishing, 3rd Edition, 2002. Malden, MA.
2. American Heart Association. Heart Disease and Stroke Statistics-2004 Update. Dallas, Tex.: American Heart Association, 2003.
3. Haffner, S. M., Lehto, S., Ronnemaa, T., et al., "Mortality from Coronary Heart Disease in Subjects with Type 2 Diabetes and in Nondiabetic Subjects with and without Prior Myocardial Infarction," *New England Journal of Medicine,* 339(4), 1998, pages 229–234.
4. Hu, F. B., Stampfer, M. J., Solomon, C. G., et al., "The Impact of Diabetes Mellitus on Mortality from All Causes and Coronary Heart Disease in Women: 20 Years of Follow-Up," *Archives of Internal Medicine,* 161(14), 2001, pages 1717–1723.
5. Balkau, B., Shipley, M., Jarrett, R. J., et al., "High Blood Glucose Concentration Is a Risk Factor for Mortality in Middle-Aged Nondiabetic Men. 20-Year Follow-up in the Whitehall Study, the Paris Prospective Study, and the Helsinki Policemen Study," *Diabetes Care,* 21(3), 1998, pages 360–367.
6. Kenchaiah, S., Evans, J. C., Levy, D., et al., "Obesity and the Risk of Heart Failure," *New England Journal of Medicine,* 347(5), 2002, pages 305–313.
7. Kirpichnikov, D., McFarlane, S. I., Sowers, J. R., "Heart Failure in Diabetic Patients: Utility of Beta-Blockade," *Journal of Cardiac Failure,* 9(4), 2003, pages 333–344.
8. Gaziano, J. M., Hennekens, C. H., O'Donnell, C. J., et al., "Fasting Triglycerides, High-Density Lipoprotein, and Risk of Myocardial Infarction," *Circulation,* 96(8), 1997, pages 2520–2525.
9. Abbasi, F., McLaughlin, T., Lamendola, C., et al., "High Carbohydrate Diets, Triglyceride-Rich Lipoproteins, and Coronary Heart

Disease Risk," *American Journal of Cardiology,* 85(1), 2000, pages 45–48.

10. Assmann, G., Schulte, H., Funke, H., et al., "The Emergence of Triglycerides as a Significant Independent Risk Factor in Coronary Artery Disease," *European Heart Journal,* 19 Suppl M, 1998, pages M8-M14.

11. St-Pierre, A. C., Ruel, I. L., Cantin, B., et al., "Comparison of Various Electrophoretic Characteristics of LDL Particles and Their Relationship to the Risk of Ischemic Heart Disease," *Circulation,* 104(19), 2001, pages 2295–2299.

12. Garvey, W. T., Kwon, S., Zheng, D., et al., "Effects of Insulin Resistance and Type 2 Diabetes on Lipoprotein Subclass Particle Size and Concentration Determined by Nuclear Magnetic Resonance," *Diabetes,* 52(2), 2003, pages 453–462.

13. Hickey, J. T., Hickey, L., Yancy, W. S. J., et al., "Clinical Use of a Carbohydrate-Restricted Diet to Treat the Dyslipidemia of the Metabolic Syndrome," *Metabolic Syndrome and Related Disorders,* 1(3), 2003, pages 227–232.

14. Westman, E. C., Yancy, W. S., Jr., Guyton, J. S., "Effect of a Low Carbohydrate Ketogenic Diet Program on Fasting Lipid Subfractions," *Circulation,* 106(19(SII)), 2002, page 727.

15. Luc, G., Bard, J. M., Arveiler, D., et al., "Lipoprotein (a) as a Predictor of Coronary Heart Disease: The Prime Study," *Atherosclerosis,* 163(2), 2002, pages 377–384.

16. Gotto, A. M., Jr., Brinton, E. A., "Assessing Low Levels of High-Density Lipoprotein Cholesterol as a Risk Factor in Coronary Heart Disease: A Working Group Report and Update," *Journal of the American College of Cardiology,* 43(5), 2004, pages 717–724.

17. Hickey, J. T., Hickey, L., Yancy, W. S. J., et al., "Clinical Use of a Carbohydrate-Restricted Diet to Treat the Dyslipidemia of the Metabolic Syndrome," *Metabolic Syndrome and Related Disorders,* 1(3), 2003, pages 227–232.

18. Westman, E. C., Mavropoulos, J., Yancy, W. S., et al., "A Review of Low-Carbohydrate Ketogenic Diets," *Current Atherosclerosis Reports,* 5(6), 2003, pages 476–483.

19. Hudgins, L. C., "Effect of High-Carbohydrate Feeding on Triglyc-

eride and Saturated Fatty Acid Synthesis," *Proceedings of the Society for Experimental Biology and Medicine,* 225(3), 2000, pages 178–183.

20. Hudgins, L. C., Hellerstein, M. K., Seidman, C. E., et al., "Relationship between Carbohydrate-Induced Hypertriglyceridemia and Fatty Acid Synthesis in Lean and Obese Subjects," *Journal of Lipid Research,* 41(4), 2000, pages 595–604.

21. Gaziano, J. M., Hennekens, C. H., O'Donnell, C. J., et al., "Fasting Triglycerides, High-Density Lipoprotein, and Risk of Myocardial Infarction," *Circulation,* 96(8), 1997, pages 2520–2525.

22. Austin, M. A., Hokanson, J. E., Edwards, K. L., "Hypertriglyceridemia as a Cardiovascular Risk Factor," *American Journal of Cardiology,* 81(4A), 1998, pages 7B-12B.

23. Expert Panel on Detection, Evaluation, And Treatment of High Blood Cholesterol In Adults, "Executive Summary of the Third Report of the National Cholesterol Education Program (NCEP) Expert Panel on Detection, Evaluation, and Treatment of High Blood Cholesterol in Adults (Adult Treatment Panel III)," *Journal of the American Medical Association,* 285(19), 2001, pages 2486–2497.

24. Ashton, E., Liew, D., Krum, H., "Should Patients with Chronic Heart Failure Be Treated with 'Statins'?" *Heart Failure Monitor,* 3(3), 2003, pages 82–86.

25. Ashton, E., Liew, D., Krum, H., "Should Patients with Chronic Heart Failure Be Treated with 'Statins'?" *Heart Failure Monitor,* 3(3), 2003, pages 82–86.

26. Westman, E. C., Mavropoulos, J., Yancy, W. S., et al., "A Review of Low-Carbohydrate Ketogenic Diets," *Current Atherosclerosis Reports,* 5(6), 2003, pages 476–483.

27. Arcaro, G., Cretti, A., Balzano, S., et al., "Insulin Causes Endothelial Dysfunction in Humans: Sites and Mechanisms," *Circulation,* 105(5), 2002, pages 576–582.

28. Festa, A., Hanley, A. J., Tracy, R. P., et al., "Inflammation in the Prediabetic State Is Related to Increased Insulin Resistance Rather Than Decreased Insulin Secretion," *Circulation,* 108(15), 2003, pages 1822–1830.

29. Caballero, A. E., "Endothelial Dysfunction in Obesity and Insulin

Resistance: A Road to Diabetes and Heart Disease," *Obesity Research*, 11(11), 2003, pages 1278–1289.

30. Expert Panel on Detection, Evaluation, And Treatment of High Blood Cholesterol In Adults, "Executive Summary of the Third Report of the National Cholesterol Education Program (NCEP) Expert Panel on Detection, Evaluation, and Treatment of High Blood Cholesterol in Adults (Adult Treatment Panel III)," *Journal of the American Medical Association*, 285(19), 2001, pages 2486–2497.

31. Fedder, D. O., Koro, C. E., L'Italien, G. J., "New National Cholesterol Education Program III Guidelines for Primary Prevention Lipid-Lowering Drug Therapy: Projected Impact on the Size, Sex, and Age Distribution of the Treatment-Eligible Population," *Circulation*, 105(2), 2002, pages 152–156.

32. Reaven, G., "Syndrome X," *Current Treatment Options in Cardiovascular Medicine*, 3(4), 2001, pages 323–332.

33. Sharman, M. J., Kraemer, W. J., Love, D. M., et al., "A Ketogenic Diet Favorably Affects Serum Biomarkers for Cardiovascular Disease in Normal-Weight Men," *Journal of Nutrition*, 132(7), 2002, pages 1879–1885.

34. Volek, J. S., Sharman, M. J., Gomez, A. L., et al., "An Isoenergetic Very Low Carbohydrate Diet Improves Serum HDL Cholesterol and Triacylglycerol Concentrations, the Total Cholesterol to HDL Cholesterol Ratio and Postprandial Pipemic Responses Compared with a Low Fat Diet in Normal Weight, Normolipidemic Women," *Journal of Nutrition*, 133(9), 2003, pages 2756–2761.

35. Hudgins, L. C., "Effect of High-Carbohydrate Feeding on Triglyceride and Saturated Fatty Acid Synthesis," *Proceedings of the Society for Experimental Biology and Medicine*, 225(3), 2000, pages 178–183.

36. Caballero, A. E., "Endothelial Dysfunction in Obesity and Insulin Resistance: A Road to Diabetes and Heart Disease," *Obesity Research*, 11(11), 2003, pages 1278–1289.

37. Hoogeveen, E. K., Kostense, P. J., Jakobs, C., et al., "Hyperhomocysteinemia Increases Risk of Death, Especially in Type 2 Diabetes: 5-Year Follow-up of the Hoorn Study," *Circulation*, 101(13), 2000, pages 1506–1511.

38. Soinio, M., Marniemi, J., Laakso, M., et al., "Elevated Plasma Homocysteine Level Is an Independent Predictor of Coronary Heart Disease Events in Patients with Type 2 Diabetes Mellitus," *Annals of Internal Medicine*, 140(2), 2004, pages 94–100.

39. Buysschaert, M., Dramais, A. S., Wallemacq, P. E., et al., "Hyperhomocysteinemia in Type 2 Diabetes: Relationship to Macroangiopathy, Nephropathy, and Insulin Resistance," *Diabetes Care*, 23(12), 2000, pages 1816–1822.

40. Ridker, P. M., Cushman, M., Stampfer, M. J., et al., "Inflammation, Aspirin, and the Risk of Cardiovascular Disease in Apparently Healthy Men," *New England Journal of Medicine*, 336(14), 1997, pages 973–979.

41. Ridker, P. M., Hennekens, C. H., Buring, J. E., et al., "C-Reactive Protein and Other Markers of Inflammation in the Prediction of Cardiovascular Disease in Women," *New England Journal of Medicine*, 342(12), 2000, pages 836–843.

42. Forouhi, N. G., Sattar, N., McKeigue, P. M., "Relation of C-Reactive Protein to Body Fat Distribution and Features of the Metabolic Syndrome in Europeans and South Asians," *International Journal of Obesity and Related Metabolic Disorders*, 25(9), 2001, pages 1327–1331.

43. Ziccardi, P., Nappo, F., Giugliano, G., et al., "Reduction of Inflammatory Cytokine Concentrations and Improvement of Endothelial Functions in Obese Women after Weight Loss Over One Year," *Circulation*, 105(7), 2002, pages 804–809.

44. Volek, J. S., Sharman, M. J., Gomez, A. L., et al., "An Isoenergetic Very Low Carbohydrate Diet Improves Serum HDL Cholesterol and Triacylglycerol Concentrations, the Total Cholesterol to HDL Cholesterol Ratio and Postprandial Pipemic Responses Compared with a Low Fat Diet in Normal Weight, Normolipidemic Women," *Journal of Nutrition*, 133(9), 2003, pages 2756–2761.

45. Ford, E. S., "The Metabolic Syndrome and C-Reactive Protein, Fibrinogen, and Leukocyte Count: Findings from the Third National Health and Nutrition Examination Survey," *Atherosclerosis*, 168(2), 2003, pages 351–358.

Chapter 10: The Atkins Blood Sugar Control Program

1. Atkins, R. C., *Dr. Atkins' New Diet Revolution,* Avon Books, 2002.
2. Atkins, R. C., *Atkins for Life,* 1st edition, St. Martin's Press, 2003.
3. Atkins Health & Medical Information Services, *The Atkins Essentials: A Two-Week Program to Jump-start Your Low Carb Lifestyle,* Avon Books, 2003.
4. Atkins, R. C., *Dr. Atkins' New Carbohydrate Gram Counter,* M. Evans & Company Inc., 2002.
5. Gandhi, T. K., Weingart, S. N., Borus, J., et al., "Adverse Drug Events in Ambulatory Care," *New England Journal of Medicine,* 348(16), 2003, pages 1556–1564.
6. Lazarou, J., Pomeranz, B. H., Corey, P. N., "Incidence of Adverse Drug Reactions in Hospitalized Patients: A Meta-Analysis of Prospective Studies," *Journal of the American Medical Association,* 279(15), 1998, pages 1200–1205.
7. Whelton, P. K., Appel, L. J., Espeland, M. A., et al., "Sodium Reduction and Weight Loss in the Treatment of Hypertension in Older Persons: A Randomized Controlled Trial of Nonpharmacologic Interventions in the Elderly (TONE). TONE Collaborative Research Group," *Journal of the American Medical Association,* 279(11), 1998, pages 839–846.

Chapter 12: The Importance of Good Fats

1. Simopoulos, A. P., "The Importance of the Ratio of Omega-6/Omega-3 Essential Fatty Acids," *Biomedicine and Pharmacotherapy,* 56(8), 2002, pages 365–379.
2. Sharman, M. J., Kraemer, W. J., Love, D. M., et al., "A Ketogenic Diet Favorably Affects Serum Biomarkers for Cardiovascular Disease in Normal-Weight Men," *Journal of Nutrition,* 132(7), 2002, pages 1879–1885.
3. Hays, J. H., Gorman, R. T., Shakir, K. M., "Results of Use of Metformin and Replacement of Starch with Saturated Fat in Diets of Patients with Type 2 Diabetes," *Endocrine Practice,* 8(3), 2002, pages 177–183.
4. Hu, F. B., Stampfer, M. J., Manson, J. E., et al., "Dietary Saturated

Fats and Their Food Sources in Relation to the Risk of Coronary Heart Disease in Women," *American Journal of Clinical Nutrition,* 70(6), 1999, pages 1001–1008.

5. He, K., Merchant, A., Rimm, E. B., et al., "Dietary Fat Intake and Risk of Stroke in Male ·US Healthcare Professionals: 14 Year Prospective Cohort Study," *British Medical Journal,* 327(7418), 2003, pages 777–782.

6. Salmeron, J., Manson, J. E., Stampfer, M. J., et al., "Dietary Fiber, Glycemic Load, and Risk of Non-Insulin-Dependent Diabetes Mellitus in Women," *Journal of the American Medical Association,* 277(6), 1997, pages 472–477.

7. Mensink, R. P., Katan, M. B., "Effect of Monounsaturated Fatty Acids Versus Complex Carbohydrates on High-Density Lipoproteins in Healthy Men and Women," *Lancet,* 1(8525), 1987, pages 122–125.

8. Lee, K. W., Lip, G. Y., "The Role of Omega-3 Fatty Acids in the Secondary Prevention of Cardiovascular Disease," *The Quarterly Journal of Medicine,* 96(7), 2003, pages 465–480.

9. Kris-Etherton, P. M., Harris, W. S., Appel, L. J., "Fish Consumption, Fish Oil, Omega-3 Fatty Acids, and Cardiovascular Disease," *Arteriosclerosis, Thrombosis, and Vascular Biology,* 23(2), 2003, pages e20–30.

10. Kris-Etherton, P. M., Harris, W. S., Appel, L. J., "Omega-3 Fatty Acids and Cardiovascular Disease: New Recommendations from the American Heart Association," *Arteriosclerosis, Thrombosis, and Vascular Biology,* 23(2), 2003, pages 151–152.

11. Erkkila, A. T., Lehto, S., Pyorala, K., et al., "N-3 Fatty Acids and 5-Y Risks of Death and Cardiovascular Disease Events in Patients with Coronary Artery Disease," *American Journal of Clinical Nutrition,* 78(1), 2003, pages 65–71.

12. Friedberg, C. E., Janssen, M. J., Heine, R. J., et al., "Fish Oil and Glycemic Control in Diabetes. A Meta-Analysis," *Diabetes Care,* 21(4), 1998, pages 494–500.

13. Lee, K. W., Lip, G. Y., "The Role of Omega-3 Fatty Acids in the Secondary Prevention of Cardiovascular Disease," *The Quarterly Journal of Medicine,* 96(7), 2003, pages 465–480.

14. Toft, I., Bonaa, K. H., Ingebretsen, O. C., et al., "Effects of N-3

Polyunsaturated Fatty Acids on Glucose Homeostasis and Blood Pressure in Essential Hypertension. A Randomized, Controlled Trial," *Annals of Internal Medicine,* 123(12), 1995, pages 911–918.

15. Foran, S. E., Flood, J. G., Lewandrowski, K. B., "Measurement of Mercury Levels in Concentrated Over-the-Counter Fish Oil Preparations: Is Fish Oil Healthier Than Fish?" *Archives of Pathology and Laboratory Medicine,* 127(12), 2003, pages 1603–1605.

16. Wen, Z. Y., Chen, F., "Heterotrophic Production of Eicosapentaenoic Acid by Microalgae," *Biotechnology Advances,* 21(4), 2003, pages 273–294.

17. Crawford, M., Galli, C., Visioli, F., et al., "Role of Plant-Derived Omega-3 Fatty Acids in Human Nutrition," *Annals of Nutrition and Metabolism,* 44(5–6), 2000, pages 263–265.

18. Ascherio, A., "Epidemiologic Studies on Dietary Fats and Coronary Heart Disease," *American Journal of Medicine,* 113(S9B), 2002, pages 9S-12S.

19. Sacks, F. M., Katan, M., "Randomized Clinical Trials on the Effects of Dietary Fat and Carbohydrate on Plasma Lipoproteins and Cardiovascular Disease," *American Journal of Medicine,* 113(S9B), 2002, pages 13S-24S.

20. Willett, W. C., Ascherio, A., "Trans Fatty Acids: Are the Effects Only Marginal?" *American Journal of Public Health,* 84(5), 1994, pages 722–724.

Chapter 13: The Importance of Protein

1. Schnohr, P., Thomsen, O. O., Riis Hansen, P., et al., "Egg Consumption and High-Density-Lipoprotein Cholesterol," *Journal of Internal Medicine,* 235(3), 1994, pages 249–251.

2. Knopp, R. H., Retzlaff, B., Fish, B., et al., "Effects of Insulin Resistance and Obesity on Lipoproteins and Sensitivity to Egg Feeding," *Arteriosclerosis, Thrombosis, and Vascular Biology,* 23(8), 2003, pages 1437–1443.

3. Reaven, G. M., Abbasi, F., Bernhart, S., et al., "Insulin Resistance, Dietary Cholesterol, and Cholesterol Concentration in Postmenopausal Women," *Metabolism: Clinical and Experimental,* 50(5), 2001, pages 594–597.

4. Layman, D. K., "The Role of Leucine in Weight Loss Diets and Glucose Homeostasis," *Journal of Nutrition*, 133(1S), 2003, pages 261S-267S.

5. Gannon, M. C., Nuttall, F. Q., Saeed, A., et al., "An Increase in Dietary Protein Improves the Blood Glucose Response in Persons with Type 2 Diabetes," *American Journal of Clinical Nutrition*, 78(4), 2003, pages 734–741.

6. Layman, D. K., Shiue, H., Sather, C., et al., "Increased Dietary Protein Modifies Glucose and Insulin Homeostasis in Adult Women During Weight Loss," *Journal of Nutrition*, 133(2), 2003, pages 405–410.

7. Layman, D. K., Baum, J. I., "Dietary Protein Impact on Glycemic Control During Weight Loss," *Journal of Nutrition*, 134(4), 2004, pages 968S-973S.

8. Hu, F. B., Stampfer, M. J., Manson, J. E., et al., "Dietary Protein and Risk of Ischemic Heart Disease in Women," *American Journal of Clinical Nutrition*, 70(2), 1999, pages 221–227.

9. Stamler, J., Elliott, P., Kesteloot, H., et al., "Inverse Relation of Dietary Protein Markers with Blood Pressure. Findings for 10,020 Men and Women in the INTERSALT Study. INTERSALT Cooperative Research Group. International Study of Salt and Blood Pressure," *Circulation*, 94(7), 1996, pages 1629–1634.

10. Facchini, F. S., Saylor, K. L., "A Low-Iron-Available, Polyphenol-Enriched, Carbohydrate-Restricted Diet to Slow Progression of Diabetic Nephropathy," *Diabetes*, 52(5), 2003, pages 1204–1209.

11. Jameel, N., Pugh, J. A., Mitchell, B. D., et al., "Dietary Protein Intake Is Not Correlated with Clinical Proteinuria in NIDDM," *Diabetes Care*, 15(2), 1992, pages 178–183.

12. Meloni, C., Morosetti, M., Suraci, C., et al., "Severe Dietary Protein Restriction in Overt Diabetic Nephropathy: Benefits or Risks?" *Journal of Renal Nutrition*, 12(2), 2002, pages 96–101.

13. Hegsted, M., Schuette, S. A., Zemel, M. B., et al., "Urinary Calcium and Calcium Balance in Young Men as Affected by Level of Protein and Phosphorus Intake," *Journal of Nutrition*, 111(3), 1981, pages 553–562.

14. Spencer, H., Kramer, L., DeBartolo, M., et al., "Further Studies of the Effect of a High Protein Diet as Meat on Calcium Metabolism,"

American Journal of Clinical Nutrition, 37(6), 1983, pages 924–929.

15. Kerstetter, J. E., O'Brien, K. O., Insogna, K. L., "Dietary Protein Affects Intestinal Calcium Absorption," *American Journal of Clinical Nutrition,* 68(4), 1998, pages 859–865.

16. Hannan, M. T., Tucker, K. L., Dawson-Hughes, B., et al., "Effect of Dietary Protein on Bone Loss in Elderly Men and Women: The Framingham Osteoporosis Study," *Journal of Bone and Mineral Research,* 15(12), 2000, pages 2504–2512.

17. Dawson-Hughes, B., Harris, S. S., "Calcium Intake Influences the Association of Protein Intake with Rates of Bone Loss in Elderly Men and Women," *American Journal of Clinical Nutrition,* 75(4), 2002, pages 773–779.

18. Dawson-Hughes, B., Harris, S. S., Rasmussen, H., et al., "Effect of Dietary Protein Supplements on Calcium Excretion in Healthy Older Men and Women," *Journal of Clinical Endocrinology and Metabolism,* 89(3), 2004, pages 1169–1173.

19. Kurzer, M. S., "Phytoestrogen Supplement Use by Women," *Journal of Nutrition,* 133(6), 2003, pages 1983S-1986S.

Chapter 14: The Atkins Glycemic Ranking

1. Jenkins, D. J., Wolever, T. M., Taylor, R. H., et al., "Glycemic Index of Foods: A Physiological Basis for Carbohydrate Exchange," *American Journal of Clinical Nutrition,* 34(3), 1981, pages 362–366.

2. Salmeron, J., Manson, J. E., Stampfer, M. J., et al., "Dietary Fiber, Glycemic Load, and Risk of Non-Insulin-Dependent Diabetes Mellitus in Women," *Journal of the American Medical Association,* 277(6), 1997, pages 472–477.

3. Ludwig, D. S., "Glycemic Load Comes of Age," *Journal of Nutrition,* 133(9), 2003, pages 2695–2696.

4. Liu, S., Willett, W. C., Stampfer, M. J., et al., "A Prospective Study of Dietary Glycemic Load, Carbohydrate Intake, and Risk of Coronary Heart Disease in US Women," *American Journal of Clinical Nutrition,* 71(6), 2000, pages 1455–1461.

5. Ford, E. S., Liu, S., "Glycemic Index and Serum High-Density

Lipoprotein Cholesterol Concentration among US Adults," *Archives of Internal Medicine,* 161(4), 2001, pages 572–576.

6. Liu, S., Manson, J. E., Stampfer, M. J., et al., "Dietary Glycemic Load Assessed by Food-Frequency Questionnaire in Relation to Plasma High-Density-Lipoprotein Cholesterol and Fasting Plasma Triacylglycerols in Postmenopausal Women," *American Journal of Clinical Nutrition,* 73(3), 2001, pages 560–566.

7. Ludwig, D. S., Majzoub, J. A., Al-Zahrani, A., et al., "High Glycemic Index Foods, Overeating, and Obesity," *Pediatrics,* 103(3), 1999, page E26:1–6.

8. Jarvi, A. E., Karlstrom, B. E., Granfeldt, Y. E., et al., "Improved Glycemic Control and Lipid Profile and Normalized Fibrinolytic Activity on a Low-Glycemic Index Diet in Type 2 Diabetic Patients," *Diabetes Care,* 22(1), 1999, pages 10–18.

Chapter 15: Fiber Facts

1. Atkins, R. C., *Dr. Atkins' New Carbohydrate Gram Counter,* M. Evans & Company Inc., 2002.

2. Institute of Medicine of the National Academies, "Dietary Reference Intakes for Energy, Carbohydrates, Fiber, Fat, Fatty Acids, Cholesterol, Protein, and Amino Acids," available at: http://books. nap. edu/books/0309085373/html/index. html, accessed on April 9, 2004.

3. Bialostosky, K., et al, "Dietary Intake of Macronutrients, Micronutrients, and Other Constituents: United States, 1988–94," *Vital Health Statistics,* 11(245), 2002.

Chapter 16: The Bountiful Harvest

1. Bazzano, L. A., He, J., Ogden, L. G., et al., "Fruit and Vegetable Intake and Risk of Cardiovascular Disease in US Adults: The First National Health and Nutrition Examination Survey Epidemiologic Follow-up Study," *American Journal of Clinical Nutrition,* 76(1), 2002, pages 93–99.

2. Bazzano, L. A., He, J., Ogden, L. G., et al., "Fruit and Vegetable Intake and Risk of Cardiovascular Disease in US Adults: The First National Health and Nutrition Examination Survey Epidemio-

logic Follow-up Study," *American Journal of Clinical Nutrition,* 76(1), 2002, pages 93–99.

3. Williams, D. E., Wareham, N. J., Cox, B. D., et al., "Frequent Salad Vegetable Consumption Is Associated with a Reduction in the Risk of Diabetes Mellitus," *Journal of Clinical Epidemiology,* 52(4), 1999, pages 329–335.

4. Johnston, C. S., Taylor, C. A., Hampl, J. S., "More Americans Are Eating '5 a Day' but Intakes of Dark Green and Cruciferous Vegetables Remain Low," *Journal of Nutrition,* 130(12), 2000, pages 3063–3067.

5. Foster-Powell, K., Holt, S. H., Brand-Miller, J. C., "International Table of Glycemic Index and Glycemic Load Values: 2002," *American Journal of Clinical Nutrition,* 76(1), 2002, pages 5–56.

6. Sullivan, M. J., Scott, R. L., "Postprandial Glycemic Response to Orange Juice and Nondiet Cola: Is There a Difference?" *Diabetes Educator,* 17(4), 1991, pages 274–278.

7. Bolton, R. P., Heaton, K. W., Burroughs, L. F., "The Role of Dietary Fiber in Satiety, Glucose, and Insulin: Studies with Fruit and Fruit Juice," *American Journal of Clinical Nutrition,* 34(2), 1981, pages 211–217.

8. Gannon, M. C., Nuttall, F. Q., Krezowski, P. A., et al., "The Serum Insulin and Plasma Glucose Responses to Milk and Fruit Products in Type 2 (Non-Insulin-Dependent) Diabetic Patients," *Diabetologia,* 29(11), 1986, pages 784–791.

9. Hayden, M. R., Tyagi, S. C., "Islet Redox Stress: The Manifold Toxicities of Insulin Resistance, Metabolic Syndrome and Amylin Derived Islet Amyloid in Type 2 Diabetes Mellitus," *Journal of the Pancreas,* 3(4), 2002, pages 86–108.

10. Hayden, M. R., Tyagi, S. C., "Islet Redox Stress: The Manifold Toxicities of Insulin Resistance, Metabolic Syndrome and Amylin Derived Islet Amyloid in Type 2 Diabetes Mellitus," *Journal of the Pancreas,* 3(4), 2002, pages 86–108.

11. Nelson, J. L., Bernstein, P. S., Schmidt, M. C., et al., "Dietary Modification and Moderate Antioxidant Supplementation Differentially Affect Serum Carotenoids, Antioxidant Levels and Markers of Oxidative Stress in Older Humans," *Journal of Nutrition,* 133(10), 2003, pages 3117–3123.

12. Ford, E. S., Mokdad, A. H., Giles, W. H., et al., "The Metabolic Syndrome and Antioxidant Concentrations: Findings from the Third National Health and Nutrition Examination Survey," *Diabetes,* 52(9), 2003, pages 2346–2352.
13. Fung, T. T., Manson, J. E., Solomon, C. G., et al., "The Association Between Magnesium Intake and Fasting Insulin Concentration in Healthy Middle-Aged Women," *Journal of the American College of Nutrition,* 22(6), 2003, pages 533–538.
14. Seddon, J. M., Ajani, U. A., Sperduto, R. D., et al., "Dietary Carotenoids, Vitamins A, C, and E, and Advanced Age-Related Macular Degeneration. Eye Disease Case-Control Study Group," *Journal of the American Medical Association,* 272(18), 1994, pages 1413–1420.

Chapter 17: Controlling Your Carbs—and Liking It

1. Wursch, P., Pi-Sunyer, F. X., "The Role of Viscous Soluble Fiber in the Metabolic Control of Diabetes. A Review with Special Emphasis on Cereals Rich in Beta-Glucan," *Diabetes Care,* 20(11), 1997, pages 1774–1780.
2. Foster-Powell, K., Holt, S. H., Brand-Miller, J. C., "International Table of Glycemic Index and Glycemic Load Values: 2002," *American Journal of Clinical Nutrition,* 76(1), 2002, pages 5–56.
3. Chiasson, J. L., Josse, R. G., Gomis, R., et al., "Acarbose for Prevention of Type 2 Diabetes Mellitus: The STOP-NIDDM Randomised Trial," *Lancet,* 359(9323), 2002, pages 2072–2077.
4. Kaiser, T., Sawicki, P. T., "Acarbose for Prevention of Diabetes, Hypertension and Cardiovascular Events? A Critical Analysis of the STOP-NIDDM Data," *Diabetologia,* 47(3), 2004, pages 575–580.

Chapter 18: Sugar Nation

1. USDA, "Major Trends in U. S. Food Supply, 1909–99," *FoodReview,* 23(1), 2000, pages 8–15.
2. Sullivan, M. J., Scott, R. L., "Postprandial Glycemic Response to Orange Juice and Nondiet Cola: Is There a Difference?" *Diabetes Educator,* 17(4), 1991, pages 274–278.

3. Natah, S. S., Hussien, K. R., Tuominen, J. A., et al., "Metabolic Response to Lactitol and Xylitol in Healthy Men," *American Journal of Clinical Nutrition*, 65(4), 1997, pages 947–950.
4. USDA, "Major Trends in U. S. Food Supply, 1909–99," *FoodReview*, 23(1), 2000, pages 8–15.
5. Elliott, S. S., Keim, N. L., Stern, J. S., et al., "Fructose, Weight Gain, and the Insulin Resistance Syndrome," *American Journal of Clinical Nutrition*, 76(5), 2002, pages 911–922.

Chapter 19: Drink to Your Health

1. Foster-Powell, K., Holt, S. H., Brand-Miller, J. C., "International Table of Glycemic Index and Glycemic Load Values: 2002," *American Journal of Clinical Nutrition*, 76(1), 2002, pages 5–56.
2. Bolton, R. P., Heaton, K. W., Burroughs, L. F., "The Role of Dietary Fiber in Satiety, Glucose, and Insulin: Studies with Fruit and Fruit Juice," *American Journal of Clinical Nutrition*, 34(2), 1981, pages 211–217.
3. Gannon, M. C., Nuttall, F. Q., Krezowski, P. A., et al., "The Serum Insulin and Plasma Glucose Responses to Milk and Fruit Products in Type 2 (Non-Insulin-Dependent) Diabetic Patients," *Diabetologia*, 29(11), 1986, pages 784–791.
4. Sullivan, M. J., Scott, R. L., "Postprandial Glycemic Response to Orange Juice and Nondiet Cola: Is There a Difference?" *Diabetes Educator*, 17(4), 1991, pages 274–278.
5. Zemel, M. B., "Role of Dietary Calcium and Dairy Products in Modulating Adiposity," *Lipids*, 38(2), 2003, pages 139–146.
6. Kerr, D., Sherwin, R. S., Pavalkis, F., et al., "Effect of Caffeine on the Recognition of and Responses to Hypoglycemia in Humans," *Annals of Internal Medicine*, 119(8), 1993, pages 799–804.
7. Keijzers, G. B., De Galan, B. E., Tack, C. J., et al., "Caffeine Can Decrease Insulin Sensitivity in Humans," *Diabetes Care*, 25(2), 2002, pages 364–369.
8. Thong, F. S., Derave, W., Kiens, B., et al., "Caffeine-Induced Impairment of Insulin Action but Not Insulin Signaling in Human Skeletal Muscle Is Reduced by Exercise," *Diabetes*, 51(3), 2002, pages 583–590.

9. Sesso, H. D., Gaziano, J. M., Buring, J. E., et al., "Coffee and Tea Intake and the Risk of Myocardial Infarction," *American Journal of Epidemiology,* 149(2), 1999, pages 162–167.

10. Hegarty, V. M., May, H. M., Khaw, K. T., "Tea Drinking and Bone Mineral Density in Older Women," *American Journal of Clinical Nutrition,* 71(4), 2000, pages 1003–1007.

11. Dulloo, A. G., Duret, C., Rohrer, D., et al., "Efficacy of a Green Tea Extract Rich in Catechin Polyphenols and Caffeine in Increasing 24-H Energy Expenditure and Fat Oxidation in Humans," *American Journal of Clinical Nutrition,* 70(6), 1999, pages 1040–1045.

12. Hosoda, K., Wang, M. F., Liao, M. L., et al., "Antihyperglycemic Effect of Oolong Tea in Type 2 Diabetes," *Diabetes Care,* 26(6), 2003, pages 1714–1718.

13. Caimi, G., Carollo, C., Lo Presti, R., "Diabetes Mellitus: Oxidative Stress and Wine," *Current Medical Research and Opinion,* 19(7), 2003, pages 581–586.

14. Avogaro, A., Sambataro, M., Marangoni, A., et al., "Moderate Alcohol Consumption, Glucose Metabolism and Lipolysis: The Effect on Adiponectin and Tumor Necrosis Factor Alpha," *Journal of Endocrinological Investigation,* 26(12), 2003, pages 1213–1218.

15. Lange, J., Arends, J., Willms, B., "Alcohol-Induced Hypoglycemia in Type I Diabetic Patients," *Medizinisohe Klinik (Munich),* 86(11), 1991, pages 551–554.

16. Swade, T. F., Emanuele, N. V., "Alcohol & Diabetes," *Comprehensive Therapy,* 23(2), 1997, pages 135–140.

17. Sacks, D. B., Bruns, D. E., Goldstein, D. E., et al., "Guidelines and Recommendations for Laboratory Analysis in the Diagnosis and Management of Diabetes Mellitus," *Clinical Chemistry,* 48(3), 2002, pages 436–472.

Chapter 20: Getting Extra Help: Supplements for Blood Sugar Control

1. Fletcher, R. H., Fairfield, K. M., "Vitamins for Chronic Disease Prevention in Adults: Clinical Applications," *Journal of the American Medical Association,* 287(23), 2002, pages 3127–3129.

2. Barringer, T. A., Kirk, J. K., Santaniello, A. C., et al., "Effect of a Multivitamin and Mineral Supplement on Infection and Quality

of Life. A Randomized, Double-Blind, Placebo-Controlled Trial," *Annals of Internal Medicine,* 138(5), 2003, pages 365–371.

3. Hayden, M. R., Tyagi, S. C., "Islet Redox Stress: The Manifold Toxicities of Insulin Resistance, Metabolic Syndrome and Amylin Derived Islet Amyloid in Type 2 Diabetes Mellitus," *Journal of the Pancreas,* 3(4), 2002, pages 86–108.

4. Jiang, R., Manson, J. E., Meigs, J. B., et al., "Body Iron Stores in Relation to Risk of Type 2 Diabetes in Apparently Healthy Women," *Journal of the American Medical Association,* 291(6), 2004, pages 711–717.

5. Hayden, M. R., Tyagi, S. C., "Islet Redox Stress: The Manifold Toxicities of Insulin Resistance, Metabolic Syndrome and Amylin Derived Islet Amyloid in Type 2 Diabetes Mellitus," *Journal of the Pancreas,* 3(4), 2002, pages 86–108.

6. Sinclair, A. J., Taylor, P. B., Lunec, J., et al., "Low Plasma Ascorbate Levels in Patients with Type 2 Diabetes Mellitus Consuming Adequate Dietary Vitamin C," *Diabetic Medicine,* 11(9), 1994, pages 893–898.

7. Sargeant, L. A., Wareham, N. J., Bingham, S., et al., "Vitamin C and Hyperglycemia in the European Prospective Investigation into Cancer—Norfolk (EPIC-Norfolk) Study: A Population-Based Study," *Diabetes Care,* 23(6), 2000, pages 726–732.

8. Natali, A., Sironi, A. M., Toschi, E., et al., "Effect of Vitamin C on Forearm Blood Flow and Glucose Metabolism in Essential Hypertension," *Arteriosclerosis, Thrombosis, and Vascular Biology,* 20(11), 2000, pages 2401–2406.

9. Ting, H. H., Timimi, F. K., Boles, K. S., et al., "Vitamin C Improves Endothelium-Dependent Vasodilation in Patients with Non-Insulin-Dependent Diabetes Mellitus," *Journal of Clinical Investigation,* 97(1), 1996, pages 22–28

10. Carr, A., Frei, B., "The Role of Natural Antioxidants in Preserving the Biological Activity of Endothelium-Derived Nitric Oxide," *Free Radical Biology and Medicine,* 28(12), 2000, pages 1806–1814.

11. Price, K. D., Price, K. S., Reynolds, R. D., " Hyperglycemia-Induced Ascorbic Acid Deficiency Promotes Endothelial Dysfunction and the Development of Atherosclerosis," *Atherosclerosis,* 158(1), 2001, pages 1–12.

12. Trumbo, P., Schlicker, S., Yates, A. A., et al., "Dietary Reference Intakes for Energy, Carbohydrate, Fiber, Fat, Fatty Acids, Cholesterol, Protein and Amino Acids," *Journal of the American Dietetic Association*, 102(11), 2002, pages 1621–1630.

13. Paolisso, G., D'Amore, A., Galzerano, D., et al., "Daily Vitamin E Supplements Improve Metabolic Control but Not Insulin Secretion in Elderly Type II Diabetic Patients," *Diabetes Care*, 16(11), 1993, pages 1433–1437.

14. Devaraj, S., Jialal, I., "Low-Density Lipoprotein Postsecretory Modification, Monocyte Function, and Circulating Adhesion Molecules in Type 2 Diabetic Patients with and without Macrovascular Complications: The Effect of Alpha-Tocopherol Supplementation," *Circulation*, 102(2), 2000, pages 191–196.

15. Trumbo, P., Schlicker, S., Yates, A. A., et al., "Dietary Reference Intakes for Energy, Carbohydrate, Fiber, Fat, Fatty Acids, Cholesterol, Protein and Amino Acids," *Journal of the American Dietetic Association*, 102(11), 2002, pages 1621–1630.

16. Ametov, A. S., Barinov, A., Dyck, P. J., et al., "The Sensory Symptoms of Diabetic Polyneuropathy Are Improved with Alpha-Lipoic Acid: The Sydney Trial," *Diabetes Care*, 26(3), 2003, pages 770–776.

17. Maebashi, M., Makino, Y., Kurukawa, Y., et al., "Therapeutic Evaluation of the Effect of Biotin on Hyperglycemia in Patients with Non-Insulin Dependent Diabetes Mellitus," *Journal of Clinical Biochemistry and Nutrition*, 14, 1993, pages 211–218.

18. McCarty, M. F., "Toward Practical Prevention of Type 2 Diabetes," *Medical Hypotheses*, 54(5), 2000, pages 786–793.

19. McCarty, M. F., "Toward a Wholly Nutritional Therapy for Type 2 Diabetes," *Medical Hypotheses*, 54(3), 2000, pages 483–487.

20. Koutsikos, D., Agroyannis, B., Tzanatos-Exarchou, H., "Biotin for Diabetic Peripheral Neuropathy," *Biomedicine and Pharmacotherapy*, 44(10), 1990, pages 511–514.

21. Maffucci, T., Brancaccio, A., Piccolo, E., et al., "Insulin Induces Phosphatidylinositol-3-Phosphate Formation through Tc10 Activation," *EMBO Journal*, 22(16), 2003, pages 4178–4189.

22. Jones, A. W., Geisbuhler, B. B., Shukla, S. D., et al., "Altered Biochemical and Functional Responses in Aorta from Hypertensive Rats," *Hypertension*, 11(6 Pt 2), 1988, pages 627–634.

23. Anderson, R. A., "Chromium, Glucose Intolerance and Diabetes," *Journal of the American College of Nutrition*, 17(6), 1998, pages 548–555.

24. Ducros, V., "Chromium Metabolism. A Literature Review," *Biological Trace Element Research*, 32, 1992, pages 65–77.

25. Anderson, R. A., Cheng, N., Bryden, N. A., et al., "Elevated Intakes of Supplemental Chromium Improve Glucose and Insulin Variables in Individuals with Type 2 Diabetes," *Diabetes*, 46(11), 1997, pages 1786–1791.

26. Anderson, R. A., "Chromium, Glucose Intolerance and Diabetes," *Journal of the American College of Nutrition*, 17(6), 1998, pages 548–555.

27. Stearns, D. M., Silveira, S. M., Wolf, K. K., et al., "Chromium(III) Tris(Picolinate) Is Mutagenic at the Hypoxanthine (Guanine) Phosphoribosyltransferase Locus in Chinese Hamster Ovary Cells," *Mutation Research*, 513(1–2), 2002, pages 135–142.

28. Kao, W. H., Folsom, A. R., Nieto, F. J., et al., "Serum and Dietary Magnesium and the Risk for Type 2 Diabetes Mellitus: The Atherosclerosis Risk in Communities Study," *Archives of Internal Medicine*, 159(18), 1999, pages 2151–2159.

29. Rodriguez-Moran, M., Guerrero-Romero, F., "Oral Magnesium Supplementation Improves Insulin Sensitivity and Metabolic Control in Type 2 Diabetic Subjects: A Randomized Double-Blind Controlled Trial," *Diabetes Care*, 26(4), 2003, pages 1147–1152.

30. White, J. R., Campbell, R. K., "Magnesium and Diabetes: A Review," *The Annals of Pharmacotherapy*, 27(6), 1993, pages 775–780.

31. Bauman, W. A., Shaw, S., Jayatilleke, E., et al., "Increased Intake of Calcium Reverses Vitamin B12 Malabsorption Induced by Metformin," *Diabetes Care*, 23(9), 2000, pages 1227–1231.

32. Trumbo, P., Schlicker, S., Yates, A. A., et al., "Dietary Reference Intakes for Energy, Carbohydrate, Fiber, Fat, Fatty Acids, Cholesterol, Protein and Amino Acids," *Journal of the American Dietetic Association*, 102(11), 2002, pages 1621–1630.

33. Zemel, M. B., "Role of Dietary Calcium and Dairy Products in Modulating Adiposity," *Lipids*, 38(2), 2003, pages 139–146.

34. DiSilvestro, R. A., "Zinc in Relation to Diabetes and Oxidative Disease," *Journal of Nutrition*, 130(5S), 2000, pages 1509S-1511S.

35. Chausmer, A. B., "Zinc, Insulin and Diabetes," *Journal of the American College of Nutrition*, 17(2), 1998, pages 109–115.

36. Fernandez-Real, J. M., Lopez-Bermejo, A., Ricart, W., "Cross-Talk between Iron Metabolism and Diabetes," *Diabetes*, 51(8), 2002, pages 2348–2354.

37. Jiang, R., Manson, J. E., Meigs, J. B., et al., "Body Iron Stores in Relation to Risk of Type 2 Diabetes in Apparently Healthy Women," *Journal of the American Medical Association*, 291(6), 2004, pages 711–717.

38. Hodgson, J. M., Watts, G. F., Playford, D. A., et al., "Coenzyme Q10 Improves Blood Pressure and Glycaemic Control: A Controlled Trial in Subjects with Type 2 Diabetes," *European Journal of Clinical Nutrition*, 56(11), 2002, pages 1137–1142.

39. van Loon, L. J., Kruijshoop, M., Menheere, P. P., et al., "Amino Acid Ingestion Strongly Enhances Insulin Secretion in Patients with Long-Term Type 2 Diabetes," *Diabetes Care*, 26(3), 2003, pages 625–630.

40. Layman, D. K., Shiue, H., Sather, C., et al., "Increased Dietary Protein Modifies Glucose and Insulin Homeostasis in Adult Women During Weight Loss," *Journal of Nutrition*, 133(2), 2003, pages 405–410.

41. Muller, D. M., Seim, H., Kiess, W., et al., "Effects of Oral L-Carnitine Supplementation on in Vivo Long-Chain Fatty Acid Oxidation in Healthy Adults," *Metabolism: Clinical and Experimental*, 51(11), 2002, pages 1389–1391.

42. Mingrone, G., Greco, A. V., Capristo, E., et al., "L-Carnitine Improves Glucose Disposal in Type 2 Diabetic Patients," *Journal of the American College of Nutrition*, 18(1), 1999, pages 77–82.

Chapter 21: Getting Extra Help: Supplements for Heart Health

1. Natali, A., Sironi, A. M., Toschi, E., et al., "Effect of Vitamin C on Forearm Blood Flow and Glucose Metabolism in Essential Hypertension," *Arteriosclerosis, Thrombosis, and Vascular Biology*, 20(11), 2000, pages 2401–2406.

2. Reaven, P. D., Herold, D. A., Barnett, J., et al., "Effects of Vitamin E on Susceptibility of Low-Density Lipoprotein and Low-Density

Lipoprotein Subfractions to Oxidation and on Protein Glycation in NIDDM," *Diabetes Care,* 18(6), 1995, pages 807–816.

3. Dreon, D. M., Fernstrom, H. A., Campos, H., et al., "Change in Dietary Saturated Fat Intake Is Correlated with Change in Mass of Large Low-Density-Lipoprotein Particles in Men," *American Journal of Clinical Nutrition,* 67(5), 1998, pages 828–836.

4. Hickey, J. T., Hickey, L., Yancy, W. S. J., et al., "Clinical Use of a Carbohydrate-Restricted Diet to Treat the Dyslipidemia of the Metabolic Syndrome," *Metabolic Syndrome and Related Disorders,* 1(3), 2003, pages 227–232.

5. Devaraj, S., Jialal, I., "Low-Density Lipoprotein Postsecretory Modification, Monocyte Function, and Circulating Adhesion Molecules in Type 2 Diabetic Patients with and without Macrovascular Complications: The Effect of Alpha-Tocopherol Supplementation," *Circulation,* 102(2), 2000, pages 191–196.

6. Hoogeveen, E. K., Kostense, P. J., Jakobs, C., et al., "Hyperhomocysteinemia Increases Risk of Death, Especially in Type 2 Diabetes: 5-Year Follow-up of the Hoorn Study," *Circulation,* 101(13), 2000, pages 1506–1511.

7. Buysschaert, M., Dramais, A. S., Wallemacq, P. E., et al., "Hyperhomocysteinemia in Type 2 Diabetes: Relationship to Macroangiopathy, Nephropathy, and Insulin Resistance," *Diabetes Care,* 23(12), 2000, pages 1816–1822.

8. Passaro, A., Calzoni, F., Volpato, S., et al., "Effect of Metabolic Control on Homocysteine Levels in Type 2 Diabetic Patients: A 3-Year Follow-Up," *Journal of Internal Medicine,* 254(3), 2003, pages 264–271.

9. Desouza, C., Keebler, M., McNamara, D. B., et al., "Drugs Affecting Homocysteine Metabolism: Impact on Cardiovascular Risk," *Drugs,* 62(4), 2002, pages 605–616.

10. Passaro, A., Calzoni, F., Volpato, S., et al., "Effect of Metabolic Control on Homocysteine Levels in Type 2 Diabetic Patients: A 3-Year Follow-Up," *Journal of Internal Medicine,* 254(3), 2003, pages 264–271.

11. Mayer, O., Filipovsky, J., Hromadka, M., et al., "Treatment of Hyperhomocysteinemia with Folic Acid: Effects on Homocysteine Levels, Coagulation Status, and Oxidative Stress Markers," *Journal of Cardiovascular Pharmacology,* 39(6), 2002, pages 851–857.

12. Lipsy, R. J., "Overview of Pharmacologic Therapy for the Treatment of Dyslipidemia," *Journal of Managed Care Pharmacy,* 9(S1), 2003, pages 9–12.

13. Wang, W., Basinger, A., Neese, R. A., et al., "Effects of Nicotinic Acid on Fatty Acid Kinetics, Fuel Selection, and Pathways of Glucose Production in Women," *American Journal of Physiology, Endocrinology and Metabolism,* 279(1), 2000, pages E50–59.

14. Prisco, D., Rogasi, P. G., Matucci, M., et al., "Effect of Oral Treatment with Pantethine on Platelet and Plasma Phospholipids in IIa Hyperlipoproteinemia," *Angiology,* 38(3), 1987, pages 241–247.

15. Klevay, L. M., Milne, D. B., "Low Dietary Magnesium Increases Supraventricular Ectopy," *American Journal of Clinical Nutrition,* 75(3), 2002, pages 550–554.

16. Rukshin, V., Shah, P. K., Cercek, B., et al., "Comparative Antithrombotic Effects of Magnesium Sulfate and the Platelet Glycoprotein IIb/IIIa Inhibitors Tirofiban and Eptifibatide in a Canine Model of Stent Thrombosis," *Circulation,* 105(16), 2002, pages 1970–1975.

17. Rude, R., Manoogian, C., Ehrlich, L., et al., "Mechanisms of Blood Pressure Regulation by Magnesium in Man," *Magnesium,* 8(5–6), 1989, pages 266–273.

18. Militante, J. D., Lombardini, J. B., "Treatment of Hypertension with Oral Taurine: Experimental and Clinical Studies," *Amino Acids,* 23(4), 2002, pages 381–393.

19. Schaffer, S. W., Lombardini, J. B., Azuma, J., "Interaction between the Actions of Taurine and Angiotensin II," *Amino Acids,* 18(4), 2000, pages 305–318.

20. Schuller-Levis, G. B., Park, E., "Taurine: New Implications for an Old Amino Acid," *FEMS Microbiology Letters,* 226(2), 2003, pages 195–202.

21. Toft, I., Bonaa, K. H., Ingebretsen, O. C., et al., "Effects of N-3 Polyunsaturated Fatty Acids on Glucose Homeostasis and Blood Pressure in Essential Hypertension. A Randomized, Controlled Trial," *Annals of Internal Medicine,* 123(12), 1995, pages 911–918.

22. Kris-Etherton, P. M., Harris, W. S., Appel, L. J., "Fish Consumption, Fish Oil, Omega-3 Fatty Acids, and Cardiovascular Disease,"

Arteriosclerosis, Thrombosis, and Vascular Biology, 23(2), 2003, pages e20–30.

23. Kris-Etherton, P. M., Harris, W. S., Appel, L. J., "Omega-3 Fatty Acids and Cardiovascular Disease: New Recommendations from the American Heart Association," *Arteriosclerosis, Thrombosis, and Vascular Biology,* 23(2), 2003, pages 151–152.

24. Friedberg, C. E., Janssen, M. J., Heine, R. J., et al., "Fish Oil and Glycemic Control in Diabetes. A Meta-Analysis," *Diabetes Care,* 21(4), 1998, pages 494–500.

25. Lee, K. W., Lip, G. Y., "The Role of Omega-3 Fatty Acids in the Secondary Prevention of Cardiovascular Disease," *QJM,* 96(7), 2003, pages 465–480.

26. Jackson, P. R., Wallis, E. J., Haq, I. U., et al., "Statins for Primary Prevention: At What Coronary Risk Is Safety Assured?" *British Journal of Clinical Pharmacology,* 52(4), 2001, pages 439–446.

Chapter 22: Walking Away from Diabetes

1. Helmrich, S. P., Ragland, D. R., Leung, R. W., et al., "Physical Activity and Reduced Occurrence of Non-Insulin-Dependent Diabetes Mellitus," *New England Journal of Medicine,* 325(3), 1991, pages 147–152.

2. Pan, X. R., Li, G. W., Hu, Y. H., et al., "Effects of Diet and Exercise in Preventing NIDDM in People with Impaired Glucose Tolerance. The Da Qing Igt and Diabetes Study," *Diabetes Care,* 20(4), 1997, pages 537–544.

3. Boule, N. G., Haddad, E., Kenny, G. P., et al., "Effects of Exercise on Glycemic Control and Body Mass in Type 2 Diabetes Mellitus: A Meta-Analysis of Controlled Clinical Trials," *Journal of the American Medical Association,* 286(10), 2001, pages 1218–1227.

4. Pate, R. R., Pratt, M., Blair, S. N., et al., "Physical Activity and Public Health. A Recommendation from the Centers for Disease Control and Prevention and the American College of Sports Medicine," *Journal of the American Medical Association,* 273(5), 1995, pages 402–407.

5. Myers, J., Prakash, M., Froelicher, V., et al., "Exercise Capacity and Mortality among Men Referred for Exercise Testing," *New England Journal of Medicine,* 346(11), 2002, pages 793–801.

6. Lee, I. M., Sesso, H. D., Oguma, Y., et al., "Relative Intensity of Physical Activity and Risk of Coronary Heart Disease," *Circulation*, 107(8), 2003, pages 1110–1116.

Chapter 23: Your Personal Exercise Program

1. Albert, C. M., Mittleman, M. A., Chae, C. U., et al., "Triggering of Sudden Death from Cardiac Causes by Vigorous Exertion," *New England Journal of Medicine*, 343(19), 2000, pages 1355–1361.
2. Hu, F. B., Sigal, R. J., Rich-Edwards, J. W., et al., "Walking Compared with Vigorous Physical Activity and Risk of Type 2 Diabetes in Women: A Prospective Study," *Journal of the American Medical Association*, 282(15), 1999, pages 1433–1439.

Chapter 24: It's Not Just Baby Fat

1. Centers for Disease Control and Prevention, CDC At a Glance: "Diabetes: Disabling, Deadly, and on the Rise 2004," available at: http://www.cdc.gov/nccdphp/aag/pdf/aag_ddt2004.pdf, accessed on April 15, 2004.
2. American Heart Association, "Obesity and Overweight in Children," available at: http://www.americanheart.org/presenter.jhtml?identifier=4670, accessed on April 15, 2004.
3. WHO Global Strategy on Diet, Physical Activity and Health, "Fact Sheet: Obesity and Overweight," 2003, available at: http://www.who.int/hpr/NPH/docs/gs_obesity.pdf, accessed on April 20, 2004.
4. Halford, J. C., Gillespie, J., Brown, V., et al., "Food Advertisements Induce Food Consumption in Both Lean and Obese Children," *Obesity Research*, 12(1), 2004, page 171.
5. Dwyer, J. T., Michell, P., Cosentino, C., et al., "Fat-Sugar See-Saw in School Lunches: Impact of a Low Fat Intervention," *Journal of Adolescent Health*, 32(6), 2003, pages 428–435.
6. American Academy of Pediatrics Committee on School Health, "Soft Drinks in Schools," *Pediatrics*, 113(1 Pt 1), 2004, pages 152–154.
7. Dews, P. B., O'Brien, C. P., Bergman, J., "Caffeine: Behavioral Effects of Withdrawal and Related Issues," *Food and Chemical Toxicology*, 40(9), 2002, pages 1257–1261.

8. Ludwig, D. S., Peterson, K. E., Gortmaker, S. L., "Relation Between Consumption of Sugar-Sweetened Drinks and Childhood Obesity: A Prospective, Observational Analysis," *Lancet,* 357(9255), 2001, pages 505–508.

9. Harnack, L., Stang, J., Story, M., "Soft Drink Consumption among US Children and Adolescents: Nutritional Consequences," *Journal of the American Dietetic Association,* 99(4), 1999, pages 436–441.

10. Caballero, B., "Global Patterns of Child Health: The Role of Nutrition," *Annals of Nutrition and Metabolism,* 46 (11S), 2002, pages 3–7.

11. Wyshak, G., "Teenaged Girls, Carbonated Beverage Consumption, and Bone Fractures," *Archives of Pediatrics and Adolescent Medicine,* 154(6), 2000, pages 610–613.

12. Nicklas, T., Johnson, R., "Position of the American Dietetic Association: Dietary Guidance for Healthy Children Ages 2 to 11 Years," *Journal of the American Dietetic Association,* 104(4), 2004, pages 660–677.

13. Block, G., Smith, J., "New Nutrition Analysis Shows Results of Kids' Simple Fruit and Vegetable Substitutions," March 2002, available at: http://www.dole5aday.com/Media/Press/RecentReleases/031602.jsp?topmenu=5, accessed on April 21, 2004.

14. Giammattei, J., Blix, G., Marshak, H. H., et al., "Television Watching and Soft Drink Consumption: Associations with Obesity in 11-to 13-Year-Old Schoolchildren," *Archives of Pediatrics and Adolescent Medicine,* 157(9), 2003, pages 882–886.

15. Guo, S. S., Wu, W., Chumlea, W. C., et al., "Predicting Overweight and Obesity in Adulthood from Body Mass Index Values in Childhood and Adolescence," *American Journal of Clinical Nutrition,* 76(3), 2002, pages 653–658.

16. Whitaker, R. C., Wright, J. A., Pepe, M. S., et al., "Predicting Obesity in Young Adulthood from Childhood and Parental Obesity," *New England Journal of Medicine,* 337(13), 1997, pages 869–873.

17. Ferraro, K. F., Thorpe, R. J., Jr., Wilkinson, J. A., "The Life Course of Severe Obesity: Does Childhood Overweight Matter?" *Journals of Gerontology. Series B, Psychological Sciences and Social Sciences,* 58(2), 2003, pages S110–119.

18. Gunnell, D. J., Frankel, S. J., Nanchahal, K., et al., "Childhood Obesity and Adult Cardiovascular Mortality: A 57-Y Follow-Up Study Based on the Boyd Orr Cohort," *American Journal of Clinical Nutrition*, 67(6), 1998, pages 1111–1118.

19. Engeland, A., Bjorge, T., Sogaard, A. J., et al., "Body Mass Index in Adolescence in Relation to Total Mortality: 32-Year Follow-Up of 227,000 Norwegian Boys and Girls," *American Journal of Epidemiology*, 157(6), 2003, pages 517–523.

20. Berenson, G. S., Wattigney, W. A., Tracy, R. E., et al., "Atherosclerosis of the Aorta and Coronary Arteries and Cardiovascular Risk Factors in Persons Aged 6 to 30 Years and Studied at Necropsy (the Bogalusa Heart Study)," *American Journal of Cardiology*, 70(9), 1992, pages 851–858.

21. Chu, N. F., Rimm, E. B., Wang, D. J., et al., "Clustering of Cardiovascular Disease Risk Factors Among Obese Schoolchildren: The Taipei Children Heart Study," *American Journal of Clinical Nutrition*, 67(6), 1998, pages 1141–1146.

22. Sorof, J. M., Lai, D., Turner, J., et al., "Overweight, Ethnicity, and the Prevalence of Hypertension in School-Aged Children," *Pediatrics*, 113(3 Pt 1), 2004, pages 475–482.

23. Cook, S., Weitzman, M., Auinger, P., et al., "Prevalence of a Metabolic Syndrome Phenotype in Adolescents: Findings from the Third National Health and Nutrition Examination Survey, 1988–1994," *Archives of Pediatrics and Adolescent Medicine*, 157(8), 2003, pages 821–827.

24. Cruz, M. L., Weigensberg, M. J., Huang, T. T., et al., "The Metabolic Syndrome in Overweight Hispanic Youth and the Role of Insulin Sensitivity," *Journal of Clinical Endocrinology and Metabolism*, 2004, 89(1), pages 108–13.

25. Sinha, R., Fisch, G., Teague, B., et al., "Prevalence of Impaired Glucose Tolerance Among Children and Adolescents with Marked Obesity," *New England Journal of Medicine*, 346(11), 2002, pages 802–810.

26. von Mutius, E., Schwartz, J., Neas, L. M., et al., "Relation of Body Mass Index to Asthma and Atopy in Children: The National Health and Nutrition Examination Study III," *Thorax*, 56(11), 2001, pages 835–838.

27. Edmunds, L., Waters, E., Elliott, E. J., "Evidence Based Pediatrics: Evidence Based Management of Childhood Obesity," *BMJ*, 323(7318), 2001, pages 916–919.
28. Bray, G. A., "Obesity and Reproduction," *Human Reproduction*, 12(1S), 1997, pages 26–32.
29. Franks, S., "Adult Polycystic Ovary Syndrome Begins in Childhood," *Best Practice Research. Clinical Endocrinology &Metabolism*, 16(2), 2002, pages 263–272.
30. Lewy, V. D., Danadian, K., Witchel, S. F., et al., "Early Metabolic Abnormalities in Adolescent Girls with Polycystic Ovarian Syndrome," *Journal of Pediatrics*, 138(1), 2001, pages 38–44.
31. Lumeng, J. C., Gannon, K., Cabral, H. J., et al., "Association Between Clinically Meaningful Behavior Problems and Overweight in Children," *Pediatrics*, 2003, 112(5), pages 1138–1145.
32. Schwimmer, J. B., Burwinkle, T. M., Varni, J. W., "Health-Related Quality of Life of Severely Obese Children and Adolescents," *Journal of the American Medical Association*, 2003, 289, pages 1813–1819.
33. Sondike, S. B., Copperman, N., Jacobson, M. S., "Effects of a Low-Carbohydrate Diet on Weight Loss and Cardiovascular Risk Factor in Overweight Adolescents," *Journal of Pediatrics*, 2003, 142(3), pages 253–258.

Chapter 25: Type 2 Diabetes and Your Child

1. American Diabetes Association, "Type 2 Diabetes in Children and Adolescents. American Diabetes Association," *Diabetes Care*, 23(3), 2000, pages 381–389.
2. American Diabetes Association, "Type 2 Diabetes in Children and Adolescents. American Diabetes Association," *Diabetes Care*, 23(3), 2000, pages 381–389.
3. Pinhas-Hamiel, O., Dolan, L. M., Daniels, S. R., et al., "Increased Incidence of Non-Insulin-Dependent Diabetes Mellitus among Adolescents," *Journal of Pediatrics*, 128(5 Pt 1), 1996, pages 608–615.

4. Fagot-Campagna, A., Pettitt, D. J., Engelgau, M. M., et al., "Type 2. Diabetes among North American Children and Adolescents: An Epidemiologic Review and a Public Health Perspective," *Journal of Pediatrics,* 136(5), 2000, pages 664–672.

5. Alberti, K. G., Zimmet, P. Z., "Definition, Diagnosis and Classification of Diabetes Mellitus and Its Complications. Part 1: Diagnosis and Classification of Diabetes Mellitus Provisional Report of a WHO Consultation," *Diabetic Medicine,* 15(7), 1998, pages 539–553.

6. American Diabetes Association, "Type 2 Diabetes in Children and Adolescents. American Diabetes Association," *Diabetes Care,* 23(3), 2000, pages 381–389.

7. Kibirige, M., Metcalf, B., Renuka, R., et al., "Testing the Accelerator Hypothesis: The Relationship Between Body Mass and Age at Diagnosis of Type 1 Diabetes," *Diabetes Care,* 26(10), 2003, pages 2865–2870.

8. Libman, I. M., Pietropaolo, M., Arslanian, S. A., et al., "Evidence for Heterogeneous Pathogenesis of Insulin-Treated Diabetes in Black and White Children," *Diabetes Care,* 26(10), 2003, pages 2876–2882.

9. Dean, H., "Diagnostic Criteria for Non-Insulin Dependent Diabetes in Youth (NIDDM-Y)," *Clinical Pediatrics,* 37(2), 1998, pages 67–71.

10. National Institute of Diabetes and Digestive and Kidney Diseases. National Diabetes Statistics Fact Sheet: General Information and National Estimates on Diabetes in the United States, 2003. Bethesda, MD: U. S. Department of Health and Human Services, National Institutes of Health, 2003.

11. Waldhor, T., Schober, E., Rami, B., et al., "The Prevalence of IDDM in the First Degree Relatives of Children Newly Diagnosed with Iddm in Austria—a Population-Based Study. Austrian Diabetes Incidence Study Group," *Experimental and Clinical Endocrinology and Diabetes,* 107(5), 1999, pages 323–327.

12. Redondo, M. J., Yu, L., Hawa, M., et al., "Heterogeneity of Type I Diabetes: Analysis of Monozygotic Twins in Great Britain and the United States," *Diabetologia,* 44(3), 2001, pages 354–362.

13. American Diabetes Association, "Type 2 Diabetes in Children and Adolescents. American Diabetes Association," *Diabetes Care,* 23(3), 2000, pages 381–389.

14. Jones, K. L., "Non-Insulin Dependent Diabetes in Children and Adolescents: The Therapeutic Challenge," *Clinical Pediatrics,* 37(2), 1998, pages 103–110.

15. Stuart, C. A., Driscoll, M. S., Lundquist, K. F., et al., "Acanthosis Nigricans," *Journal of Basic and Clinical Physiology and Pharmacology,* 9(2–4), 1998, pages 407–418.

16. Smith, C. P., Archibald, H. R., Thomas, J. M., et al., "Basal and Stimulated Insulin Levels Rise with Advancing Puberty," *Clinical Endocrinology,* 28(1), 1988, pages 7–14.

17. Onyemere, K. U., Lipton, R. B., "Parental History and Early-Onset Type 2 Diabetes in African Americans and Latinos in Chicago," *Journal of Pediatrics,* 141(6), 2002, pages 825–829.

18. Svensson, M., Sundkvist, G., Arnqvist, H. J., et al., "Signs of Nephropathy May Occur Early in Young Adults with Diabetes Despite Modern Diabetes Management: Results from the Nationwide Population-Based Diabetes Incidence Study in Sweden (DISS)," *Diabetes Care,* 26(10), 2003, pages 2903–2909.

19. Henricsson, M., Nystrom, L., Blohme, G., et al., "The Incidence of Retinopathy 10 Years after Diagnosis in Young Adult People with Diabetes: Results from the Nationwide Population-Based Diabetes Incidence Study in Sweden (DISS)," *Diabetes Care,* 26(2), 2003, pages 349–354.

20. Hillier, T. A., Pedula, K. L., "Complications in Young Adults with Early-Onset Type 2 Diabetes: Losing the Relative Protection of Youth," *Diabetes Care,* 26(11), 2003, pages 2999–3005.

21. Hillier, T. A., Pedula, K. L., "Complications in Young Adults with Early-Onset Type 2 Diabetes: Losing the Relative Protection of Youth," *Diabetes Care,* 26(11), 2003, pages 2999–3005.

22. Dean, H., Flett, B., "Natural History of Type 2 Diabetes Diagnosed in Childhood: Long-Term Follow-Up in Young Adult Years," Diabetes, 51(S2), 2002, Abstract 99-OR, pages A24-A25.

23. Bray, G. A., "Obesity and Reproduction," *Human Reproduction,* 12(S1), 1997, pages 26–32.

Subject Index

Recipe Index